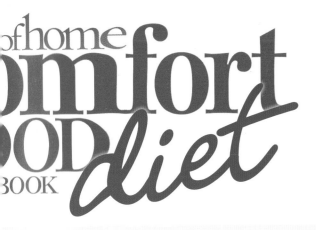

ofhome
omfort
ood *diet*
BOOK

…be slimmer and healthier even
…ve comfort food and lead a busy
…h this comprehensive third
…of our best-selling book, you'll
…satisfying new recipes. Many
…k and easy to make. Paired with
…ips and tools here, they can help
…ow this simple, proven approach
…t loss and healthy living. Start
…What have **you** got to lose?

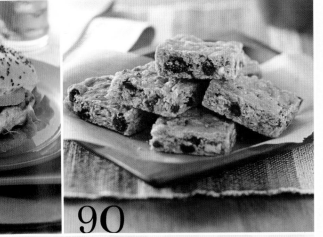

90

A TASTE OF HOME/READER'S DIGEST BOOK

© 2011 Reiman Media Group, LLC
5400 S. 60th St., Greendale WI 53129
All rights reserved.

Taste of Home and Reader's Digest are registered trademarks of
The Reader's Digest Association, Inc.

Editor-in-Chief: Catherine Cassidy
Vice President, Executive Editor/Books: Heidi Reuter Lloyd
Creative Director: Howard Greenberg
North American Chief Marketing Officer: Lisa Karpinski
Food Director: Diane Werner, RD
Food Editor: Peggy Woodward, RD
Senior Editor/Retail Books: Faithann Stoner
Associate Creative Director: Edwin Robles Jr.
Art Director: Rudy Krochalk
Content Production Manager: Julie Wagner
Layout Designers: Emma Acevedo, Catherine Fletcher
Production Assistant: Kathryn Pieters

Project Editors: Jan Briggs, Ellie Martin Cliffe, Andrea Mesalk,
Barbara Schuetz, Victoria Soukup Jensen, Julie Schnittka
Copy Chief: Deb Warlaumont Mulvey
Copy Editors: Alysse Gear, Dulcie Shoener
Recipe Asset System Manager: Coleen Martin
Recipe Testing & Editing: Taste of Home Test Kitchen
Food Photography: Taste of Home Photo Studio
Administrative Assistant: Barb Czysz

THE READER'S DIGEST ASSOCIATION, INC.
President and Chief Executive Officer: Tom Williams
Executive Vice President, RDA, & President, North America:
Dan Lagani
President/Publisher, Trade Publishing: Harold Clarke
Associate Publisher: Rosanne McManus
Vice President, Sales and Marketing: Stacey Ashton

For other Taste of Home books and products, visit tasteofhome.com.
For more Reader's Digest products and information,
visit rd.com (in the United States) or rd.ca (in Canada).

International Standard Book Number (10): 0-89821-910-8
International Standard Book Number (13): 978-0-89821-910-4
Library of Congress Control Number: 2011934910

COVER PHOTOGRAPHY
Photographer: Dan Roberts
Food Stylist: Kathryn Conrad
Set Stylist: Stephanie Marchese

Pictured on front cover: Country Chicken with Gravy (p. 278), Low-Fat
Macaroni and Cheese (p. 205) and Dijon Green Beans (p. 174).

Pictured on back cover from left to right: Tex-Mex Beef Barbecues
(p. 232), Coconut-Cherry Cream Squares (p. 214) and
Ratatouille With Polenta (p. 271).

Printed in China
1 3 5 7 9 10 8 6 4 2

eating right never tasted so good!

As a *Taste of Home Healthy Cooking* subscriber, you'll look forward to:

- 100+ healthy recipes & tips that help you cook, eat, live BETTER!

- Healthy makeovers of all your favorites

- Luscious dishes, light on calories, big on taste

- Easy-to-follow recipes, everyday ingredients

- Practical, proven live-well advice

- Mouthwatering color photos throughout

- Exclusive eNewsletter with bonus recipes and special subscriber-only offers.

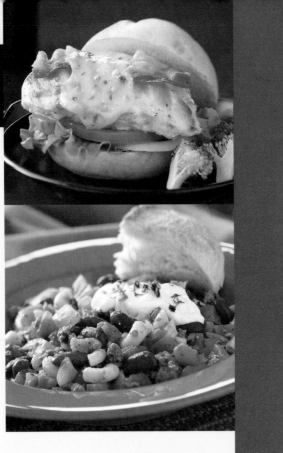

MAIL THIS CARD TODAY!

FROM: _____

_____

PLACE
STAMP
HERE

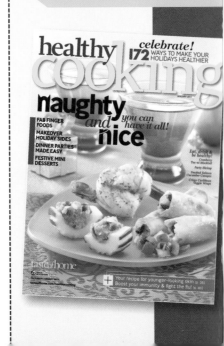

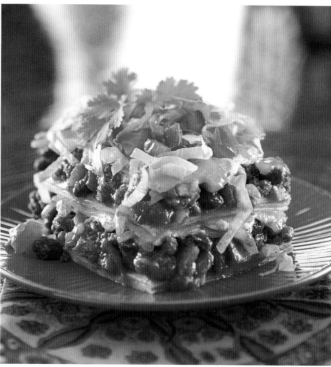

taste of home comfort FOOD diet COOKBOOK

ENCHILADA CASSER-OLÉ!, PAGE 159

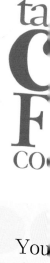

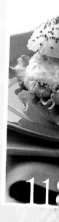

You
if yo
life!
editi
find
are c
all th
you f
to we
today

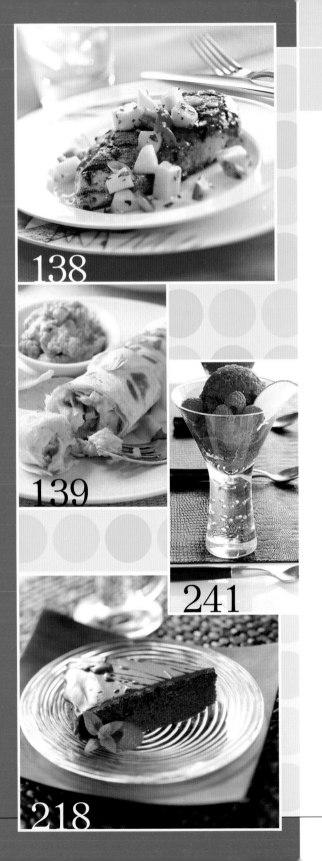

138

139

241

218

table of contents

Making It Work for You.......................... 6

Comfort Food Diet Basics 8

    Step 1... 9

    Step 2... 10

    Steps 3 and 4 11

Success! Dramatic Weight-Loss Stories........... 12

Company Loses 650 Pounds......................... 20

Bring Balance to Your Diet 26

New USDA MyPlate Guidelines 28

Portion Control 30

Get the (Nutrition) Facts 31

Shopping Smart 32

Lighten Up Your Family Favorites 35

Out of the Kitchen, Not Out of Control 36

Basics of Freezing Foods 38

What's Eating You? 42

Super Foods....................................... 44

Move It and Lose It............................... 46

Free Foods Round Out Your Meals................. 52

Six-Week Meal Planner............................ 54

Snacks 76

Breakfasts.. 86

Lunches... 100

Dinners... 122

Side Dishes....................................... 172

Desserts.. 206

Bonus: Slow Cooker Favorites 226

Bonus: 8-Ingredient or Less Recipes............. 236

Bonus: 20-Minute or Less Prep Recipes........ 264

Meal Planning Worksheets......................... 294

Indexes... 296

Comfort Food Diet is
changing lives for the better

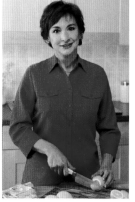

You can lose weight, live a healthy life and still eat the satisfying comfort foods you crave with the **Taste of Home Comfort Food Diet!**

Due to the overwhelming popularity of our delicious and effective diet plan, the editors at *Taste of Home* are thrilled to bring you this third edition—*Comfort Food Diet Cookbook: Quick and Easy Favorites.*

Many diet plans revolve around costly packaged foods or fads that don't live up to expectations and lead you back to your old, unhealthy ways sooner or later. The Comfort Food Diet is a sensible approach to weight loss that's easy, affordable and, most importantly, livable and satisfying for life.

The plan is simple: Eat three complete meals and two snacks a day for a total of 1,400 calories. Watch your portion sizes, and go for regular walks. You'll see the pounds drop off.

This plan provides hundreds of lightened-up recipes for your all-time favorite foods. If you crave cheesy casseroles, hearty sandwiches or rich chocolate cupcakes, they are on the menu. We cut the calories from classic dishes, tested every recipe, calculated all of the Nutrition Facts and ran everything past a registered dietitian for approval. All you need to do is enjoy the satisfying meals, snacks and desserts in this book.

Grab this new *Comfort Food Diet Cookbook* and make a great change for you and your family! Get started right away, and you'll remember this as the first day of your new healthy life!

To help yourself succeed at your goals, check out the Comfort Food Diet website. You'll find interactive meal and fitness plans and the ability to connect with other Comfort Food Diet members. Visit tasteofhome.com/cfdiet.

I find that the job I do as Food Director of *Taste of Home* requires plenty of eating and tasting. All the recipes in this book are tested in our Test Kitchen to make sure they work for you every time you prepare them. And we make a special effort to taste each recipe. We want to guarantee the recipe you serve your family will quickly become a favorite.

So do what I do, and enjoy serving your family these comforting, lightened-up recipes that are sure to please.

Diane Werner

—Diane Werner, RD
Food Director, *Taste of Home*

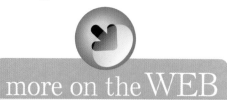

more on the WEB

To help with your weight-loss and healthful-lifestyle goals, check out these tools on the web. Visit the Comfort Food Diet Cookbook website at tasteofhome.com/cfdiet to get started. Sign up for the Comfort Food Diet monthly newsletter at tasteofhome.com/cfdnewsletter. Each month you'll receive a new menu plan, expert tips and more.

Quick and Easy
meals without any guilt

Believe it! The words "comfort food" and "diet" actually do go together. The *Taste of Home Comfort Food Diet Cookbook* offers a healthy way to slim down without giving up the foods you adore.

As a working mom, I'm delighted that this third edition focuses on foods that are quick and easy. You can have it all: luscious foods your family will love, portion sizes that leave you satisfied but within a sensible calorie range, and easy preparation so even on your busiest days you don't have to resort to the fast-food drive-thru.

These recipes aren't tricky to prepare, but if extra-fast fare is what you need, check out our three bonus chapters: Slow Cooker Favorites, 8-Ingredient or Less Recipes and 20-Minute Prep or Less Recipes. If you want healthful meals in a hurry, you don't have to rely on prepackaged frozen dinners anymore.

Plus, you'll save time with all the family-friendly recipes here. You won't have to prepare one thing for your family and another light dish for yourself.

This new edition also includes prep and cook times with each recipe, so you can match up the ingredients you have on hand with a dish that suits the amount of time you have to spend in the kitchen.

Losing weight has never been easier...or tastier. In the *Taste of Home Comfort Food Diet Cookbook: Quick and Easy Favorites,* you'll find:

- *380 incredible recipes that pare down calories and fat.*
- *A six-week meal guide that takes menu planning off your shoulders.*
- *Nutrition Facts plus prep and cook times with every recipe.*

In addition, we've added a **for 2** icon to recipes that are perfectly portioned to serve two people. If you're trying to cook for one or two, you'll find these smaller-yield recipes are just what you need.

I hope you enjoy this wonderful new edition of the *Comfort Food Diet Cookbook*. Dig right in, and you'll see just how delicious losing weight can be!

Peggy Woodward

—Peggy Woodward, RD
   Food Editor, *Taste of Home*

making it work
FOR YOU!

A Simple Plan with Impressive Results

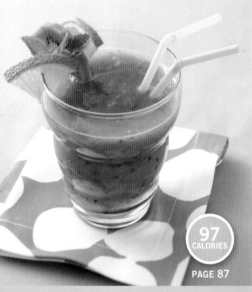

97 CALORIES

PAGE 87

What can the Comfort Food Diet do for YOU? Are you trying to lose weight, improve your health or just feel and look your best? This easy-to-follow plan combines a commonsense approach to healthy eating with the tools you need to succeed. Plus, a series of inspirational success stories and great tips from readers provide motivation and support.

I've lost a good amount of weight in 16 weeks following the Comfort Food Diet. I am down several clothing sizes, feel so much better and have more energy. I've completely changed how I view and eat food. And after being overweight for 25+ years, this is the first time I am truly excited about a diet and its results. …Tami Kuehl, Nebraska

Every one of the 380 recipes in this cookbook includes a complete set of Nutrition Facts, and many list Diabetic Exchanges when applicable. Don't let the lean numbers listed there fool you. No matter how light the recipes are, your family will be too busy savoring the tempting meals you serve to realize that they are eating healthy.

This program is great because the recipes are family-friendly. My husband has loved all the recipes I've tried. It's not hard to make the healthier choice with all the good things we can eat. …Andrea Johnson, Illinois

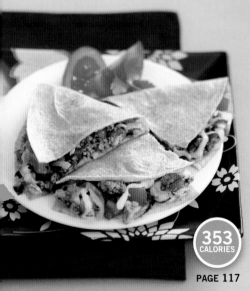

353 CALORIES

PAGE 117

It's true. The recipes in the *Comfort Food Diet Cookbook* offer all the hearty, satisfying goodness you'd expect from a classic home-cooked meal.

These dishes are already a hit with families because they were shared by cooks who submitted their favorites recipes to *Taste of Home* magazine or one of its sister publications. And now you can enjoy these wonderful recipes, too!

I am dropping pounds following the Comfort Food Diet. I find the recipes to be very good, and even my husband is losing weight! ...Anne Merrill, New York

This third edition focuses on quick and easy recipes. Not only has each recipe been evaluated by a registered dietitian, but they also have all passed a review in the Taste of Home Test Kitchen, so you know they'll be healthy and delicious. You'll find prep and cook times and special chapters of extra-speedy fare so you can fit healthy eating into your busy schedule.

Plus, the recipes go together easily with everyday ingredients you probably already have in your kitchen. You'll also discover no-fuss menu additions (with calorie counts) throughout the chapters to round out your meals.

My family and I have tried at least 40 recipes from the Comfort Food Diet Cookbook! I've lost pounds and inches by combining the new recipes with daily workouts. We haven't forfeited taste for weight loss, which is the best part of this plan! ...Lisa Miller, Connecticut

You'll also find tips for exercise, hints for getting the most out of grocery shopping and secrets to lighten your own recipes for favorite comfort foods. Get ready to be inspired! Eating right has never tasted so good.

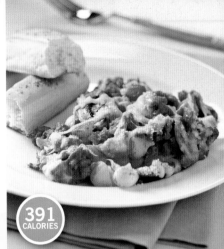

391 CALORIES

PAGE 166

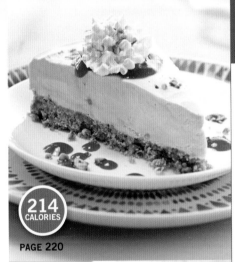

214 CALORIES

PAGE 220

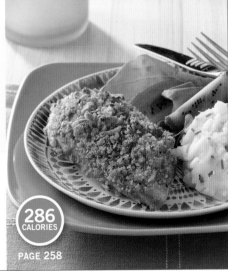

286 CALORIES

PAGE 258

This PROVEN PLAN is your key to a healthier lifestyle and trimmer figure—even if your days are busy!

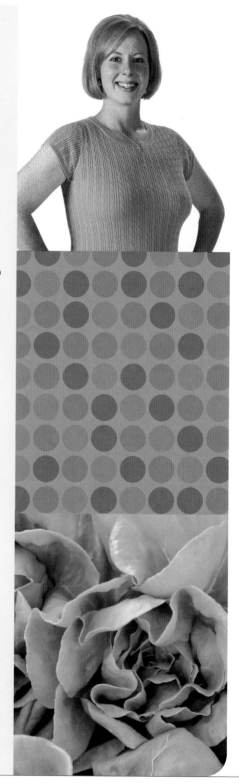

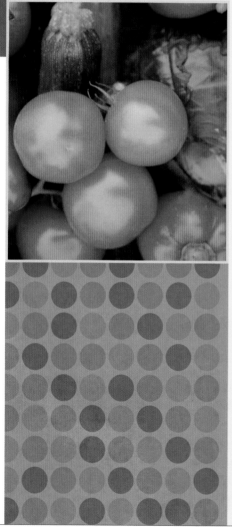

Some other weight-loss plans expect that you can squeeze group meetings into your already hectic days. We know how busy you are. The Comfort Food Diet is simple and has easy, commonsense tools built in to help you stay on track and shed pounds without taking up a lot of time. In this new edition of the *Comfort Food Diet Cookbook*, we've added the prep and cook times to every recipe, so you can quickly match up your calorie needs with the amount of time you have available to cook.

Each chapter is arranged in calorie order so you can quickly find a recipe to meet your calorie needs without searching around. Plus, we have three new bonus chapters filled with time-saving recipes: Slow Cooker Favorites, 8-Ingredient or Less Recipes and 20-Minute or Less Prep Recipes.

As you'll see on the coming pages, the basics behind the Comfort Food Diet are simple: watch your portion sizes, count your calories and get moving every day to help burn them. But it's the idea that you can eat foods that you and your family will love, maintain your busy schedule and still lose weight that makes this program a winner!

COMFORT FOOD DIET BASICS

Cooking healthy meals and keeping your family happy is easy with recipes from the Comfort Food Diet. Familiar dishes and flavors here won't seem light to them, but they are! Enjoy a healthier lifestyle and a satisfied family with the help of this book. You'll slim down by following the four simple steps outlined here.

1 Eat three meals and two snacks a day for a total of 1,400 calories.

If you're a woman, shoot for a total calorie consumption of 1,400 calories per day. Men should consume 1,500 calories per day. Check with your doctor before you begin this plan to see if this calorie guideline is appropriate for you. Then consider the Six-Week Meal Plan on pages 54-75. There you'll find detailed menus that total roughly 1,400 calories per day.

Use the following guide to distribute calories through the day:

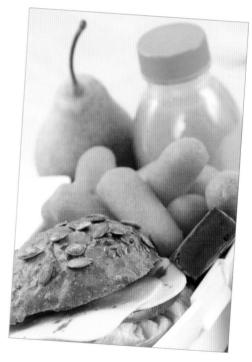

- 350 calories for breakfast

- 450 calories for lunch

- 500 calories for dinner

- Two 50-calorie or two 100-calorie snacks, depending on the total calories you're aiming for per day. You can consume more or less calories in a snack or meal than what is suggested here as long as your daily total is 1,400 or 1,500 calories.

2 Start a food diary to keep track of everything you eat. See pages 294-295 for blank Do-It-Yourself Meal-Planning Worksheets.

Keeping a food diary is a key to success on the Comfort Food Diet. By writing down everything you eat, you can easily identify eating habits you hadn't noticed previously. You're also less likely to cheat if you know you'll have to jot down that sundae you had at lunch or the extra cookie you snuck in after dinner.

Use your food journal or the Meal-Planning Worksheets to help you plan menus in advance as well. Browse through this cookbook and decide which of the hearty dishes you plan to make. Map out menus and snacks for an entire day in advance, then go back and record what you actually ate.

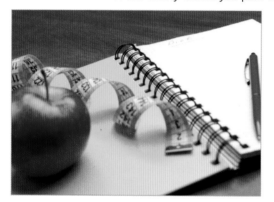

Always remember to watch portion sizes, and review the Nutrition Facts at the end of each recipe to learn what a serving size is. If you increase the serving size, the amount of calories (and nutrients) will obviously increase as well.

It's also important to understand that you can mix and match foods however you'd like as long as you stay within the 1,400 or 1,500 daily calorie limit.

For instance, let's say you enjoy Greek Pizza (p. 155) for lunch. Note that the recipe makes four individual pizzas, but the serving size and Nutrition Facts are based on one pizza. As such, you can enjoy one pizza and serve the others to family members or refrigerate them for a handy lunch or dinner tomorrow.

The guideline for lunch is 450 calories, and one Greek Pizza weighs in at 320 calories. This means you can also enjoy ½ cup of 1% chocolate milk (85 calories) and carrots (free food) for a lunch that totals only 405 calories. You can add another food that is about 45 calories, or you can spend those calories later in the day. It's up to you—as long as your daily caloric intake meets the 1,400 or 1,500 goal.

3 See the Smart Snacks List (p. 77-78), the Free Foods Chart (p. 53) and the calorie breakdowns before each chapter when pairing foods with entrees.

The lunch example covered in Step 2 noted that ½ cup of 1% chocolate milk was 85 calories. How would you know that? Simply turn to pages 77-78 for the Smart Snacks list. There you'll find 79 ideas for low-calorie bites that don't require a recipe. These items are great for snacking, and they also make tasty additions to meals as demonstrated by the lunch example. While these items come in at 100 calories or less, you still need to write them down in your food diary.

Similarly, the Free Foods Chart offers dozens of items that you can enjoy without guilt. In fact, these foods are so light, there's no need to worry about their calorie content as long as you follow any portion restrictions they might offer.

The chapters in the *Comfort Food Diet Cookbook* are broken down into Snacks, Breakfasts, Lunches, Dinners, Side Dishes, Desserts, Slow Cooker Favorites, 8-Ingredient or Less Recipes and 20-Minute or Less Prep Recipes. Every chapter begins with lower-calorie staples and ends with higher-calorie specialties.

If you ate a lunch below the 450 calorie guideline, you may want to consider a higher-calorie dinner. If you enjoyed a high-calorie breakfast and morning snack, you may want to stick with a lunch that's a bit lighter.

Many of the chapters overlap a little, making meal planning easy! For example, some of the higher-calorie lunches would make wonderful low-calorie dinners. You could also look at the calorie breakdown at the beginning of the side dish chapter and choose one of those recipes for a meat-free lunch or substantial snack.

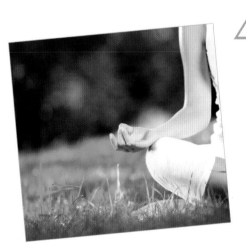

4 Add exercise to burn extra calories

Find a form of exercise that you would enjoy doing every day or on a regular basis. Walking is a great way to start exercising. Walking with family or friends is a great motivator to keep you going.

Swimming, yoga, biking or a dance fitness program are fun ways to exercise. These activities can also be done alone or with family and friends. Choosing an activity that keeps you interested will make you want to exercise. You may have to change activities every few months to maintain that spark.

I WALKED AWAY
From My Sedentary Lifestyle!

The Comfort Food Diet helped me lose more than half my body weight and got me moving again!

By Pam Holmes
Lincoln, Nebraska

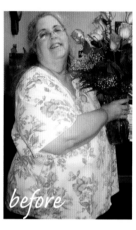

before

I remember being eight years old, wearing one of the many beautiful hand-sewn dresses my mother made for me and thinking that if I cinched the belt tighter, I wouldn't look so fat.

Things changed after I had been married for a few years. The pounds piled on after each of my three sons was born. I was no longer fat; I was morbidly obese. In July 2009, my doctor weighed me at 328 pounds. Before that visit, I had no idea how much I weighed. I didn't own a scale.

In my career, I had earned my bachelor's degree in elementary education. But I took a sedentary desk job as an administrative assistant at a university, so I got little exercise and brought a lot of unhealthy snacks to work with me. I snacked all day in front of my computer.

And for 30 years, I ate anything and everything I wanted. I love food, and I never limited myself, even though I was battling high blood pressure for the last 15 years. My doctor had me on five different medications, and it was still borderline high.

At home, I just wanted to sit in my chair and watch TV. My kitchen chair had wheels, and I would roll around in it while I prepared and cleaned up meals. It just hurt my legs too much to stand or walk.

Vacations and other fun activities were limited because I couldn't walk very far. Physical activity of any sort was completely out of the question.

I started half-heartedly to lose some weight after that eye-opening visit to the doctor in July 2009. Giving up my beloved carbonated full-sugar soft drinks helped me lose 24 pounds. But it was not enough.

SCARY NEWS

In December 2009, I went to the doctor complaining

after

that my heart was pounding hard after even the slightest physical exertion. The doctor ordered an EKG and told me the test seemed to show that I had already had a heart attack. Even though subsequent tests with a cardiologist proved that my heart was fine, his words finally got my attention. It was now or never.

So I launched a "get healthy for life" campaign. If I wanted to maintain any serious weight loss, I knew I couldn't do a short-term "fix" but needed a lifestyle change.

To start, I simply cut back on my overall food intake by eliminating between-meal snacks and eating only one helping of the food I prepared for my family. As the pounds came off, I got more motivated and started cooking and eating healthier foods like fruits, vegetables, lean beef, chicken and fish.

I found many wonderful low-fat and low-calorie recipes in the *Comfort Food*

Diet Cookbook and loved that the nutritional facts were listed for each recipe. It was easy for me to monitor my calorie intake. My husband and son even enjoyed (and still enjoy) the recipes I prepare from the cookbook, too—and they're both real meat-and-potato guys.

I also started walking. Running was not a possibility for me since my knee and hip joints are bad. But I knew that if I didn't start moving, I would lose my ability to get around. I was almost 60 years old and afraid I was going to lose my mobility.

The end of my steep, quarter-mile-long driveway became my first walking goal. My husband, Duane, walked with me a few times. I was always huffing and puffing; he was not. That motivated me to walk a little farther down the road every night.

The first time I made it to the end of our road—1.25 miles—I felt like Rocky, and I did a little dance. I still tell people that spot is where I had my "Rocky moment."

I walk a lot farther now, and I also took up bicycling again. What a joy it is after not being on a bike in 30 years!

LOSING WEIGHT AND MAINTAINING IT!

Through my path to weight loss, I set interim goals as I shed pounds. I wanted to get into the 240s before a friend's wedding and to the 220s before my 40th wedding anniversary. I especially wanted to weigh less than 200 pounds by my 60th birthday. And two months before the big 6-0, I weighed in at 199.6 pounds. I was officially in ONE-derland!

A year and a half after beginning my "get healthy for life" campaign, I reached my ultimate goal of weighing

160 pounds. My total weight loss was 172 pounds, and I am now less than half the size I used to be!

Currently, I weigh 150 pounds. My blood pressure has returned to normal, and my doctor is slowly weaning me off all the medications. I went from a size 5X to an extra-large or large in blouses, and I now wear a size 10 in jeans. Never in my adult life have I been this small.

To maintain my weight, I eat breakfast again after skipping that meal for years. I eat a lot of salads for lunch. I love them with grilled chicken breast and a drizzle of low-fat dressing. Fruit is my favorite snack—I eat grapes like candy! For dinner, I usually eat whatever I prepare for my family, but I give myself a smaller portion. And fruit makes a great dessert!

I still love home-style comfort food, and I find that it's not too tricky to swap ingredients to make dishes healthier with little or no difference in taste. I still make recipes from the *Comfort Food Diet Cookbook*. And I still eat out sometimes, but I make healthier choices. I look on the restaurant's website beforehand so I can pick a wholesome dish to order and avoid less healthy options.

MY ACTIVE LIFE

Now I can do anything! I can literally walk for miles. My house is cleaner, too, because I have more energy to do housework.

My grandchildren and I also have so much fun together now, because I can stay active for longer periods of time. I can't wait to go to the amusement park with them! (That was a great motivator to lose weight.)

Counted cross-stitch is something I enjoy again,

Pam's favorite ways to exercise

- **WALKING.** I started out slow but gained so much strength and speed that I now walk for miles at a time.

- **BIKING.** It is low-impact, which is good for my knees and hips. I'll ride my bike while my son runs next to me.

- **DVDS.** When the roads are covered with ice and snow in the winter, I use walking DVDs to stay active.

- **HOUSEWORK.** It may not be your favorite thing, but it keeps me moving—and I can see my progress!

too. It's a satisfying hobby and not just because of the lovely things I'm making. When my fingers and mind are busy, it keeps me out of the kitchen.

I can't even name all of the differences this weight loss has made in my life. I can get a regular-sized bath towel around me after a shower. I can cross my legs. I don't have to ask for a seat belt extender on an airplane, and I can sit in a lawn chair! I have confidence and self-esteem; I feel like a first-class citizen again.

There are no great secrets to weight loss. It's hard work, and it takes discipline. But you will never regret the day you decided to get healthy, and that turning point will ring in your memory as a great one. By losing half of myself—178 pounds—I regained my whole life.

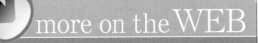

more on the WEB

Having success on the Comfort Food Diet? Share your story at Comfortfooddiet@tasteofhome.com.

I Love Being an
ACTIVE MOM!

My new healthy lifestyle and being 56 pounds lighter let me enjoy more quality family time than ever.

By Tami Kuehl
Loup City, Nebraska

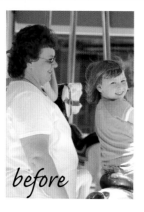

before

I have always grappled with my weight—even as a child. And like many newlywed women, once I walked down the aisle, I stopped worrying about managing my eating habits and let myself go. Then I gained even more weight while pregnant with my daughter, Bailey, as well as during the postpartum depression that followed. I had trouble keeping up with my active little girl.

One of the hobbies Bailey and I enjoyed together was scrapbooking. But something important was missing from our early projects: pictures of the two of us. Self-conscious about my weight, I shied away from cameras. I realized that not only was my lifestyle unfair to Bailey, I was cheating myself as well.

My daughter began to ask questions in the kitchen and take an interest in cooking and baking. I knew I had to change my bad habits so she would learn how to make healthier choices

and avoid the struggles that I'd endured my entire life.

CHANGING MY LIFE

In January 2011, my life changed when I started to follow Taste of Home's Comfort Food Diet. I quickly developed the tools I need to live more healthfully. It isn't like any other diet I've been on; I can eat real food, and it tastes good.

I like to plan my meals in advance and cook up a storm on weekends so I can reheat dishes during the week. Choosing recipes that include similar ingredients and incorporating ones that freeze or store well has helped save time and money.

Keeping track of my calorie intake also hugely impacted my weight loss journey. Now that I'm good at

after

estimating calories, I realize I used to consume more than 5,000 on some days. To help with the calorie counting, I have relied on the *Comfort Food Diet Cookbook: Family Classics Collection* as well as a calorie-listing book. In fact, I have two copies: one in the house and one in the car so I can quickly check nutrition facts at restaurants and make better menu choices.

The more my weight drops, the more active I want to be. My best piece of workout equipment is Max, our West Highland terrier, because I cannot put him in the closet when I get tired of him. The two of us walk four times a day, totaling up to a mile each, weather permitting. And since I'm so much more energetic, Bailey and my husband, Shane, and I enjoy frequent bike rides and Nintendo Wii Fit competitions on family game nights.

Exercise is built into my work life, too. My family home is close to both of my seasonal part-time jobs, so I typically walk to and from work. During the day, I also walk to the post office and the bank as well as home for lunch with Shane. According to my pedometer, I average between 8,000 and 9,000 steps each day. I can hardly believe the impact this increased activity has had on both my body and lifestyle.

OVERCOMING OBSTACLES

Along with all these successes, I've had to navigate some challenges, too. For one, I need to make a big effort to steer clear of those tempting, ooey-gooey sweets at the office, church events and family gatherings. I satisfy my sweet tooth with just a bite or two, or with 100-calorie snacks from the supermarket. In the end, it's all about choices. I still have the occasional ice cream bar, a serving of dessert or a miniature candy bar, but I adjust my calories for that day to include them.

I've also worked hard to drink more water and consume the nutrients I need. Now, I take a water bottle everywhere. So I can have a larger supper, my days include many smaller, nutrient- and fiber-filled meals and snacks. Lately, I've been enjoying granola bars, fruit, popcorn, and green salads topped with ingredients like chicken, nuts, apples and chickpeas, plus a tasty low-calorie dressing.

Lastly, I've had to deal with some physical issues, including arthritis in my right ankle, which used to be an easy excuse for inactivity. Finding shoes that fit well was key. The right equipment and professional help when needed have allowed me to overcome my biggest physical challenge.

LOOKING FORWARD

I can honestly say it took me just three months to lose the "baby weight" that I had been packing on during the seven years since Bailey was born. In the first 12 weeks of dieting, I lost 35 pounds, and now I'm down 56 pounds. I'm currently at 220 pounds and I'd like to lose about 45 more. The progress I've made toward my goal has built up so much energy that I'm practically bursting at the seams to move. My walking pace is nearly a jog, and Max has a hard time keeping up. I used to call that pace my "ticked-off strut," but since starting the Comfort Food Diet, it has become my normal gait.

It's clear that my new lifestyle is beginning to have an effect on Bailey, too, because she frequently asks about calories and makes comments about unhealthy foods. Sometimes she holds up her hands and says, "Mommy, you used to be this wide, but now you are only this wide."

My weight-loss journey has been made simple with a few small, complementary changes: reducing my calorie intake and increasing my activity. I don't feel like I'm on a "diet" or sacrificing, and the excitement of losing those pounds keeps me motivated. I am sleeping better, my joints don't ache as much as they used to, and I'm almost always smiling. Though I'm usually on the go, I do let myself slow down when I walk by a store window—just to catch a glimpse of my reflection.

Top 5 Restaurant Tricks

Eating away from home can be nerve-racking when you don't have control over every ingredient that goes into a meal. Here are five rules of thumb that help me stay on track.

1. Just because it's called a salad doesn't mean it's good for you. Opt for lots of greens with grilled meat instead of the fried stuff. Ask for the dressing on the side, and, if it's available, go for light vinaigrette—you'll be glad you did.

2. Order from the kids' menu. These portions satisfy and keep me from returning to "super size." At many fast-food restaurants, the kids' meals also include a side of fresh fruit and smaller desserts.

3. Get the (nutrition) facts. Most chain restaurants publish nutritional information, and many local ones do, too. Ask the cashier or your server for a copy; many are also available online.

4. Skip the breads, rolls and buns. These pack in a lot of extra calories. If you're having a sandwich, go open-faced, or order without the bread so you can splurge on dessert.

5. "Save" your calories. If I know I'm eating supper at a restaurant, I'll fix a light breakfast and lunch so I can really enjoy dinner, without feeling the need to order the lightest choice. I may have fruit, granola and yogurt for breakfast and a green salad with apple for lunch and drink lots of water throughout the day. That leaves me with plenty of calories for supper!

more on the WEB

For more recipes like the ones in this *Comfort Food Diet Cookbook*, check out tasteofhome.com/cfdiet.

Rewriting My Own History as
'IN SHAPE' NOT 'OVERWEIGHT'

I lost 65 pounds in a year and gained better health and the confidence to take control of my life!

By Richelle Fry
Springdale, Arkansas

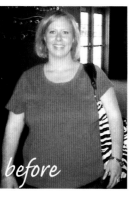

before

I have struggled with my weight all my life. When I was growing up, I was always a little bit bigger than the other kids. And I continued to gain weight into my 20s until 215 pounds were packed onto my 5-foot-one-inch frame. When I was 23, I had to have back surgery. At 26, I had back surgery again. The extra weight I was carrying continued to be a big problem.

A few years ago, I lost almost 70 pounds in a very short time and in a very unhealthy way. Around that time, I met my best friend and husband, Terry, and I gained all the weight back. I lost my job and I wasn't sure what my next step was going to be. Terry encouraged me to pursue my lifelong dream of earning my college degree in history, which I love.

For the first time, I felt happy. I had a happy home, a wonderful husband who found me beautiful and a great new direction in my life. I knew I weighed too much, but I wasn't inspired to do anything about it.

BABY STEPS TOWARD SUCCESS

When I returned to college, I was determined to succeed, so I worked really hard. But that left me with little time for eating. Each day, I ended up having one large, unhealthy meal late in the evening. That's when I realized that my habits had to stop. I wouldn't be able to do my best in any area of my life if I wasn't feeling my best. So I decided to make some healthy changes.

I started by incorporating more fruits, vegetables and yogurt into my diet. Rather than one huge meal a day, I tried to eat several small meals. I drank less diet soda—which was very difficult for me—and more water.

after

Exercise is not my favorite thing, but I made a conscious decision to walk more, especially around campus. Then Terry and I started walking through our neighborhood in the evenings; this is something we still do. Our walks serve two great purposes: we get daily exercise, and we have a chance to reconnect after a busy day. Even when I'm tired or don't feel like walking, Terry encourages me to go with him since it's a great way to spend time together.

Terry's mother also lives with us. As I started losing weight and wanted to continue, we made the effort to eat better as a family. We shared big salads loaded with vegetables. We ate leaner meats. Now, chicken shows up on our menu at least four times a week. Terry makes the best

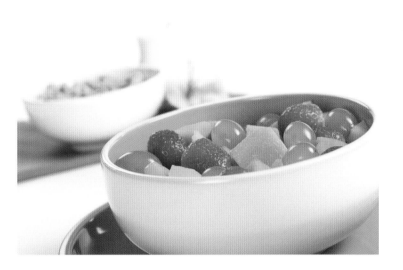

Richelle's Easy Changes

Find someone to encourage you

Drink less soda

Drink more water

Put flavor packets in your water to keep your taste buds interested

Cook with lean meats

Go for a walk—relax and exercise at the same time

Indulge only a little bit

Don't be hard on yourself

meat loaf, so we switched out the ground beef for lean ground turkey. Now we have a lighter way to enjoy our favorite comfort food. We avoid fatty foods and all fast food.

Even snacking got healthier. My current favorite snack is popcorn, especially when it's air-popped. I often put some fat-free butter and cheese seasonings on it, but it's also great plain. And I find that I really do love salads. I usually eat a small salad four times a day or whenever my stomach starts rumbling. And my top way to get going in the morning is with a serving of oatmeal sprinkled with a pinch of cinnamon.

LITTLE INDULGENCES

My sweet tooth has been an obstacle along the way, despite my newfound love for salads. I adore cookies and desserts, so it's hard for me to walk through our kitchen and not indulge in the sweets. I have to ask myself if I really want the cookie or if I just want it because I see it. It's kind of like going to the grocery store when you are hungry—you don't need all that junk food, but you see it and it

looks good, so you buy it. Then you get home and instantly regret going overboard.

I strongly believe that you should not deprive yourself. When I want a cookie, I break off a small piece to satisfy my craving—and that's it. Having a small portion of what you are craving will not ruin your day or throw you off your healthy path. If you've watched your food choices and portion sizes the last few days, a little indulgence will not be the end of the world. If I have a weak moment and eat too many calories, I try not to beat myself up over it. I'm human and make mistakes. I just get back on my healthy path again the next day.

In one year, I have lost 65 pounds and know that I've done it gradually by watching what I eat and working exercise into my day. Now I have tons of confidence and higher self-esteem. My back feels better than ever. I'm happy to know that Terry and I can continue to have fun visiting many historical sites since our healthy lifestyle will ensure a long life together.

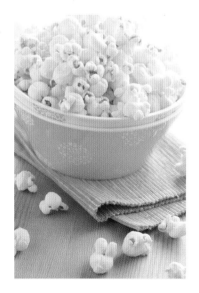

LOSING WEIGHT
For Real This Time!

Having a full, busy life distracted me from taking care of myself and losing weight—until I got serious.

By Kim Bennett
Jackson, Tennessee

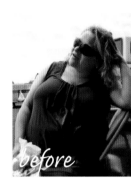

before

Following fad diet plans has never really worked out well for me. Having been plump since I was a toddler, I started my first "diet" before seventh grade. The weight came off quickly, but I gained it back just as fast. A year after my son was born, I weighed the same as I did the day I brought him home from the hospital. When I put on a bathing suit in the summer of 2010, I held 198 pounds on my 5-foot-3-inch frame and was totally disheartened. I was shocked when I looked at photos of myself—was I really that big?

During the year, my job as a sixth grade language arts teacher is stressful, and I work more than full time. I also have a 6-year-old daughter and a 2-year-old son, and my parents have both been ill. For a long time, I didn't have good coping skills to help me deal with feeling sad or stressed. So I ate. That overstuffed feeling became normal for me, and the pounds kept piling on.

I was tired of feeling this way, and so was my husband. He has always been supportive, and we were ready to make some serious changes together.

THREE KEY ELEMENTS

So I said, "good-bye, diet mentality." This time, I approached weight loss as a new lifestyle instead of a short-term fix. I found that weight loss is basically a mathematical formula. Bottom line: I had to eat less and move more if I wanted to see any sort of change.

There were three integral elements to my weight loss success. The first was nutrition. Instead of talking about a "diet," my daughter and I worked on healthy eating, and we learned how to make better choices. Fruit and vegetable portions increased, and our intake of simple

after

carbohydrates decreased. I made sure we were eating enough protein, too. The recipes in the *Comfort Food Diet Cookbook* were really great, because they helped me modify our meals but were family-friendly so everyone passed them around the table with pleasure.

The second element was movement. I had to create a caloric deficit by moving more. I didn't always need to exercise formally since I am a middle school teacher and a mother of two. My days are always busy, so I am not sitting much—but I still needed to move more. So I started to wear a pedometer and aim for 15,000 steps every day. It was so easy to take a few extra steps here and there, and the pedometer made it simple to see my progress.

The third element of my weight loss was the emotional component. I had to figure out what made me eat poorly. I identified my triggers and found ways to subvert them. If I knew I was going to be sad or stressed, such as when my husband was out of town for several weeks, I made sure to plan some relaxation for myself. Sometimes it was as simple as a hot bath after the kids were asleep or finding a babysitter for a few hours to devote some time to myself. I started to listen to my body and not my emotions when it came to hunger. Then I could be smart and more deliberate about my actions.

PLANNING AHEAD AND SAVING CALORIES

Planning meals was another key to staying on track. Though it was a big challenge for me, I've integrated it into my daily life. Instead of not having a plan, I now make sure that we have two or three servings of fish each week and that we eat a rainbow of produce. Every week we have a family outing to the farmers market, so we eat lots of fresh produce and get our vitamins and nutrients.

And when I get up each day, I reach for a yogurt, my new staple breakfast food. Sometimes I make extra breakfast items on the weekend to heat up throughout the week, such as individual ham and cheese frittatas, a recipe I got from an earlier version of the *Comfort Food Diet Cookbook*.

As much as I try to plan each dinner, that time of day can quickly go awry. So I have a stash of quick-and-easy meal ideas that I can whip up if necessary. It's no trouble to keep meal-size portions of browned lean ground beef or turkey in the freezer. That way, I can pull it out and reheat it on really hectic evenings.

Another speedy idea: I mix the cooked ground meat with low-fat, low-sugar spaghetti sauce and serve it over Shirataki noodles, thin Japanese noodles that are low in calories.

I also freeze casseroles or casserole ingredients for fast dinner prep. A deli rotisserie chicken weighed out in portions is easily paired with fresh or frozen vegetables as a dinner.

Slow cookers are my new friends, too! I put an entree in one, and two vegetable sides in other ones. When I get home, a hot meal is ready.

My snacks are also important, because I need to keep my energy level up and my hunger low. I love string cheese, nuts, seeds, vegetable sticks with Greek yogurt dip and hard-boiled eggs. I portion out items at home; I don't snack continuously from the big package at work.

In the evening, I like to indulge in a small dessert. I keep healthy, individual desserts around the house for the whole family. When I make a dessert, I portion it and store it in containers right away. Then it's a conscious decision to get another whole dessert instead of scooping out "just a little more." When I'm tempted to eat more, I head to bed.

EVERY STEP COUNTS

All of these changes in the last year have helped me lose 63 pounds. I now weigh in at 135 pounds, which is a healthy weight for my frame. My wonderful husband, who was enthusiastic as I implemented this new style of eating for our family, has lost 45 pounds, too!

I will maintain my weight loss by monitoring calories and keeping up my activity level. I take my kids outside to ride bikes and play, or we stay inside and compete in fun, active video games. I use my elliptical machine, and I try to take the stairs instead of the elevator. I walk to the store instead of driving.

Kim's Healthy Substitutes

1. Greek yogurt is a great substitute for sour cream. It works well in dip mixes.

2. Instead of using spray oil, I use a pastry brush to spread oil evenly. It's also easier to measure.

3. Being Southern, I drink a lot of iced tea. I sweeten it with sugar substitute.

4. Instead of flavored coffee creamer, I use unsweetened vanilla almond milk. It makes my coffee rich and creamy without added sugar.

But I do occasionally stray. I've even gained a few pounds here and there. When that happens, I am disappointed but not discouraged. I just take a deep breath and dive back into my healthy lifestyle.

PERMANENT CHANGES

My family, neighbors and coworkers have been my cheering section. I get compliments daily and requests for weight loss advice. My husband has been so supportive, and I could not have achieved this goal without him.

I am now much healthier and happier and better equipped to keep up with my kids, my house and my job. The side benefits are greater confidence and self-esteem. I'm thrilled to be making positive, permanent changes that improve my life and the lives of everyone around me.

more on the WEB

For additional Comfort Food Diet tools and tips, check tasteofhome.com/cfdiet.

Take a Group Mentality to
WEIGHT-LOSS

The Taste of Home staff switches one type of comfort food for another and loses a combined total of 650 pounds!

It is surely only a matter of minutes into each employee's first day before he or she is warned of that 10 extra pounds looming on his or her waistline of the future. Many laugh such comments off, but it's not long before they admit to having extended their belts a notch or two.

No one blames them. After all, it's nearly impossible to resist the incredible tastes that bombard the staff every day.

That trend halted when Taste of Home published the *Comfort Food Diet Cookbook*.

PUTTING IT TOGETHER

With the success of the *Comfort Food Diet Cookbook*, employees began to look at their own eating and exercise habits. They decided it was time to make a change. It was January, after all, and keeping weight-loss resolutions is nearly always a challenge in the winter. Why not tackle this year's healthy-living promise with a group of coworkers who understood the problems we all seem to face?

A small team of organizers reached out to staff members, gauging interest in an office-wide program based on Taste of Home's *Comfort Food Diet Cookbook*. To everyone's surprise, a whopping 62 people eagerly signed up!

Hearty casseroles, cheesy dips and spreads, golden pastries and gooey chocolate cakes smothered in luscious frosting. These are just a few of the items up for grabs any day of the week at the Milwaukee office of Reader's Digest.

While the building may be home to the team behind the *Comfort Food Diet Cookbook*, it's also the spot where *Taste of Home* magazine and a slew of other titles are published. And because all Taste of Home recipes are tested and photographed in the Milwaukee office, there's an assortment of mouthwatering delights waiting around nearly every corner nearly any time of day. Even desserts quietly placed in the cafeteria at 10 a.m. mysteriously disappear within the hour.

Working for the Taste of Home brand clearly has its share of delicious perks. Reader's Digest veterans never tire of platters of freshly baked cookies set out by the Test Kitchen staff, and new employees stare wide-eyed at the variety of succulent delights coming from the Photo Studio, everything free to anyone who'd like to try a bite.

Registered dietitian and *Comfort Food Diet Cookbook* editor Peggy Woodward outlined a 16-week strategy following the book's weight-loss plan. She also created a series of motivational topics. Weekly thirty-minute meetings were scheduled during the workday, so participants wouldn't have to worry about missing get-togethers due to obligations at home.

At the first meeting, each group member received a copy of the *Comfort Food Diet Cookbook* and an inexpensive pedometer. Peggy reviewed the plan's four main principles: Eat five times per day within a total range of 1,400 or 1,500 calories; keep a food diary; take advantage of the diet's Free Foods and Smart Snacks; and work in some exercise.

The energetic meeting ended with each participant weighing in on a scale set up in a private area of the building. Each member logged their weight onto a spreadsheet under a previously established code name. This allowed everyone to be honest without exposing their weights to the entire office. As participants documented their weights each week, a group facilitator tracked the code names and calculated the group's overall weight loss.

AWAY WE GO!

The meetings that followed proved to be fun and exciting for everyone. Weekly topics ranged from emotional eating to making smart choices at the grocery store. Guest speakers offered presentations on exercising and meal planning, and Peggy shared her personal food diary with the group.

In addition, the building's facilities department mapped out a walking track—eight times around the route added up to 1 mile—and the office cafeteria added several options from the *Comfort Food Diet Cookbook* to the menu. Best of all, bowls of free fruit were set out daily to help group participants avoid the buttery sensations and sugary temptations that lingered around the office.

To keep everyone motivated further, members were given punch cards. People earned punches for hitting the walking track three times per week, keeping up their food journals or reviewing recipes from the *Comfort Food Diet Cookbook*. Once a card was full, a small prize was awarded!

It wasn't long before group members started to see their efforts pay off. In fact, after the first three weeks, the group had lost a total of 220 pounds!

TEAM WORK MAKES THE DREAM WORK

Group-wide goals were also set for total pounds lost. When those goals were met, everyone received a prize such as a blank food journal, plastic water bottle or 3-pound weight set.

Halfway through the program, the group was separated into two teams, creating a friendly, lively air of competition. Folks earned punches on their cards if their team won fun-filled games about calories and fitness. Punches were also allotted to the team that lost the most weight over a week's time.

Things were working! People were sticking to the diet, losing weight and meeting their personal health goals—all while eating the foods they loved!

Members happily shared their favorite recipes with one another and discussed weight-loss tips they discovered. A "Suggestion Box" helped guarantee that weekly meetings covered relevant topics, and emails summarizing the group's statuses kept everyone in the loop even when their workload prevented them from attending a meeting.

At the end of the 16-week program, the participating employees had lost a total of 650 pounds! Some members were excited to have reached their goal of a 10- or 20-pound loss; others dropped 30, 40 or even 60 pounds over the four-month program and were thrilled. Folks were feeling better, living healthier and still feeding their families the meals they craved—without a lot of extra calories, fat and sodium.

Though the employee program has ended, many staff members continue to use the building's walking track, keep a food diary and rely on the cookbook for weekly menu planning. And while the Reader's Digest-Milwaukee office continues to test mouthwatering recipes every day, we're all feeling a lot healthier thanks to everything we learned from the *Comfort Food Diet Cookbook*!

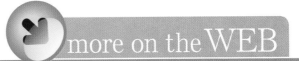
more on the WEB

Why not start a *Comfort Food Diet Cookbook* group for your office or company—or even with friends or extended family? Check out the additional recipes, tools and motivation at tasteofhome.com/cfdiet.

New Love of Lighter Foods and Exercise
MEANS A HEALTHY LIFE

Eating more fruits and vegetables and moving more helped me lose 75 pounds!

By Jim Palmen
Reader's Digest Employee

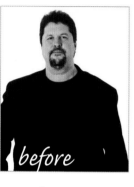

before

I've worked for the world's largest food and entertaining magazine for the past 15 years. Being creative director for creative marketing is the perfect fit for me—but until the Comfort Food Diet, not all of my clothes were.

Over the years, I gained a few pounds here and there. Over time, it added up to more than 100.

After a long, hard day at work, I'd come home, eat an unhealthy dinner, plop down in front of the TV and think about what I wanted for dessert. It was an easy—and sometimes delicious—pattern to fall into. But my energy was so low that I breathed heavily just putting my socks on for the day.

I also found myself eating for two. I'm a pretty thrifty guy, and I never like to waste food. So when my kids didn't finish their meals, I was the first to help them out. That is the quickest way to pack on the pounds.

With these habits, I lacked energy and felt tired all the time. I knew I was shortening my life because of my food choices and lack of exercise. I wanted to make a change; I wanted

to have more energy and be able to enjoy life with my wife of 22 years, Lynn, and our two great children, Melissa and Mat.

The *Comfort Food Diet Cookbook* weight loss program was introduced at work at the perfect time for me. It was a good opportunity for me to stay focused, set goals and finally shed those extra pounds.

I wanted to commit to the diet, and that was easy when my co-worker, Widdy, served as my motivator. We had the same goal—to live healthier lives—and we used each other to stay motivated, share diet tips and walk at lunch. I had plenty of days when I almost lost focus, but I could always count on Widdy to keep me on track—sometimes literally.

after

USING COMFORT FOOD DIET TOOLS

When I started the diet, I wrote down everything that I ate. I used the daily calorie sheets in the cookbook to reflect on my food choices, and it forced me to make smart decisions. I also ate more slowly. My busy lifestyle caused me to rush when I ate, and I would eat so fast that I consumed twice as much food as I should have. The food was unhealthy, too.

By slowing down, I actually tasted what I was eating. I discovered new flavors, and I started to eat things I never would have tried before.

Using better portion control also helped me understand how I had gained weight over the years. I purchased smaller dinner plates so I could eat smaller portions of food without realizing it. It was a psychological thing for me to see a full plate, no matter how big the plate was.

Now, when my kids don't finish their meals, I take the leftovers for lunch the next day instead of doubling my dinner portions. I still allow myself to eat some high-calorie foods, but I combine them with healthier options. I'll have a bite of pizza with two bites of salad. I'll eat an apple and then have a cookie. And I drink a lot more water.

I drink a lot of coffee, too, so I know I am consuming my daily amount of fluids. But when I find myself craving a snack or feeling hungry, I drink a glass of water to ease those hunger pangs, and it helps.

About three months into the diet, I had a wonderful realization. One morning, a huge crash came from my closet. The shelves on which I store my clothes fell to the floor, and my clothes were scattered everywhere. I decided to try everything on and get rid of the stuff that didn't fit anymore. I ended up donating almost half of my clothes. They were too big!

SMART SNACKING

On my path to better fitness, popcorn has been a key snack. My family munches on popcorn five days a week. We used to make it with oil in a pan and top it with loads of butter, but now we enjoy air-popped popcorn. And instead of real butter with tons of calories, I use zero-calorie butter spray and sprinkle on grated Parmesan cheese, spices or a bit of sea salt. (That butter spray is tasty on vegetables and toast, too.) Craving conquered.

Salsa became another good friend on the Comfort Food Diet. I was amazed by its added flavor on eggs or vegetables. The bonus: Salsa is "free" calories! I've learned to take advantage of free foods and eat the proper portions of them.

Another craving buster—and free food—is pickles. When I find myself looking in the refrigerator for something to munch, I dip into the pickle jar. It's a "free" way to calm my craving for a satisfying, salty crunch.

STAY AWAY FROM FAST FOOD!

Another obstacle in my path was the ease of hitting the drive-thru on my way home from work. Most things on fast food menus are three times the portion a person needs, and they're high in calories. Grab a sugar-laden soft drink to go with your meal, and you've ruined your diet for more than just that day. If the drive-thru is your only option, however, look on the restaurant's website for the best foods available. Most restaurants have nutritional information online, so you can abide by your diet and choose something you will not regret down the road.

Avoiding the drive-thru is easy if you get into the habit of preparing meals at home. It's easier to control portions, cook healthy choices and eat more delicious food.

Taste of Home's website also has great resources for planning meals. The Meal Planning Worksheet and Grocery List features allow easy shopping to plan a menu for the week. I definitely take advantage of these online tools.

Jim's favorite low-cal snacks

- BANANA
- APPLE
- CHEWING GUM
- GRAPES
- SALSA
- MILLER GENUINE DRAFT 64

NEW HOBBIES

Overall, the *Comfort Food Diet Cookbook* helped me learn that healthy foods actually taste pretty darn good! The book has a great variety of recipes to choose from, and it helped me easily plan meals along my journey to weight loss.

The last six months of my weight-loss plan have had one recurring theme: set a goal. By setting big and small goals and continually setting new ones, I have lost 75 pounds. I also competed in two 5K runs and will run a third one soon.

In fact, I love exercising now. I consider it one of my hobbies along with going to baseball games and entertaining my friends and family.

We even have a stationary bike as a permanent fixture in our living room now. Any time I'm watching TV, I hop on and get a lot of exercise without even really noticing.

I have so much more energy to do these things, and I accomplish more every day since I lost so much weight. I am 48, and I feel younger than ever. Maybe 50 isn't so scary!

Out With the Old,
IN WITH THE SKINNY

With the support of my husband and coworkers, losing weight and eating healthy foods became fun and rewarding.

By Marie Parker
Reader's Digest Employee

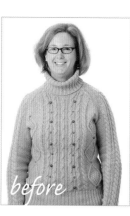

before

For me, weight loss was never much of an issue. But since I had children, I have gained and lost the same 10 pounds countless times.

I always have two sizes in my closet, and I never know which one is going to fit. Nothing ever fits like I want it to, especially my cute party clothes. Those ten pounds may not be much, but they make themselves known—at just the wrong times.

My husband, Andrew, and I have two sons, Maxwell and Grayson. They both attend the same college in Las Vegas. Last fall, while we were helping move them into school, I suffered a horrible open fracture of my toe. It was awful. I was in pain for months and couldn't exercise. I was at the mercy of my husband to feed me—and he's no healthy eater.

I gained about a pound a week. I think I ended up weighing even more than when I was pregnant. Soon, out of my two-size closet, I had no clothes that fit. So I hobbled on my crutches to the store and bought new, bigger pants. I was not happy about that.

MAKING CHANGES

The Comfort Food Diet Club began at work at just the right time for me. My toe was beginning to heal, and I could finally walk on the treadmill a bit. But I knew I needed something more to motivate me in my weight loss.

I really enjoyed the structure of weighing in and attending meetings at work. The club kept us moving and engaged us in the program by using incentives and setting goals. Walking on the indoor track at lunch was easy and just plain fun. I felt—and still feel—so much stronger than I did before my toe injury.

Combining exercise and calorie counting was the golden ticket for my weight

after

loss. Following recipes from the *Comfort Food Diet Cookbook* made healthy eating so much easier, because I could track the calories in each meal.

The diet taught me that I was eating too much protein and not enough grains; you can tell what kind of diet I was on in the past. I was also eating too much between meals, such as cake samples in the Test Kitchen or a handful of nuts from my desk drawer here and there. Those snacks added up, and I didn't realize it.

Now, I love salads. I switch up their bases, but they're usually spinach, red and green leaf lettuce or spring mix. I cut up a few days' worth of vegetables to add color and flavor to my salads, too. I'll prep carrots, broccoli, cucumbers and more! Sometimes I even blanch the veggies for a different texture.

However, I don't buy reduced-fat salad dressings. I learned that fat is usually replaced with sugar in those. Instead, I opt for olive oil-based dressings. Slimmer waistline, here I come!

FEELING ENERGIZED

I feel so much better now that I consume less protein and more grains. I count calories now, so I know exactly how much is too much. On the Comfort Food Diet, every day is broken up into three meals of a certain calorie count, and that is so easy for me to follow. I love this plan, because it includes food I like to cook and eat—but it's all made in a healthy way.

Counting calories also makes it easy to go out to eat and fit those kinds of meals into my diet. So many restaurant websites tell you the calories in each dish! It's so cool to think that I lost weight eating enchiladas, burgers and casseroles. And I can surely continue that! If I do gain some weight back, I'm not afraid, because I have a plan—and tons of deliciously light recipes. At any given time, I have about ten recipes that I am waiting to try.

I've lost 33½ pounds in six months, and I have so much energy. I take a body toning class once a week, do arm exercises with weights two or three times a week and do lots of sit-ups. At least three times a week, I walk for 30 to 45 minutes. And a few times every month, I also go for a giant walk for an hour or two. My husband occasionally walks with me, which makes exercise more fun.

I was a size 12; now I'm a size 6. It was so much fun to get rid of my size 12 clothes. Then size 10. Then size 8! It was mind-blowing to think I could fit into anything I wanted to wear from my closet—even my cute stuff. Then, boom! Nothing fit. This time, I went shopping for skinny clothes! I donated 12 bags of clothes to a local thrift store.

I'm 5 feet 4 inches and I now weigh 127 pounds. I've reached my goal. And I reached this point while eating my favorite comfort foods. What an amazing feeling!

Marie's Favorite Comfort Food Diet Recipes

(These recipes appear in the Family Classics edition of the *Comfort Food Diet Cookbook*)

- Turkey Breakfast Sausage Patties
- Blueberry Oat Pancakes
- Slow-Cooked Pork Tacos
- Fully Loaded Chili
- Asian Chicken Dinner
- Bravo Broccoli
- Black Bean Veggie Enchiladas

Marie's daily food outline

- **BREAKFAST.** I usually have a grain and fruit for breakfast, like oatmeal and a banana. Or I'll eat a protein and a grain, such as a veggie omelet with toast.

- **LUNCH.** Salad or leftovers from dinner the night before are my go-to lunch choices. I like spinach salads and eat only olive oil-based dressings.

- **DINNER.** I love trying new recipes from the *Comfort Food Diet Cookbook* at dinner. My coworkers and I swap our best-loved recipes from the diet.

- **SNACKS.** I have two snacks a day, and I mostly reach for fruit, yogurt or both. I recently got hooked on almond butter and rice cakes, too.

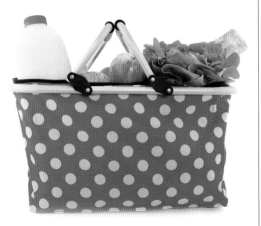

BRING BALANCE
& variety to your diet

Counting your calories may be the key to losing weight, but it's still important
(and not tricky) to make sure you're getting good nutrition to fuel your body so you can
be more active—and have more fun. Here's how to achieve a balanced diet.

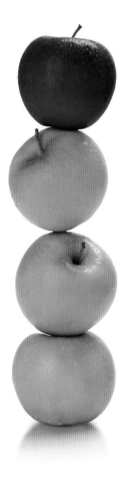

FIBER

Most Americans do not eat as much fiber as they should. Your daily fiber goal
should be 20 to 30 grams, which includes soluble and insoluble fiber.

Insoluble fiber can be found in whole wheat and brown rice, while soluble
fiber is a part of oatmeal, beans and barley. Soluble fiber helps to lower
cholesterol, and insoluble fiber keeps your digestive tract healthy.

Along with aiding digestion, consuming the right amount of fiber each day
can help lower your risk of heart disease and diabetes. The best part? Fiber
helps keep you feeling full, which can help prevent you from overeating and
keep you on track with your diet.

tips to help boost your fiber

- Making soup? Add extra veggies.
- Add wheat germ or oat bran to yogurt and casseroles. You won't notice
  the difference.
- Add a tablespoon or two of ground flaxseed to your morning smoothie.
- Leave the skins on when you eat fruits and vegetables.
- Toss some garbanzo beans or kidney beans in your salad.
- Choose whole grain breads and crackers. Whole wheat or whole grain
  flour should be listed as the first ingredient on the food label.

PROTEIN

The body needs a constant supply of protein to repair and rebuild cells
that are worn or damaged. About half of the protein we consume creates
enzymes, which help cells carry out necessary chemical reactions.
Proteins also transport oxygen to cells, help muscles contract and produce
antibodies. Men should consume about 55 grams of protein a day, while
women should consume about 45 grams per day.

CARBOHYDRATES

Moderation is key when consuming carbohydrates. Carbs shouldn't be feared when you're on a diet, because they energize your body, which is necessary for your daily exercise.

There are two types of carbohydrates: sugar and starch. Sugars are in fruit, milk and granulated sugar, and starches include grains and potatoes. Your body converts all sugars and starches to glucose—a source of energy.

Positive carbohydrate choices include whole grains, reduced-fat dairy products and a variety of fruits and vegetables. Want to eliminate empty calories? Cut out packaged cakes, pies and cookies. These choices are highly processed and don't contribute to a healthy diet.

CHOLESTEROL

Although saturated and trans fats have a larger effect on blood cholesterol than eating foods high in cholesterol, you should still limit your daily intake of cholesterol to 300 mg. Cholesterol is found in foods from animals, such as eggs, meat and dairy products.

FAT

Believe it: There are some healthy fats! Monounsaturated and polyunsaturated fats, which are found in olive and canola oils and nuts and seeds, are all healthier options. Adults should limit fat to about 30% of their calories each day. This means you should be eating no more than 50 grams of fat daily if you are consuming 1,400 to 1,500 calories per day.

SATURATED FAT

While saturated fat is found mostly in high-fat meats and dairy foods, it is also found in coconut oil, palm kernel oil and some processed foods. Consume only 17 grams of saturated fat per day, which is 10% of calories following a 1,400 to 1,500 calorie-a-day diet.

TRANS FAT

LDL (bad) cholesterol increases with saturated fat and trans fat, increasing your risk of coronary artery disease. Trans fats can also decrease HDL (good) cholesterol. Limit trans fat as often as you can, and try to stay below 1.5 to 2.0 grams per day. Foods that commonly contain trans fat include vegetable shortening, stick margarine, fried foods, processed foods and store-bought baked goods.

SODIUM

Restrict sodium to no more than 2,300 mg a day—equivalent to about one teaspoon of table salt. The best way to reduce salt is to cut back on restaurant and processed foods like canned vegetables, deli meat and condiments. Generally, a food product that has been prepared for you to buy—such as frozen dinners and convenience products—will contain a high amount of sodium.

Refer to the section on freezing foods (p. 38-41) to plan ahead and freeze healthy meals so you won't be tempted by high-sodium packaged foods.

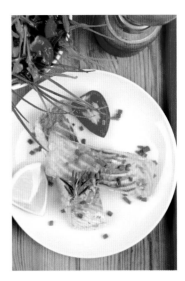

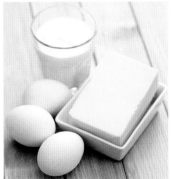

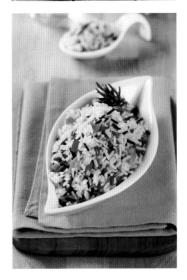

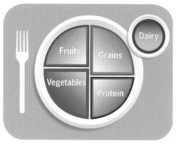

THE DISH on MyPlate

Step up to the USDA's new plate (or MyPlate) and change your eating habits for the better

It's easier to eat right, thanks to the U.S. Department of Agriculture (USDA). The government agency that built the long-standing Food Guide Pyramid has replaced it with a dinner plate in an effort to make following a healthy diet a no-brainer.

The aptly named MyPlate symbol (shown above left) is divided into four sections—fruits, vegetables, grains and protein—with a "cup" on the side to represent dairy. What immediately catches your eye is that fruits and veggies fill half the plate, with protein making up the smallest portion.

If that isn't the way your plate looks during dinner time, prepare for an appetite adjustment.

How can the MyPlate symbol make healthy eating easier? Instead of encouraging you to figure out how many servings of this and that you should eat each day, as in the old pyramid, the plate helps you visualize the symbol when you dish up your meal. Figure out how to make your plate look more like MyPlate. Maybe it's trading the potato chips for cut-up fresh fruit or splitting that huge steak with your spouse. You can even apply the symbol to a fast-food meal!

The key messages of the USDA's revised dietary guidelines are:
- Enjoy food, but eat less
- Avoid oversized portions
- Make half your plate fruit and vegetables
- Make at least half your grains whole grains
- Drink water instead of sugary drinks
- Choose fat-free or 1% (low-fat) milk
- Check the sodium in foods—and aim low

More ways to save on calories and fat when eating out:
- Ask for condiments on the side
- Choose packets of light dressings
- Skip the salt and fat (like bacon and cheese)
- Avoid supersized portions and buffets
- Don't eat on the run
- Check out fast-food restaurants' nutritional information for their menu items on their websites before you go

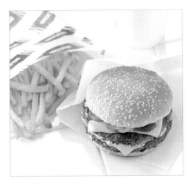

Say your typical drive-thru dinner consists of a hearty double cheeseburger, fries and a soda.

Instead of eating from the bag, assemble it on a dinner plate and see how it compares to MyPlate. The bun and burger (grains and protein) may fill one half of the plate, but the cheese adds extra fat and sodium. The fries spill over the entire other half, and though they're potatoes, they're loaded with fat, calories and sodium—hardly a nutritious choice.

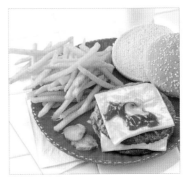

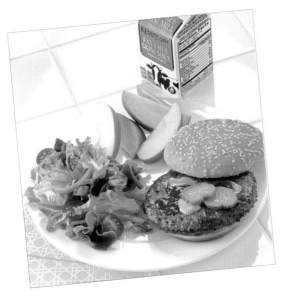

How do you make that fast-food meal look like MyPlate? You can still choose a burger and bun; just downsize to a single patty, skip the cheese and opt for a whole grain bun if it's available. For the other half of the plate, order a side salad. Some fast-food restaurants also offer fruit choices. Don't forget to swap out soda for milk. You'll cut the fat, calories and sodium, add nutrients and jumpstart a habit that will do your body good.

Want to learn more about the USDA's guidelines and how to make them work for you? Visit **choosemyplate.gov.**

portion size
CHART

Large restaurant portions and super-sized fast food meals make it hard to remember how big a standard healthy serving really is. Keep these visuals in mind when estimating a proper portion size.

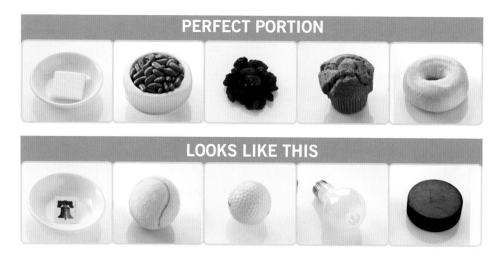

PERFECT PORTION

LOOKS LIKE THIS

- **1 teaspoon butter,** a postage stamp or the tip of your thumb
- **1 cup beans,** a tennis ball or a cupped handful
- **2 tablespoons dried fruit or nuts,** a golf ball or a small cupped handful
- **1 small muffin,** the round part of a light bulb
- **1 small bagel,** a hockey puck (3" diameter)
- **3 ounces meat,** a purse pack of tissues or your outstretched palm
- **1 dinner roll,** a bar of soap or half your palm
- **1 pancake,** a music CD
- **1 tablespoon salad dressing,** a silver dollar
- **1 cup chips,** a tennis ball or a cupped handful
- **1 3x3-inch piece of cake,** a tennis ball

get your (nutrition)
FACTS STRAIGHT!

Nutrition Facts

Serving Size 1/4 Cup (30g)
Servings Per Container About 38

Amount Per Serving

Calories 200   Calories from Fat 150

	% Daily Value*
Total Fat 17g	**26%**
Saturated Fat 2.5g	**13%**
Trans Fat 0g	
Cholesterol 0mg	**0%**
Sodium 120mg	**5%**
Total Carbohydrate 7g	**2%**
Dietary Fiber 2g	**8%**
Sugars 1g	
Protein 5g	

Vitamin A 0%	•	Vitamin C 0%
Calcium 4%	•	Iron 8%

*Percent Daily Values are based on a 2,000 calorie diet.

The nutrition information found on packaged foods makes it easy to buy the healthiest food for your family.

Regulated by the Food Safety and Inspection Service and the Food and Drug Administration, Nutrition Facts panels are found on nearly every item in the grocery store. And while food labels can be a bit confusing, they're not impossible to translate once you understand them.

SERVING SIZE

The top of the Nutrition Facts panel (see example above) lists serving information. Food manufacturers follow guidelines that ensure the serving sizes of like products are comparable. This makes it a cinch for shoppers to determine which brand of orange juice offers the most vitamin C per serving, which spaghetti sauce has the least calories and so on.

CALORIES. The panel lists the number of calories each serving contains—and how many of those calories come from fat. In the example above, there are 200 calories in one serving, and 150 of them come from fat. Remember, however, that if you ate 1/2 cup (or 2 servings), you'd take in 400 calories, of which 300 would be fat.

FATS. Also listed is the total number of fat grams per serving and how many of those grams come from saturated and trans fats (the "bad" fats).

CARBOHYDRATES. The "Total Carbohydrate" figure lists all of the carbs contained in the item. Since dietary fiber and sugars are of special interest to consumers, their amounts are highlighted individually as well as being included in the total carb number.

The "sugars" listed include those that occur naturally in foods, such as lactose in milk, as well as sugars that are added during processing.

PERCENT DAILY VALUE

The Percent Daily Value listed on the nutrition panel indicates how much each component in the product contributes to a 2,000-calorie-per-day eating plan. In the example at left, the total fat for a serving comprises 26% of the daily value, whereas the sodium comprises 5%.

Manufacturers must list the Percent Daily Value of vitamin A, vitamin C, calcium and iron on every food label so that consumers will know how the product fits into a well-balanced diet. Other vitamins and minerals may also be listed, depending on the space on the label and the manufacturer's preference.

If the Daily Value for calcium, iron, vitamin A, etc. is more than 10%, the product is generally considered to be a good source of that particular nutrient.

At the end of the nutrition label, you'll find an ingredients list—a requirement on all food products that contain more than one ingredient. Ingredients are listed in order, with the most major component (based on weight) of the product listed first and other ingredients following in decreasing order.

SHOPPING SMART
for family groceries
A new way of grocery shopping that will help you choose healthy foods!

The grocery store can feel like a foreign country when you're trying to eat healthier.

Learning your way around the healthy options is easier than you think. You could probably find the soda, frozen pizza and packaged cookies with your eyes closed. But mapping out the nutritious, fresh foods is simple, too.

Spend less time in the middle of the store, looking through row upon row of processed foods. Instead, allocate most of your time and money on the outer aisles, where the gems like fresh fruits and vegetables are kept.

Yes, many of the foods that are the best choices for healthy eaters are on the perimeter of the store. That includes produce, dairy and the butcher section, with its array of fresh meat and fish.

Getting to know these parts of the store is beneficial because many of your meals can follow this formula: choose your protein, then add vegetables, fruit and a whole grain to make a meal. You'll still need to go to the middle of the store for pasta, rice, frozen foods and other items. But avoid the big sections of processed foods like chips, meals in a box or a can, cookies and candy that beckoned to you in the past.

It's tempting to blame your busy lifestyle for preventing you from having the time to shop for healthy foods. But it doesn't take any longer to shop for healthy foods than it does for unhealthy ones. Save yourself some time at the grocery store by planning your meals and writing out grocery lists. You'll save time in the kitchen, too, because you won't be staring into your refrigerator, wondering what to make for dinner.

Shopping healthy is all about choosing the right foods for your meal plan: lean, unprocessed meat and fish, high-quality fruits and vegetables, whole grains and low-fat dairy. Eating healthy means taking these basic starters and preparing them for your family without adding unnecessary fat and calories.

ABOUT PRODUCE

When it comes to good-for-you staples, fresh produce is best, followed closely by frozen fruits or vegetables. Canned products are a distant third.

Spend a lot of time in the fresh produce section and get to know your naturally healthy foods. You recognize your old favorites—carrots, celery, potatoes...but what about jicama? Or kale? Your new favorite food could be right in front of you, and you don't even know it yet!

Trying new produce is one of the fun parts of healthy eating. Give yourself the goal of trying a new fruit or vegetable every week. Have your family members take turns at picking a new fresh food, and try it together. If you like it, find a way to incorporate it into your meals.

The produce manager can explain individual produce items and how they're best prepared. Ask questions; these folks like to share their knowledge—but make sure to ask for healthy ways to make your newfound favorites.

Fresh produce is even fresher at the farmers market. If there's one near you, get there early so you're guaranteed the best selection. Talk to the farmers who grow the produce you're buying. They are used to eating what they grow, so they often have simple recipes and healthy preparation tips to share.

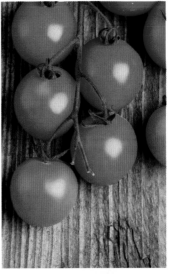

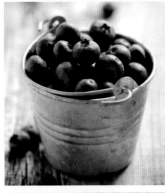

ABOUT MEAT & FISH

When you're at the meat counter, avoid processed meats like sausage. They're often made with high-fat ingredients and a number of additives. Instead, look for fresh chicken and turkey with the occasional lean cuts of beef and pork.

When buying your chicken or turkey, either buy skinless or remove the skin and fat at home so your pieces are lean. The breast is leanest. When buying ground turkey, make sure it is ground breast, not turkey pieces; those "pieces" can include skin and have as much fat as regular ground beef!

For red meat, cuts that include the word "round" or "loin" are generally leaner. Look for firm meat that smells and looks fresh with no off-color areas. Read the packages to make sure your meat wasn't injected with water, flavorings or preservatives.

And if you're buying fish, choose fresh, firm fish that doesn't smell fishy. It's OK to ask when it was delivered to the store. If the fresh fish looks or smells iffy, go for frozen seafood instead.

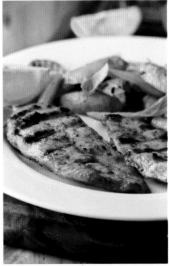

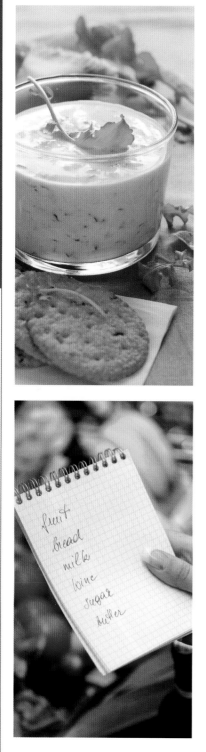

KNOWING THE INS & OUTS

While sticking to the perimeter of the store can help you pick healthy items, you will need to venture into the aisles for some packaged and canned foods. When choosing these foods, get into the habit of checking Nutrition Facts labels (see the guide on page 31).

Look for foods that don't get many of their calories from fat, and aim for items that are low in saturated fat. Consider non-fat or low-fat options at the dairy case.

When the carbohydrate total on the label is more than twice the amount of sugar, the food is usually loaded with complex carbohydrates that are good for you. Consider making these items a part of your family's weekly menu plan.

Many items found in the deli or bakery, however, are not required to provide nutrition facts. Luckily, many of today's supermarkets make this information available upon request. When in doubt, ask. You'd be surprised at how often nutrition information is available.

Here's another important tip for successful healthy shopping: Don't go to the grocery store when you're hungry. And if your kids are looking for a snack, this may not be the best time to bring them along. You'll be tempted to give in to instant gratification (junk food), and you won't stick to your healthy eating plan either. Eat something substantial and satisfying before you leave the house.

And finally, the best shopping advice: if it's not good for you, simply don't put it in your cart. That way you can't take it home and eat it!

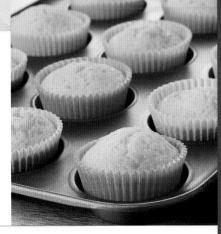

LIGHTEN UP
your family favorites!

Keep your family satisfied and healthy
by tweaking your favorite recipes just a bit.

DINNER STANDBYS:

- When serving pasta and rice, pay attention to portion sizes. A serving of cooked rice is 1/2 or 2/3 cup, while pasta is usually 1-1/2 ounces, uncooked, per serving.

- A serving of meat is considered 4 ounces, uncooked.

- Ten-inch flour tortillas have about 200 calories before any fillings are added. To go lighter, choose 6- or 8-inch tortillas instead.

- See the Portion Size Chart on page 30 for visual cues of common portion sizes.

- Until you get a feel for typical serving sizes, measure portions with measuring cups and spoons. It will help you keep on track.

- Choose lean meat when cooking. Look for skinless white-meat poultry, pork with "loin" in the name and beef with "loin" or "round" in the name.

- Consider low-sodium/no-sodium alternatives when cooking with packaged foods, boxed mixes, olives, cheese and savory seasoning mixes. Instead of canned products, choose fresh or frozen corn, sliced mushrooms, green beans and others.

- Cut back on adding high-calorie ingredients such as olives, cheese and avocado.

DESSERT FAVORITES:

- When adding chopped mix-ins such as nuts, chips, raisins or coconut to desserts, decrease the amount a bit. Try using mini chips. Toast nuts and coconut so smaller amounts have stronger flavor.

- Reduce the amount of frosting. You can usually cut the amount by 1/4 or 1/3 without missing out.

- When making frosting, confectioners' sugar can almost always be decreased without losing any of the sweetness. One tablespoon of confectioners' sugar equals 29 calories.

- Using reduced-fat butter and reduced-fat cream cheese works well in homemade frosting. Since these lighter products tend to be soft-set, the recipe may need less liquid.

- When baking, replace 1/4 or 1/2 of the butter or oil in a recipe with unsweetened applesauce. But keep in mind that applesauce is a better replacement for oil than it is for butter.

- If you're substituting a substantial amount (1/2 to 1 cup) of applesauce for fat, you can cut down on sugar a bit due to the natural sweetness of the applesauce.

- Instead of using all whole eggs in baked products, use some egg whites as a replacement. Do not use all egg whites (unless the recipe specifies to do so), as the resulting item may be spongy and tough.

- Oftentimes, sugar can be decreased slightly without making a difference in the recipe. This is especially true for recipes that are over 40 years old since they tend to be disproportionately high in sugar.

- One tablespoon of sugar equals 48 calories—so be careful when adding it to any of your baked goods.

- If your lightened-up cakes turn out tough with a dense texture, try substituting cake flour for all-purpose flour the next time you prepare them.

- It's rather difficult to lighten cookie recipes successfully and keep the original shape and texture. The best option is to prepare your little treats as usual and savor a single serving.

OUT OF THE KITCHEN
...not out of control

Don't leave your diet goals at home when you go out.
Keep your healthy-eating momentum when you eat at...

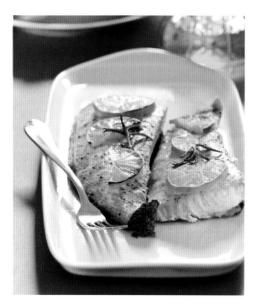

A RESTAURANT

Go fish! Most family restaurants have a number of fish and seafood options from which we can choose. Resist the urge to order fried shrimp or anything with a cream or butter sauce.

If seafood's not your thing, there are other smart options. Stir-fries, lean cuts of meat and baked chicken dishes are healthier than other menu items. Look for items that are baked, roasted, poached, broiled or steamed. Avoid those that are fried or come with a heavy sauce.

Check out the appetizers, and you might find something that makes an ideal low-calorie entree at a normal portion size. Grilled vegetable platters and side salads (with the dressing on the side) are great options. But if you order a normal entree, watch your portion size and try to save half for leftovers the next day.

THE VENDING MACHINE

Vending machines seem like a great idea when hunger comes calling. Whether at work or cheering the kids on at an after-school activity, vending machines promise comforting nibbles—but deliver few rewards.

If you need to drop a few coins into a vending machine, spend them on baked chips or pretzels. Similarly, small bags of snack mix and plain animal crackers are decent snacks. Many machines offer an assortment of mints and low-sugar gum. Give these options a try, as the strong flavor of peppermint will often curb any cravings.

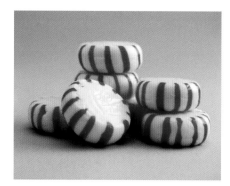

A PARTY

Family celebrations mean good people, good times and good food—that may not be good FOR you. That mile-long buffet is probably stocked with high-calorie foods that can easily tempt you.

Look for items such as veggie and fruit platters, boiled shrimp and whole wheat crackers. Decide which items you really have to try and which you can do without. Stay clear of fried foods and be leery of thick dips and spreads. Try a salsa or chutney instead.

The best way to avoid overindulging at a party is to eat something healthy before you arrive. If your stomach is full, you'll spend less time at the buffet and more time having fun!

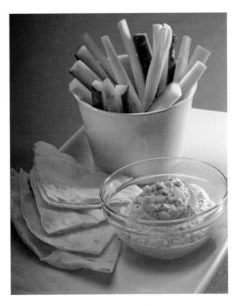

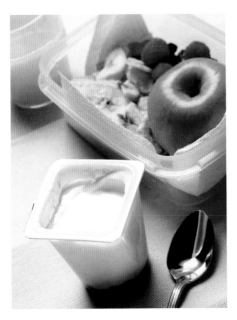

THE OFFICE

Home cooks are often so busy packing lunches for the kids they forget to fill a brown bag for themselves. Bring your own lunch to work, and you can easily keep your caloric goals intact and avoid the vending machine.

Bring a few snacks to work, too. For many people, the lure of high-calorie snacks is greatest at the workplace. Keep a container of nuts or low-calorie snack mix in your office, or whip up a batch of Granola-to-Go Bars (p. 88) or Cafe Mocha Mini Muffins (p. 266) to keep on hand when you're on the job.

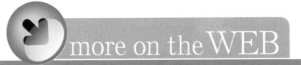

more on the WEB

Visit tasteofhome.com/cfdiet to find lots of tips and tools to help you learn more about a healthy diet and ways to work exercise into your day plus lots more comforting lower-calorie recipes like the ones here.

Basics of FREEZING FOOD

Save time, money and calories by planning ahead and freezing food.

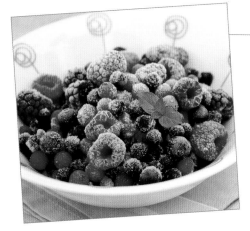

STOCKING UP

Your freezer likely houses a variety of uncooked ingredients and foods you use most often, such as ground meat, chicken breast, pork chops and frozen vegetables. These foods help simplify menu planning and speed up dinner preparation on days you cook from scratch.

But on busy days or when you just don't feel like cooking, your freezer can become a gold mine for quick meals that simply need to be thawed, reheated and enjoyed!

The next time you are making muffins, a casserole, soup or one of many other Comfort Food Diet ideas, double the recipe and freeze half to use another day or for lunches. (See page 41 for a list of recipes in this book that freeze well.) With those meals waiting for you in your freezer, it will be easy to eat healthy and stick to your calorie budget when you come home tired and hungry after a long workout or stressful day at work.

In addition, your freezer can help you take advantage of weekly sales and bulk pricing—a bonus for your diet and wallet!

WHAT CAN I FREEZE?

Almost any food can be frozen, but some maintain their quality better than others. Raw meat and poultry hold up very well in the freezer and can be good money-savers if you purchase them in bulk or on sale. Soups and stews freeze well and are easily defrosted. Baked goods are easy to freeze when you want to enjoy a cookie or two and store the rest.

Fruits like bananas (without the peel), strawberries, blueberries and raspberries do well in the freezer, and they come in very handy when you want to whip up a nutritious smoothie for breakfast. Fill a glass with frozen fruit, pour juice over it and blend it all together. You will have the exact amount of smoothie that you want and easily get a few servings of fruit for the day.

Lots of things can be frozen. So the more important question is: What will defrost well and still be edible and appetizing?

WHAT NOT TO FREEZE

- **CASSEROLES** made with mayonnaise, sour cream, yogurt or cream cheese, as well as gravies and cream-based sauces. These items will separate after thawing and the casserole will have a watery or curdled appearance.

- **RAW PRODUCE WITH A HIGH WATER CONTENT,** such as cabbage, celery, lettuce, other leafy greens, cucumbers, radishes, watermelon, tomatoes and citrus fruits. They become limp and waterlogged after thawing.

- **COOKED POTATOES** used in dishes like salads, soups or stews. They become soft, mealy and waterlogged after thawing. Consider cooking raw potatoes while you're thawing a soup or stew to add when it is reheated. However, mashed and twice-baked potatoes do freeze well.
- **DAIRY ITEMS** like cream sauces, sour cream, yogurt, mayonnaise and sauces and gravies thickened with flour and cornstarch. They will separate during defrosting.
- **COOKED PASTA** can be soft and mushy after defrosting. For the best results, undercook pasta before freezing or cook pasta while the sauce or vegetables are thawing.

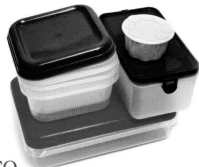

HOW TO PACKAGE THE FOOD

The materials used to store food in the freezer need to protect their edible contents from the harsh climate while maintaining quality and moisture content. Use materials that are durable, freezer-safe and moisture- and vapor-proof.

Suitable materials for freezing food are: plastic freezer jars, freezer bags, strong plastic freezer containers, plastic wrap, vacuum-sealed packages, heavy-duty foil and freezer paper. Meat and poultry may be frozen in the wrapping from the butcher for short-term freezing—but only for up to a month.

Avoid freezing food in glass jars from food products (like a spaghetti sauce jar or pickle jar), margarine tubs, cottage cheese tubs and milk cartons.

FREEZING LIKE A CHAMP

When freezing foods, always start with fresh, high quality food. Remember that foods past their prime will not improve upon freezing. That's why commercial produce is frozen at the peak of freshness—so it will be of the highest quality when you reheat it at home.

For convenience and faster reheating, package the food in single-meal or single-serving portions. This will also help you control how much you eat and keep track of calories.

Use plastic freezer jars and rigid containers for soups, stews and other liquid items. Leave some space at the top of the container to give the food space to expand as it freezes. Liquid items can also be stored in freezer bags to save space. You can lay them flat and stack them when they're frozen.

If you want to freeze a casserole or lasagna, line the casserole dish with heavy-duty foil before placing food in it. Be generous with the foil and leave big flaps around the outside of the dish. Once the food is frozen, use the foil flaps to remove it from the dish and wrap the flaps securely around the food and store it back in the freezer. For added protection, put it in a resealable plastic freezer bag.

Remove as much air as possible when packaging the food. Label and date each package so you remember what it is. Stack the packages when they are completely frozen to help keep your freezer neat and organized.

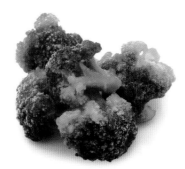

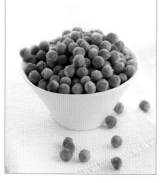

DEALING WITH FREEZER BURN

Freezer burn is not a food safety issue, but it certainly is a food quality issue. It occurs when food is not wrapped properly and is exposed to the frigid 0° air for too long. The food gets dried out and icy and may not taste the same.

Freezer burn appears as dry, leathery, off-colored areas on meat and poultry. The freezer-burned areas can be cut off before or after cooking. Any vegetables or fruit that are icy or shriveled should be discarded. To prevent this and keep your food tasty and long-lasting, be extra careful next time to remove as much of the air as possible.

DEFROSTING

Even when your food is sealed and dated, there are just three safe ways to defrost food—and many unsafe ways to do it. For example, don't defrost food at room temperature on the kitchen counter, in warm water or outdoors. The exception to this is baked goods like breads, cakes and cookies. Just unwrap these items while they thaw to prevent them from getting soggy.

These are the three safe ways to defrost food:

1. **REFRIGERATOR DEFROSTING** is safe and fuss-free, but it is the slowest method, so planning ahead is key. Most items take one or two days. Small items like a pound of ground beef can be defrosted overnight, but bulky, large items will take even longer to thaw. Allow three to five hours per pound for a small beef or pork roast and five to seven hours per pound for a large roast. A whole turkey or large whole chicken will need an entire day for every four to five pounds. When defrosting in the refrigerator, place each item in a bowl or on a plate to catch any liquid or juices.

2. **COLD WATER DEFROSTING** takes less time than thawing in the refrigerator but requires more attention. To defrost in cold water, place food in a watertight plastic storage bag. If the bag leaks, the food will absorb the water, which will affect its texture and may expose it to bacteria. Place the bag in cold water and change the water every 30 minutes until the food is thawed.

3. **MICROWAVE DEFROSTING** is suitable for last-minute thawing of small items. To defrost something in the microwave, unwrap the food and place it on a microwave-safe dish. Follow the manufacturer's recommended time and settings based on the weight of the food. Microwave defrosting can cause some areas to actually cook, so plan on preparing the food immediately after defrosting.

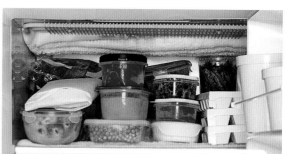

KEEP IT ORGANIZED

Along with dating your frozen treats, prevent your freezer from turning into the lost land of frozen surprises by keeping a list of what's in it. List the item and the date it was placed in the freezer. As the item is used, cross it off the list and add new items as you freeze them.

Another easy way to keep your freezer organized is to label and date your frozen treasures on the containers themselves. Use masking tape that can be easily removed as you eat the food and reuse the container.

WHAT TO FREEZE FROM THE COMFORT FOOD DIET

It's easy to stay on track if you plan ahead and have healthy, nutritious food available at all times by storing some items in the freezer. You won't be left wondering what to make for dinner, and you'll be less tempted to hit up the drive-thru or order some take-out.

Here is a list of recipes from the *Comfort Food Diet Cookbook* that will hold up in the freezer and be as delicious when reheated as they were when made fresh.

BREAKFASTS
Apple Walnut Pancakes, 95
Blueberry Oatmeal Pancakes, 270
Cafe Mocha Mini Muffins, 266
Caramel Cream Crepes, 94
Festive French Pancakes, 89
Granola-To-Go Bars, 88
Homemade Pancake Mix, 281
Turkey Breakfast Sausage, 267
Whole Grain Waffle Mix, 99

DESSERTS/SNACKS
Blondies with Chips, 213
Chocolate Chip Cookies, 209
Colorful Frozen Yogurt, 215
Frozen Fruit Cups, 237
Frozen Pistachio Dessert with Raspberry Sauce, 220
Frozen Yogurt Cookie Dessert, 255
Fruit Juice Pops, 217
Lemon Sorbet, 242
Makeover Oatmeal Bars, 211
Peanut Butter-Chocolate Chip Cookies, 208
Peanut Butter S'mores Bars, 253
Rich Peach Ice Cream, 213
Strawberry-Raspberry Ice, 241

ENTREES
Applesauce-Glazed Pork Chops, 259
Apricot-Almond Chicken Breasts, 262
Baked Barbecued Brisket, 247
Baked Chicken Fajitas, 286
Best-Ever Lamb Chops, 246
Black Bean Taco Pizza, 108
Braised Southwest Beef Roast, 136
Cajun Beef Tenderloin, 124
Cheesy Rigatoni Bake, 144
Cranberry-Orange Turkey Cutlets, 166
Dijon-Peach Pork Chops, 289
Glazed Pork Chops, 256
Grilled Pork Tenderloin, 250
Herbed Beef Tenderloin, 253
Homemade Spaghetti Sauce, 133
Honey-Grilled Pork Tenderloin, 260
Honey-Lime Roasted Chicken, 252
Hot 'n' Spicy Flank Steak, 128
Hungarian Goulash, 151

Italian Cheese-Stuffed Shells, 158
Light Chicken Cordon Bleu, 150
Mustard-Herb Chicken Breasts, 248
Onion-Dijon Pork Chops, 278
Portobello Burgundy Beef, 278
Red Clam Sauce, 232
Savory Baked Chicken, 272
Tarragon-Lemon Turkey Breast, 247
Whiskey Sirloin Steak for Two, 248
Zippy Spaghetti Sauce, 230

SANDWICHES
Barbecued Pork Sandwiches, 259
Beef Sandwiches, 233
Garden Turkey Burgers, 269
Mexican-Inspired Turkey Burgers, 282
Spinach-Feta Chicken Rolls, 109
Tex-Mex Beef Barbecues, 232
Turkey Sloppy Joes, 231

SOUPS
Burgundy Beef Stew, 234
Chili con Carne, 113
Family-Pleasing Turkey Chili, 233
Hearty Chipotle Chicken Soup, 110
Italian Sausage Bean Soup, 115
Italian Vegetable Soup, 102
One-Pot Chili, 121
Pineapple Peach Soup, 184
Sausage Kale Soup, 252
Simple Chicken Soup, 104
Southwestern Beef Stew, 131
Turkey Meatball Soup, 106
White Bean Soup, 108
Zippy Slow-Cooked Chili, 231
Zippy Three-Bean Chili, 142

FREEZER TIPS

- Use a freezer thermometer to monitor the air temperature. It should read 0° to preserve food quality.
- Keep the freezer 2/3 full for the best energy efficiency.
- Leave some space around the packages so air can circulate.
- Avoid overtaxing the freezer. Whatever is placed in the freezer should be solidly frozen within 24 hours. Adding too much food at one time will increase freezing time.
- Keep good inventory and follow the "first in, first out" rule. Use the items that have been in the freezer the longest first.
- Before freezing, cool food quickly and evenly. Transfer warm or hot foods to shallower pans or divide the food among several small, shallow containers. Help hot liquids like soups and sauces cool by stirring them frequently.

What's EATING YOU?

How to avoid emotional overeating.

If a bad day at work or home sends you straight to the refrigerator to cope, you already know something about emotional eating.

If you haven't ever downed a carton of ice cream, a bag of chips or a package of cookies in response to frustration in your life, you probably aren't an emotional eater. Consider yourself lucky.

There's nothing wrong with eating a modest amount of a favorite food because it makes you feel content. After all, comfort food is what this book is all about.

But when stress, anxiety or sadness drives you to eat more and more, or you're so preoccupied with negative feelings that you don't even notice what you're eating, it's time to confront the problem and deal with it.

Emotional eating can quickly sabotage a sensible eating plan. Here are the symptoms to help determine if you are an emotional eater.

- You eat to try to make yourself feel better rather than because you are hungry.

- It's hard to find food that is satisfying, so you don't stop eating when you're full. You keep looking for that one food that will "hit the spot."

- You eat while doing something routine such as watching TV, surfing the Internet or folding laundry. When the package suddenly hits empty, you can't believe you mindlessly ate it all.

- You get a craving for a specific food, and it seems to be related to feeling bored, lonely, angry, hopeless, underappreciated or some other negative emotion.

Finding out what makes you overeat is the key to stopping it. You cannot skip this step if you want long-term success in reaching and maintaining a healthy, comfortable body weight.

The emotional eating cycle starts with a brief period of pleasure while you're eating, followed by a feeling of failure and a promise to eat healthy going forward.

Unfortunately, though, the whole loop usually starts again. Stepping off the roller coaster and onto stable ground requires determining the "why."

The trick is not to make yourself feel worse by trying to smother those emotions with food. There are better ways to process those feelings—without wrecking your weight-loss goals. Try one (or more) of these:

- **WRITE IT DOWN.** Keeping a food journal is a powerful way to track and control what you eat. Here's a way to make it even more effective: Don't just keep a food diary—keep a mood diary, too.

  When you write down what you're eating—and remember, you have to be honest and include the wayward treats and binges—take a moment to note how you're feeling, too.

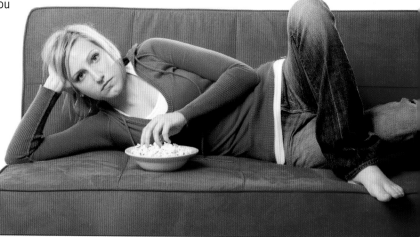

You may start to see patterns between your food choices and your emotional state. Spotting patterns is the first step to changing them.

- **BREAK THE CHAIN.** Once you identify your emotional-eating triggers, you can deal with them in more constructive ways.

  This may mean asking yourself some tough questions: What needs aren't being met, or what feelings aren't being expressed? Can you vent them in a more constructive way than heading to the fridge? Breaking the chain of events or feelings that leads to emotional eating may be as simple as picking up the phone (instead of a bag of chips) and calling a friend. Or taking the dog for a walk. Or doing something fun until the craving passes.

- **STOP AND THINK.** Now that you're more mindful of your emotional state, you'll be able to assess your situation honestly.

  When you catch yourself at the pantry door, stop and ask: Am I hungry? Is my body telling me it needs more fuel—or is my head saying there's some emotional need that isn't being met? Why do I really want to eat? What can I do instead of eating?

- **BE FOOD-CONSCIOUS.** As you become aware of your own food/mood connections, it's easy to overreact and cut yourself off from eating food you love. Don't.

Watching what you eat shouldn't be an exercise in deprivation. Shoot for moderation instead: Eat slowly so you can hear your body telling you when it's physically satisfied by food.

Don't eat in front of the TV or computer, or while you're doing something else. Focus on the food. Savor it.

And by all means, keep some favorite foods in the house, but in smaller quantities so that you're not tempted to overdo it.

GRAB A PEN:

- Make a list of all the things you'll do when you meet your weight-loss goal.

- Write a letter describing why you are sad, angry, frustrated—whatever the feeling is that you are trying to forget by eating. Tear the letter up or keep it to look at later. (Or deliver it, but not before at least 24 hours of thought.)

COUNT PLUSES:

- How many people told you how great you looked this week?

- How did you feel when you stepped on the scale and realized you had lost weight?

- How close are you to getting back into those jeans that used to fit?

DISTRACT YOURSELF:

- Fight boredom at all costs. Pick up a library book or even a trashy novel.

- Hone your mental sharpness by working your way through a crossword puzzle or something similar.

- If you hear the kitchen calling you when you know it shouldn't, head to the bathroom instead. A hot bath will relax you and get your mind off eating.

- Listen to relaxing music, your favorite CD or your iPod. Enjoy some "me" time.

BE GOOD TO YOUR BODY:

- Is the fridge calling? Go to bed early. Your body will appreciate extra sleep more than extra calories.

- Drink a glass of water or two. You might be thirsty rather than hungry, or the feeling of fullness from the water may take your mind off eating.

- Exercise boosts your mood. So walk up and down the steps at home or do other light exercise. Pull out your favorite CD and dance to the music. Get moving!

LOOK AHEAD:

- Plan your wardrobe. What can you pull from your closet that you haven't worn in years? What new piece of clothing should you buy yourself for losing 15 pounds? What's the first new thing you'll try on when you've reached your goal?

- Plan—and take—a vacation. Losing weight is hard work. Keeping it off is even harder. When you feel like you might actually consider wearing a swimsuit, start planning a vacation that lets you do it.

- To help fund your vacation or new wardrobe, reward yourself for each good choice. Put $1 in a money jar each time you avoid emotional eating. Start today!

supercharge your diet with
10 SUPER FOODS

Work these wonders into your day and get the biggest
nutritional bang for your caloric buck!

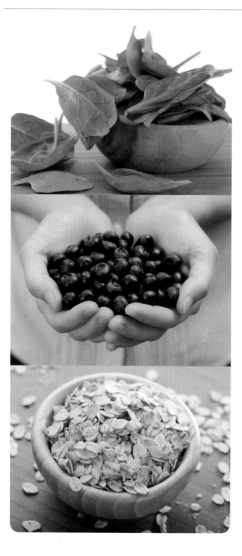

BEANS. Beans, especially the red, pinto and dark varieties, are a great way to add fiber to your diet. One cup of beans has an average of 16 g dietary fiber, which is more than half of the recommended 25 g you should be consuming daily. When combined with grains such as oats or barley, beans provide the necessary amino acids to make a complete protein. Southwest Black Bean Soup (p. 109) and Garbanzo Bean Pitas (p. 105) are sure to become favorites with your gang.

BLUEBERRIES. Talk about a super food! This list wouldn't be complete without these tiny gems that pack a powerful punch. Blueberries are loaded with antioxidants, which can protect your cells against free radicals, keeping cells healthy. A handful of blueberries also provides your body with flavonoids, vitamin K and vitamin C. When choosing your berries, remember: The deeper the color, the more chock-full of antioxidants they are. Blueberry-Stuffed French Toast (p. 92) and Triple-Berry Cobbler (p. 222) are great ways to start and end your day.

BROCCOLI. Enjoy cooked broccoli as a side dish or raw broccoli as a snack. Either way, a cup of this versatile vegetable contains a substantial amount of vitamin K, folic acid and vitamin C. The green veggie also helps boost the immune system, working toward keeping you healthy every day. Consider Broccoli-Cheese Stuffed Pizza (p. 134) and Broccoli Brown Rice Pilaf (p. 198) when adding this classic veggie to your menu plan.

EGGS. Eggs are a very nutritious and equally as versatile super food. One large egg has 6 g protein, making it a great start to your day. They are a good source of choline, an essential nutrient that helps with brain and memory development. The good news keeps coming: Eggs provide your body with vitamin D and vitamin A, aiding in bone health and good vision. Enjoy this comforting super food in Potato Egg Bake (p. 98) or simply as Hard-Cooked Eggs (p. 239) while still meeting your calorie goals.

NUTS. Nuts of all kinds are good sources of heart-healthy monounsaturated and polyunsaturated fats that may help lower cholesterol. But serving size is very important with nuts, because they can easily put you over your daily calorie intake in one snack. By adding more nuts into your diet, you will benefit from increased fiber, protein and essential fatty acids. Walnuts, almonds, pistachios and cashews are among the lower-calorie nuts–but remember to keep your portion around 1 ounce and to choose lightly salted or unsalted nuts. Nut 'n' Corn Clusters (p. 79) and Turkey Pecan Enchiladas (p. 139) are great ways to incorporate nuts into your diet.

OATS. The pure goodness of oats make them a natural for this list; they're loaded with thiamine and healthy doses of magnesium, phosphorus and zinc. Oats also provide decent amounts of fiber and protein and help lower cholesterol and risk of heart disease. In addition, enjoying oatmeal on a regular basis may decrease insulin resistance and help stabilize blood sugar. Whip up some Chewy Granola Bars (p. 90) or Apple-Cinnamon Oatmeal Mix (p. 94) and experience the goodness oats have to offer.

PLAIN YOGURT. Forget sugary breakfast cereals—plain yogurt is an ideal way to start your day. It is a lean source of protein that can become a super, super food when you mix in some blueberries for the antioxidants. Yogurt is also an excellent source of calcium and vitamin D, which help maintain healthy bones. Power up for the day with delicious Orange Fruit Cups (p. 87).

SPINACH. Add some spinach to your leafy green salad, and you'll pump up the health benefits enormously. In fact, spinach is tough to beat for the amount of vitamin K it offers. It might be hard to get kids to eat spinach, but once you incorporate it into your family's diet, the health benefits are worth it. Give Spinach-Feta Chicken Rolls (p. 109) and Wilted Garlic Spinach (p. 177) a try!

SWEET POTATOES. Think of them as "super" potatoes. Sweet potatoes are an excellent source of vitamins B6 and C. The bright orange flesh is thanks to beta-carotene, which your body converts into vitamin A, an essential nutrient and powerful antioxidant. One large sweet potato has 3 g protein, 6 g fiber and almost a quarter of your daily potassium needs. Power up your diet with sweet potatoes when you make Chipotle Sweet Potato and Spiced Apple Purees (p. 255) or Coconut-Pecan Sweet Potatoes (p. 229).

TOMATOES. These plump favorites are an exceptional source of vitamin C and lycopene, an antioxidant that can boost your immune system. So toss some chopped tomato into a pot of simmering soup, sprinkle them over your eggs at breakfast or try these Comfort Food Diet recipes: Ragu Bolognese (p. 171) and Sauteed Corn with Tomatoes and Basil (p. 182).

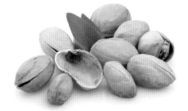

more on the WEB

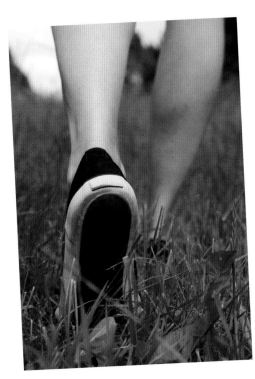

MOVE IT
and lose it!

Combine exercise with healthy eating to burn more calories and lose more weight.

The Comfort Food Diet suggests adding exercise to your week for surefire calorie-burning success. And while it might seem intimidating at first, it's easier than you think to take that first step—literally.

Whatever activity you choose should be easy, affordable and, most of all, fun! Try to find a form of exercise that you'd enjoy doing every day…or at least on a very regular basis. Consider options that fit into your schedule and meet with your doctor's approval. Look for opportunities to work out with a spouse, family member or friend. Then grab your walking shoes and take that first step!

WALK IT OFF!

Walking is a perfect way to start an exercise routine. After all, you can burn roughly 100 calories by briskly walking a mile. In addition, walking lowers blood pressure and improves cholesterol.

If you're new to fitness walking, begin with a daily 10-minute stroll. Those 10 minutes will likely turn into 20 minutes or more in a matter of days. Set a goal for yourself to walk every day for one week. Get out there and enjoy a walk around the neighborhood!

During the next week, pay attention to the speed with which you move. The average walking speed is between 1½ and 2½ mph, but a good walking speed is 3 to 4 mph. Start using short strides with quick heel-to-toe movements. Long strides may cause your front foot to act like a brake, jarring your joints and slowing you down.

Using a pedometer, start increasing your steps by 10 to 20 percent per week. You are at a great level when you've reached 10,000 steps per day or 70,000 steps per week.

Your muscles need oxygen, so don't forget to inhale deeply and exhale fully, both to a count of three. When possible, walk on soft surfaces such as dirt, sand or grass—these areas are gentle on your joints. Always stretch before and after walking to prevent muscles from tightening or cramping.

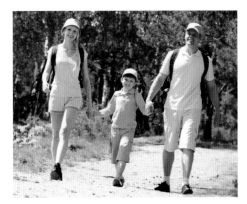

One of the benefits of walking is that you can fit in a long walk once during the day, or you can walk for short bursts throughout the day and still burn calories. In other words, if you can't fit in a 45-minute walk, you can take three 15-minute walks instead.

Walking with a buddy can make the time fly, motivate you to stick with it and push you to increase your pace. Better yet, grab your family and take a relaxing walk together.

- Enjoy a family walk before dinner to discuss the day's events.

- Make walking a special event by taking the gang to the zoo, a museum or a shopping mall.

- When the kids are frustrated, walk around the block with them. They'll burn off the stress, and you'll all burn calories.

Regardless of how you work this activity into your day, be sure to carve out walking time in your schedule. Remember, the ultimate goal is to lose weight, feel good and become the best you can be. Commit to walking regularly, and with a little dedication and perseverance, you'll take a big step in the right direction.

get MOVING!

In a landmark Harvard study of some 40,000 women over the age of 45, those who walked as little as one hour a week—even at a stroll—were half as likely to have heart attacks or blocked coronary arteries as those who rarely walked for exercise. Walking is easier with good form, so follow these easy tips for proper posture to start your path to healthier tomorrows!

HEAD
Imagine a string attached to the top of your head, pulling it straight toward the sky. Keep your chin lifted and your ears in line with your shoulders.

SHOULDERS
Keep them relaxed, down and slightly back. If they start hunching up toward your ears, take a deep breath and drop them back again.

ARMS
Elbows should be bent at about 90-degree angles, hands slightly cupped. Relax your arms and pump them forward and back as you walk; they should not crisscross in front of you. Walking with light hand weights can help build muscle and burn calories, but too much weight will strain the elbows and shoulders.

CHEST
Yoga practitioners sometimes refer to the breastbone area as your "heart light." Keep your heart light lifted and shining straight ahead.

ABDOMINALS
Pull your belly button toward your spine as if you were zipping up a snug pair of jeans. Keep those abs firm and tight as you walk.

FEET
With each step, plant your heel, roll onto the ball of your foot, and push off with your toes. Avoid rolling your foot inward or outward. To protect your feet and joints, wear good walking shoes. A proper fit means they feel great right out of the box. Make sure there's a finger width between the end of your longest toe and the inside of the front of the shoe.

BEFORE & after

Two of the most critical parts of a workout—the warm-up and cooldown—are also two of the most misunderstood

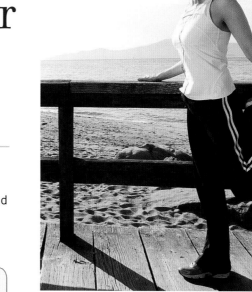

Few things have evolved as dramatically in the field of exercise science as the understanding of proper warm-ups and cooldowns. Done correctly, they make exercise safer and more enjoyable. Are you doing them the right way? Here's what you need to know.

WARMING UP

Think back to high school gym class. The typical warm-up was probably a few bouncy stretches, and if you're still warming up that way, it's time to change. Research has repeatedly shown that stretching before you exercise does nothing to increase flexibility or prevent injuries.

Instead, the best warm-up is a slow, gentle version of the activity you're about to do. For example, if you're planning a run, start with a brisk walk. Before playing tennis, make some slow practice swings. Warming up this way slowly raises your heart rate, moves blood to your muscles and warms ligaments and tendons. These important physiological changes reduce your risk of injury and make your workout more comfortable, which means you'll be more likely to do it again.

COOLING DOWN

Cooling down is just as important as warming up because it gradually decreases your heart rate and body temperature and helps prevent muscle cramping and soreness. To cool down, simply follow the guidelines for a good warm-up and continue the same physical activity at a slower pace. After a 30- to 40-minute workout, spend 5 to 10 minutes cooling down.

Once you finish your cooldown, it's time to stretch. Warm muscles will stretch more easily, and frequent stretching increases your range of motion, reducing your chance of injury.

WORK OUT RIGHT

Warm-up and cooldown suggestions for popular activities:

PHYSICAL ACTIVITY	METHOD
AEROBICS	5-10 minutes at low intensity on a stair-climber
WEIGHT TRAINING	Walking on a treadmill for 5-10 minutes. Also, do a few repetitions with light weights before moving to your full load.
RUNNING	Walking or slow jogging
SWIMMING	Slow crawl
CYCLING	Flat terrain in lower gears
HIKING	Hike on flat terrain at minimal altitude
RACQUETBALL	Brisk walk or light jog and graduated-tempo volleying
ELLIPTICAL/ STAIR-CLIMBER	Light aerobic activity, such as walking, or low-tempo step exercise

hints for
SAFER HIKING

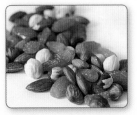

Prevent dehydration and fatigue by bringing water and nonperishable snacks, such as peanut butter and jelly sandwiches, granola and trail mix.

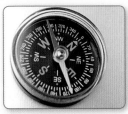

Bring a compass and cell phone as well as a clearly marked map of the area to keep you on track. Always tell someone who won't be with you where you are going.

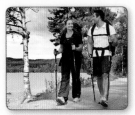

Add trekking poles to prevent injury. They help maintain balance and take strain off of your knees and ankles.

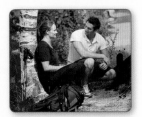

When you get tired take a break. Stumbles and falls happen more often when you've overdone it. Stretch a little, have a drink and snack, then get back to it.

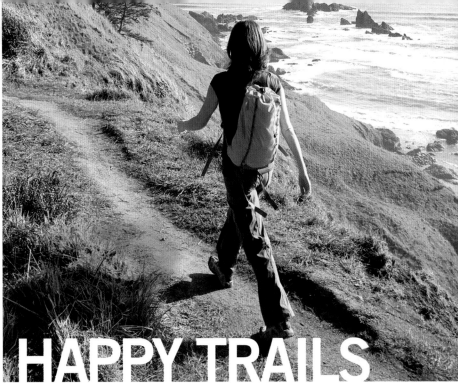

HAPPY TRAILS

HIT THE HILLS FOR A HIGH-INTENSITY, LOW-IMPACT WORKOUT

When you need a change of pace from the gym, look outdoors for a new way to tone up. Hiking burns calories, costs next to nothing and has a way of clearing your head. So read our tips and get outside. Mother Nature's a great workout partner!

WHY HIKE?

Compared to walking, hiking increases your workout's intensity. Your core abdominal and back muscles work harder as they stabilize you over uneven surfaces. And if you're hiking up a hill, all of your muscles—including your heart—get a better workout. Hiking on a steep grade and rough terrain also works hip flexors, quads, hamstrings, calves and glutes, so you get a firmer backside.

GET GOING

- Start out slowly and keep a consistent pace to help preserve your energy.
- Ask park rangers about trail elevation and layout to gauge your hike's intensity before you go. Search your state's Department of Natural Resources website for local trails.
- Consider your socks. The wrong pair can leave you blistered and miserable. Opt for

two layers. Start with a thin polyester liner that wicks moisture, and top those with thicker, warmer socks. Bring a fresh pair of both types to change midway through long hikes.

- Make a smart shoe choice. If you'll be on a well-groomed trail, opt for light and comfortable cross-trainers. A rocky, off-the-beaten path area requires good-fitting boots with a sturdy toe.
- Layer up in colder months. Start with modern performance underwear made from moisture-wicking polyester or polypropylene. Top with polyester fleece to trap warmth without making clothes soggy from sweat. Add wind- and water-resistant pants, gloves, and a coat and hat, if needed.

CLEAN UP slim down

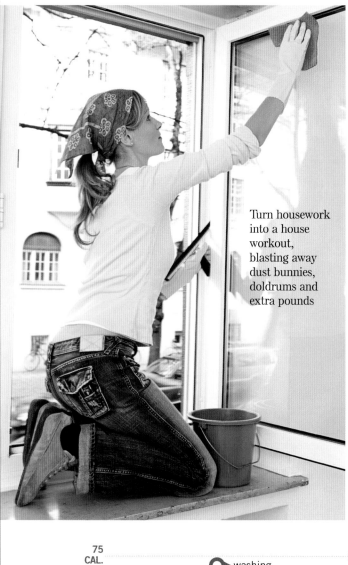

Turn housework into a house workout, blasting away dust bunnies, doldrums and extra pounds

Don't worry about pricey gym memberships or hiring a personal trainer to shape up. You have all the exercise equipment you need in the broom closet. Unless your idea of housework is to sweep the room with a glance, everyday chores are good exercise... just check out the chart below.

Spend 10 minutes doing the following tasks around your home and yard, and you'll burn more calories than you might think. Then try some of our easy ideas for making the most of cleaning chores.

EVERY MINUTE COUNTS!

A study done by Mayo Clinic scientists comparing activity levels of overweight and slim "couch potatoes" found that lean people were on their feet, moving around, for 152 more minutes per day than the others.

So, instead of using commercials to grab a snack from the fridge, get up and empty a wastebasket, run downstairs and put in a load of wash, or scrub out a casserole dish that's been soaking in the sink. You'll save all kinds of calories and your house will be shipshape.

You can turn other everyday activities into calorie-burners, too. Talk on the phone while standing up or moving around. Chop veggies by hand; mix batter with a wooden spoon; use that heavy cast-iron skillet more often; wash the floor on your hands and knees (but keep those stomach muscles tight); hang the family's sheets out to dry on the line, where they'll soak up sunshine and fresh air.

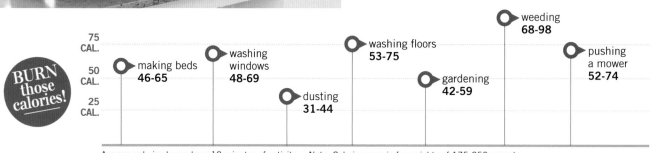

BURN those calories!

	CAL.		
75 CAL.			weeding 68-98
	washing windows 48-69	washing floors 53-75	pushing a mower 52-74
50 CAL.	making beds 46-65		
		gardening 42-59	
25 CAL.	dusting 31-44		

Average calories burned per 10 minutes of activity • Note: Calorie range is for weights of 175-250 pounds.

Exercise UNLEASHED!

FIDO FITNESS

Exercising with your dog does you both a world of good. According to the Association for Pet Obesity Prevention, pets struggle with the same epidemic weight problems as the rest of America. Excess weight exposes your dog to such health risks as diabetes, arthritis, organ failure and more. So grab that leash and hit the bricks. But keep these tips in mind as you head out the door.

START SLOW. If your dog's exercise has been limited to quick pit stops in the backyard, go easy on him. "Start in your neighborhood. Pick a flat, easy-to-walk path—around the block or just to the park and back," says Gerald Endress, fitness manager for the Duke University Diet and Fitness Center in Durham, North Carolina. When you walk, try to get in at least 10 minutes. If you walk your dog three times a day, that's a half-hour of exercise right there.

TRY SOME INTERVALS. As you and your dog build up strength and stamina—or if you already do plenty of walking but would like to step things up—try some interval training. Endress suggests about five minutes of regular strolling alternating with one minute of brisk walking or jogging. Gradually work up to the point where your dog can do five minutes at a brisk walk, then give him a minute to slow down and sniff.

MIX IT UP. Walking is great, but you can change things up with some activities in the backyard (or even in the house, if the weather's bad). Play fetch. Rolling a ball across the floor or throwing a disc across the lawn is ideal exercise for your dog. To make it more of a workout for you, hold onto the ball or disc once in a while and get him to chase you.

PLAY IT SAFE. Don't let your dog overexert itself—remember, Fido has to exercise with that fur coat on. Watch for limping or signs of difficulty with breathing. And keep the water bowl topped off at home so the dog can drink before and after your workout. If it's hot or you're going on a long walk, bring plenty of water for the two of you—and a small collapsible bowl, if you don't want the dog drinking out of your hands.

After a heart attack convinced her to get serious about her health, reader Carol Newsom, from San Leandro, California, got what she considers the best piece of "fitness equipment" ever: her dog, Whiskey. "You can't put her away in the closet and forget her," Carol says. "She's ready to go at the same time every day and she won't take no for an answer. She doesn't care if my favorite program is on or if I'm having a bad day—she wants her walk."

You certainly don't have to wait for something as serious as a heart attack to make four-legged fitness a part of your life. As Carol found, dogs can be powerful workout buddies. According to researchers at Michigan State University, dog owners are not only more likely to take regular walks (one of the simplest ways to work exercise into your day), but those who walk their dogs are more physically active in general than people who don't have a pooch.

Carol's living proof. "Whiskey has kept me on the straight and narrow," she says. "Together we have gone from walking around the block to a mile and a half. Not bad!"

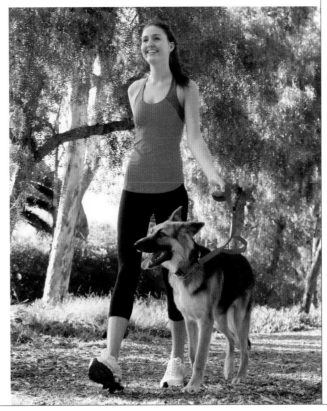

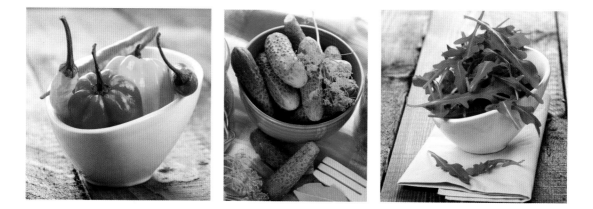

FREE foods chart
Add these foods to your menu plan without worry!

Listed at right are items considered "free foods" on the *Taste of Home* Comfort Food Diet. A free food is an item that has fewer than 20 calories and 5 or less grams of carbohydrates per serving. Whether you add these items to your meal plan, rely on them for snacks or simply use them to enhance the flavors of your favorite dishes, feel free to enjoy as many free foods as you'd like.

Free foods are an ideal way to fill you up because they are mostly non-starchy vegetables. When you make a low-calorie turkey sandwich, for instance, give it a bit of crunch with sliced cucumber, pickles or even radishes. Or pump up the flavor with fresh herbs, horseradish or hot pepper sauce...and don't worry about adding up any calories these items might contain.

On the far right, you'll find a section that offers more free foods and lists their specific portion sizes. Feel free to enjoy a serving of these items and not count the calories— but if you eat them in portion sizes larger than what's noted in the chart, the calories will have to count toward your daily goal.

EAT ALL YOU WANT

- Artichoke
- Artichoke hearts
- Asparagus
- Baby corn
- Bamboo shoots
- Bean sprouts
- Beans (green, wax, Italian)
- Beets
- Broccoli
- Broth or bouillon
- Brussels sprouts
- Cauliflower
- Carrots
- Celery
- Cucumber
- Eggplant
- Flavored sugar-free gelatin
- Garlic
- Green onions or scallions
- Greens (collard, kale, mustard, turnip)
- Hearts of palm
- Herbs (fresh or dried)
- Horseradish
- Hot pepper sauce
- Jicama
- Kohlrabi
- Leeks
- Lemon juice
- Mixed vegetables (without corn, peas or pasta)
- Mushrooms (fresh)
- Mustard
- Okra
- Onions
- Pea pods
- Pickles
- Radishes
- Rutabaga
- Salad greens (lettuce, romaine, chicory, endive, escarole, arugula, radicchio, watercress)
- Sauerkraut
- Spices
- Spinach
- Squash (summer, crookneck, zucchini)
- Sugar snap peas
- Swiss chard
- Tomato (fresh or canned)
- Turnips
- Vinegar
- Water chestnuts
- Worcestershire sauce

FREE FOODS AND BEVERAGES— DRINK AS MUCH AS YOU WANT

- Carbonated or mineral water
- Club soda
- Coffee (unsweetened or with sugar substitute)
- Diet soft drinks
- Drink mixes (sugar-free)
- Flavored water (20 calories or less)
- Tea (unsweetened or with sugar substitute)
- Tonic water (diet)
- Water

FREE FOODS WITH RESTRICTED PORTIONS

- Barbecue sauce, *2 teaspoons*
- Cream cheese (fat-free), *1 tablespoon (1/2 ounce)*
- Creamer: Nondairy, liquid, *1 tablespoon* Nondairy, powdered, *2 teaspoons*
- Honey mustard, *1 tablespoon*
- Jam or jelly (light or no sugar added), *2 teaspoons*
- Ketchup, *1 tablespoon*
- Margarine spread: Fat-free, *1 tablespoon* Reduced-fat, *1 teaspoon*

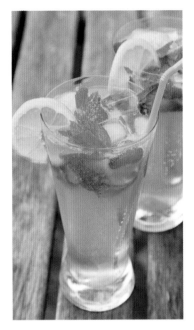

- Mayonnaise: Fat-free, *1 tablespoon* Reduced-fat, *1 teaspoon*
- Parmesan cheese (freshly grated), *1 tablespoon*
- Pickle relish, *1 tablespoon*
- Salad dressing: Fat-free or low-fat, *1 tablespoon* Fat-free Italian, *2 tablespoons*
- Salsa, *1/4 cup*
- Sour cream: Fat-free or reduced-fat, *1 tablespoon*
- Sweet and sour sauce, *2 teaspoons*
- Soy sauce, *1 tablespoon*
- Sweet chili sauce, *1 tablespoon*
- Syrup (sugar-free), *2 tablespoons*
- Taco sauce, *1 tablespoon*
- Whipped topping: Light or fat-free, *2 tablespoons* Regular, *1 tablespoon*

six-week MEAL PLAN

The following pages take the work out of calorie counting. They offer a complete six-week meal plan. Each day's guidelines suggest three meals and two snacks, totaling roughly 1,400 calories. Feel free to substitute foods or mix and match the meals from various days. Be sure, however, to pay attention to calories. To plan future weeks, record what you're eating and track calories using the blank Do-It-Yourself worksheets found on pages 294-295.

Comfort Food Diet Strategies:

- The great thing about the Comfort Food Diet is that you can serve incredible meals to your family members, who won't even realize they're eating healthy. Look through the recipes in this book, and immediately begin the meal plan by swapping in the dishes you know they'll enjoy most.

- The Comfort Food Diet tracks calories per day to make it easier to stay within the 1,400 calorie guideline. If you should exceed that limit one day, however, simply plan on consuming fewer calories the following day. Keeping a food/calorie journal will help you track such instances.

- Consider making extras and freezing leftovers for busy days or work lunches. When preparing large-batch recipes, stash a few in the freezer for low-calorie snacks and desserts.

- Review the items on the Free Foods Chart (p. 53), and use them to satisfy hunger between meals. They're also tasty ways to round out a menu without adding too many calories.

- Try to get the most nutrients from calories. In other words, a couple tablespoons of chocolate-covered raisins have nearly the same amount of calories as four dates. The dates offer more health benefits than the chocolate treats, but feel free to enjoy the raisins if your sweet tooth is begging for a little attention.

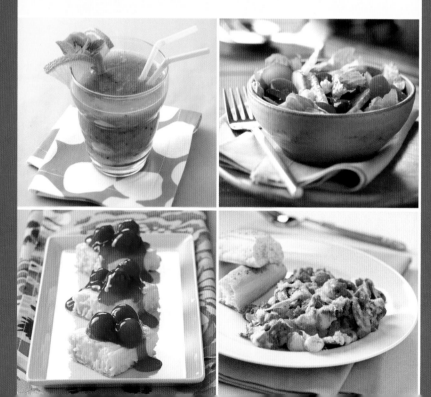

day 1

BREAKFAST:

- Mushroom Quiche (p. 245)
  154 CALORIES

- 2 slices whole wheat toast
  138 CALORIES

- with 1 teaspoon reduced-fat margarine spread
  FREE FOOD

- 1/2 cup orange juice
  55 CALORIES

BREAKFAST TOTAL: 347 CALORIES

LUNCH:

- Hot Swiss Chicken Sandwiches (p. 104)
  218 CALORIES

- Baby carrots
  FREE FOOD

- 1 Blondie with Chips (p. 213)
  133 CALORIES

- 1 cup fat-free milk
  86 CALORIES

LUNCH TOTAL: 437 CALORIES

DINNER & DESSERT:

- 1 cup Hungarian Goulash (p. 151)
  310 CALORIES

- 1/2 cup cooked egg noodles
  111 CALORIES

- Pretty Almond Green Beans (p. 179)
  78 CALORIES

- Coffee (with sugar substitute and liquid non-dairy creamer if desired)
  FREE FOOD

DINNER TOTAL: 499 CALORIES

SNACKS:

- 1/2 cup broccoli florets with 1 tablespoon fat-free ranch salad dressing
  FREE FOOD

- 1 cup cubed watermelon
  40 CALORIES

- 1/2 piece string cheese
  40 CALORIES

- 1/2 cup cubed fresh pineapple
  43 CALORIES

WEEK 1, DAY 1, TOTAL: 1,406 CALORIES

day 2

BREAKFAST:

- 1 serving French Toast with Apple Topping (p. 96)
  219 CALORIES

- 1/2 medium banana
  50 CALORIES

- Hot tea (with sugar substitute if desired)
  FREE FOOD

- 1 cup fat-free milk
  86 CALORIES

BREAKFAST TOTAL: 355 CALORIES

LUNCH:

- 3/4 cup Mediterranean Salad (p. 101)
  69 CALORIES

- 1 cup White Bean Soup (p. 108)
  270 CALORIES

- 1 whole wheat dinner roll
  76 CALORIES

- with 1 teaspoon reduced-fat margarine spread
  FREE FOOD

- 1 clementine
  35 CALORIES

- Diet soft drink
  FREE FOOD

LUNCH TOTAL: 450 CALORIES

DINNER & DESSERT:

- 1-1/4 cups Hearty Pasta Casserole (p. 171)
  416 CALORIES

- 1 big green salad (see Free Foods Chart on p. 53) with 1 tablespoon reduced-fat salad dressing
  FREE FOOD

- 1 cup fat-free milk
  86 CALORIES

DINNER TOTAL: 502 CALORIES

SNACKS:

- 3/4 cup air-popped popcorn
  24 CALORIES

- 1 medium apple
  72 CALORIES

- Baby carrots
  FREE FOOD

WEEK 1, DAY 2, TOTAL: 1,403 CALORIES

meal plan | THE COMFORT FOOD DIET

day 3

BREAKFAST:

- 3/4 cup Banana Blueberry Smoothies (p. 88)
  99 CALORIES
- 1 large scrambled egg
  101 CALORIES
- 1 slice whole wheat toast
  69 CALORIES
- with 1 teaspoon reduced-fat margarine spread
  FREE FOOD
- 1 cup fat-free milk
  86 CALORIES

BREAKFAST TOTAL: 355 CALORIES

LUNCH:

- 1 Grilled Pork Tenderloin Sandwich (p. 121)
  382 CALORIES
- 1/3 cup red grapes
  43 CALORIES
- Sugar-free flavored water
  FREE FOOD

LUNCH TOTAL: 425 CALORIES

DINNER & DESSERT:

- 1 serving Fettuccine with Black Bean Sauce (p. 288)
  350 CALORIES
- Steamed fresh broccoli florets
  FREE FOOD
- 1 big green salad (see Free Foods Chart on p. 53) with 1 tablespoon reduced-fat salad dressing
  FREE FOOD
- 1 cup fat-free milk
  86 CALORIES
- 1 Ladyfinger Cream Sandwich (p. 212)
  65 CALORIES
- Coffee (with sugar substitute and liquid non-dairy creamer if desired)
  FREE FOOD

DINNER TOTAL: 501 CALORIES

SNACKS:

- 1/2 small apple with 1 tablespoon fat-free caramel ice cream topping
  65 CALORIES
- 9 tiny twist fat-free pretzels 50 CALORIES

WEEK 1, DAY 3, TOTAL: 1,396 CALORIES

day 4

BREAKFAST:

- 1/2 cup Apple-Cinnamon Oatmeal Mix (p. 94)
  176 CALORIES
- 1/2 cup cubed fresh pineapple
  37 CALORIES
- 1 cup fat-free milk
  86 CALORIES

BREAKFAST TOTAL: 299 CALORIES

LUNCH:

- 1 cup Turkey Meatball Soup (p. 106)
  258 CALORIES
- 1 whole wheat dinner roll
  76 CALORIES
- with 1 teaspoon reduced-fat margarine spread
  FREE FOOD
- 1 medium pear
  96 CALORIES
- Coffee (with sugar substitute and liquid non-dairy creamer if desired)
  FREE FOOD

LUNCH TOTAL: 430 CALORIES

DINNER & DESSERT:

- 1 serving Hearty Salisbury Steaks (p. 275)
  233 CALORIES
- 3/4 cup Flavorful Mashed Potatoes (p. 192)
  146 CALORIES
- 2/3 cup Glazed Orange Carrots (p. 191)
  132 CALORIES
- 1 cup fat-free milk
  86 CALORIES

DINNER TOTAL: 597 CALORIES

SNACKS:

- 1 cup prepared sugar-free gelatin
  8 CALORIES
- 1 Lemon Anise Biscotti (p. 208)
  66 CALORIES

WEEK 1, DAY 4, TOTAL: 1,400 CALORIES

In order to best fit your schedule, feel free to move meals around on this daily planner.

day 5

BREAKFAST:

- 1 large scrambled egg
  101 CALORIES
- 1 slice whole wheat toast
  69 CALORIES
- with 1 teaspoon reduced-fat margarine spread
  FREE FOOD
- 1 medium grapefruit
  92 CALORIES
- 1 cup fat-free milk
  86 CALORIES

BREAKFAST TOTAL: **348 CALORIES**

LUNCH:

- 1 Grandma's French Tuna Salad Wrap (p. 114)
  328 CALORIES
- 1/3 cup red grapes
  43 CALORIES
- Celery sticks with 1 tablespoon fat-free ranch salad dressing
  FREE FOOD
- 1/2 piece string cheese
  40 CALORIES
- Mineral water
  FREE FOOD

LUNCH TOTAL: **411 CALORIES**

DINNER & DESSERT:

- 1 serving Bow Ties with Chicken & Shrimp (p. 168)
  399 CALORIES
- 1 big green salad (see Free Foods Chart on p. 53) with 1 tablespoon reduced-fat salad dressing
  FREE FOOD
- 1 cup fat-free milk
  86 CALORIES
- 1 serving Broiled Fruit Dessert (p. 209)
  80 CALORIES
- Hot tea (with sugar substitute if desired)
  FREE FOOD

DINNER TOTAL: **565 CALORIES**

SNACKS:

- 1 medium plum
  40 CALORIES
- 3/4 cup skinny latte (made with fat-free milk)
  60 CALORIES

WEEK 1, DAY 5, TOTAL: 1,424 CALORIES

day 6

BREAKFAST:

- 1 serving Festive French Pancakes (p. 89)
  163 CALORIES
- 1 Turkey Breakfast Sausage (p. 267)
  85 CALORIES
- 1 cup fat-free milk
  86 CALORIES
- 1/2 medium banana
  50 CALORIES
- Hot tea (with sugar substitute if desired)
  FREE FOOD

BREAKFAST TOTAL: **384 CALORIES**

LUNCH:

- 1 serving Raspberry Chicken Salad (p. 283)
  320 CALORIES
- 1 whole wheat dinner roll
  76 CALORIES
- with 1 teaspoon reduced-fat margarine spread
  FREE FOOD
- Hot tea (with sugar substitute if desired)
  FREE FOOD

LUNCH TOTAL: **396 CALORIES**

DINNER & DESSERT:

- 1 serving Dijon-Peach Pork Chops (p. 289)
  360 CALORIES
- 1 big green salad (see Free Foods Chart on p. 53) with 1 tablespoon reduced-fat salad dressing
  FREE FOOD
- 1 cup fat-free milk
  86 CALORIES
- 1 Pecan Kiss (p. 265)
  46 CALORIES
- Coffee (with sugar substitute and liquid non-dairy creamer if desired)
  FREE FOOD

DINNER TOTAL: **492 CALORIES**

SNACKS:

- 1/2 cup sugar-free chocolate pudding (prepared with fat-free milk) topped with a crushed chocolate wafer
  99 CALORIES
- 1/2 cup fresh blueberries
  41 CALORIES

WEEK 1, DAY 6, TOTAL: 1,412 CALORIES

day 7

BREAKFAST:

- 1 cup Cheerios with 1/2 cup fat-free milk
  154 CALORIES
- 1/2 small banana with 2 teaspooons reduced-fat creamy peanut butter
  99 CALORIES
- 1/2 cup orange juice
  55 CALORIES

BREAKFAST TOTAL: **308 CALORIES**

LUNCH:

- 1-1/2 cups Fruity Crab Pasta Salad (p. 283)
  322 CALORIES
- 1 whole wheat dinner roll
  69 CALORIES
- with 1 teaspoon reduced-fat margarine spread
  FREE FOOD
- 1 dill pickle spear
  FREE FOOD
- 1 cup fat-free milk
  86 CALORIES

LUNCH TOTAL: **477 CALORIES**

DINNER & DESSERT:

- 1 serving Easy Beef Stroganoff with noodles (p. 285)
  326 CALORIES
- 1 big green salad (see Free Foods Chart on p. 53) with 1 tablespoon reduced-fat salad dressing
  FREE FOOD
- 1 cup fat-free milk
  86 CALORIES
- 1 slice Peach-Topped Cake (p. 210)
  121 CALORIES

DINNER TOTAL: **533 CALORIES**

SNACKS:

- Carrot and celery sticks with 1 tablespoon reduced-fat ranch salad dressing
  FREE FOOD
- 1 clementine
  35 CALORIES

WEEK 1, DAY 7, TOTAL: 1,401 CALORIES

day 1

BREAKFAST:

- 1 serving Baked Eggs with Cheddar & Bacon (p. 267)
  107 CALORIES
- 1 mini bagel
  72 CALORIES
- with 1 tablespoon fat-free cream cheese
  FREE FOOD
- 2/3 cup red grapes
  86 CALORIES
- 1/2 cup orange juice
  55 CALORIES
- Hot tea (with sugar substitute if desired)
  FREE FOOD

BREAKFAST TOTAL: **320 CALORIES**

LUNCH:

- 1-1/3 cups Lasagna Soup (p. 280)
  280 CALORIES
- 1 whole wheat dinner roll
  69 CALORIES
- with 1 teaspoon reduced-fat margarine spread
  FREE FOOD
- 1 cup fat-free milk
  86 CALORIES

LUNCH TOTAL: **435 CALORIES**

DINNER & DESSERT:

- 1 Tex-Mex Beef Barbecue sandwich (p. 232)
  294 CALORIES
- Steamed green beans
  FREE FOOD
- Ice water
  FREE FOOD
- 1 serving Cranberry Apple Tart (p. 218)
  183 CALORIES

DINNER TOTAL: **477 CALORIES**

SNACKS:

- 3/4 cup skinny latte (made with fat-free milk)
  60 CALORIES
- 1 Apple Skewer (p. 265)
  80 CALORIES

WEEK 2, DAY 1, TOTAL: 1,372 CALORIES

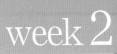

day 2

BREAKFAST:

- 1 Scrambled Egg Muffin (p. 286)
  133 CALORIES
- 1/2 cup Orange Fruit Cup (p. 87)
  80 CALORIES
- 1 cup fat-free milk
  86 CALORIES
- Hot tea (with sugar substitute if desired)
  FREE FOOD

  BREAKFAST TOTAL: 299 CALORIES

LUNCH:

- 2/3 cup Brunch Risotto (p. 258)
  279 CALORIES
- 3/4 cup fresh blueberries
  62 CALORIES
- 1 whole wheat dinner roll
  69 CALORIES
- with 1 teaspoon reduced-fat margarine spread
  FREE FOOD
- Sugar-free flavored water
  FREE FOOD

  LUNCH TOTAL: 410 CALORIES

DINNER & DESSERT:

- 1 Lime-Marinated Orange Roughy fillet (p. 270)
  169 CALORIES
- 1 medium baked russet potato
  161 CALORIES
- 1 big green salad (see Free Foods Chart on p. 53) with 1 tablespoon reduced-fat salad dressing
  FREE FOOD
- 1 cup fat-free milk
  86 CALORIES
- 1 Cherry Chocolate Parfait (p. 244)
  146 CALORIES
- Coffee (with sugar substitute and liquid non-dairy creamer if desired)
  FREE FOOD

  DINNER TOTAL: 562 CALORIES

SNACKS:

- 1 cup Parmesan Popcorn (p. 81)
  49 CALORIES
- 1 cup cubed watermelon
  40 CALORIES

WEEK 2, DAY 2, TOTAL: 1,360 CALORIES

day 3

BREAKFAST:

- 3/4 cup prepared oatmeal (made with water)
  109 CALORIES
- with 2 tablespoons raisins
  54 CALORIES
- 1 medium banana
  100 CALORIES
- 1 cup fat-free milk
  86 CALORIES
- Coffee (with sugar substitute and liquid non-dairy creamer if desired)
  FREE FOOD

  BREAKFAST TOTAL: 349 CALORIES

LUNCH:

- 1 sandwich made with 2 pieces whole wheat bread and 4 slices deli smoked turkey breast spread with 2 teaspoons fat-free mayonnaise
  178 CALORIES
- Baby carrots
  FREE FOOD
- 1 cup red grapes
  129 CALORIES
- 1 cup fat-free milk
  86 CALORIES

  LUNCH TOTAL: 393 CALORIES

DINNER & DESSERT:

- 1 serving Country Chicken with Gravy (p. 278)
  274 CALORIES
- 1/2 cup prepared brown rice
  108 CALORIES
- 1/2 cup Wilted Garlic Spinach (p. 177)
  66 CALORIES
- 2 chocolate kisses
  49 CALORIES
- Hot tea (with sugar substitute if desired)
  FREE FOOD

  DINNER TOTAL: 497 CALORIES

SNACKS:

- 1 Granola-To-Go Bar (p. 88)
  130 CALORIES
- Red and green pepper strips with 1 tablespoon reduced-fat ranch salad dressing
  FREE FOOD
- 1/2 cup sliced fresh strawberries
  27 CALORIES
- 1 cup prepared sugar-free gelatin
  8 CALORIES

WEEK 2, DAY 3, TOTAL: 1,404 CALORIES

day 4

BREAKFAST:

- 1 Colorful Cheese Omelet (p. 91)
  167 CALORIES
- 1 medium apple
  72 CALORIES
- 1 cup fat-free milk
  86 CALORIES

BREAKFAST TOTAL: 325 CALORIES

LUNCH:

- 1-1/2 cups Fruity Crab Pasta Salad (p. 283)
  322 CALORIES
- 1 whole wheat dinner roll
  69 CALORIES
- with 1 teaspoon reduced-fat margarine spread
  FREE FOOD
- 1/3 cup red grapes
  43 CALORIES
- Sugar-free flavored water
  FREE FOOD

LUNCH TOTAL: 434 CALORIES

DINNER & DESSERT:

- 1 serving Stuffed Steak Spirals (p. 130)
  214 CALORIES
- 3/4 cup Seasoned Yukon Gold Wedges (p. 190)
  121 CALORIES
- Steamed green beans with 1 teaspoon reduced-fat margarine spread
  FREE FOOD
- Iced tea (with sugar substitute if desired)
  FREE FOOD
- 1 Pina Colada Pudding Cup (p. 250)
  171 CALORIES
- 1 cup coffee (with sugar substitute and 1 tablespoon liquid non-dairy creamer if desired)
  FREE FOOD

DINNER TOTAL: 506 CALORIES

SNACKS:

- 1/2 cup chocolate soy milk
  67 CALORIES
- 1 medium plum
  40 CALORIES
- 1/2 piece string cheese
  40 CALORIES

WEEK 2, DAY 4, TOTAL: 1,412 CALORIES

day 5

BREAKFAST:

- 1/2 cup Apple-Cinnamon Oatmeal Mix (p. 94)
  176 CALORIES
- with 1 tablespoon maple syrup
  52 CALORIES
- 1/2 cup blueberries
  41 CALORIES
- 1 cup fat-free milk
  86 CALORIES

BREAKFAST TOTAL: 355 CALORIES

LUNCH:

- 1 slice Chicken Alfredo Veggie Pizza (p. 113)
  317 CALORIES
- 1 medium peach
  40 CALORIES
- Mineral water
  FREE FOOD

LUNCH TOTAL: 357 CALORIES

DINNER & DESSERT:

- 1 serving Broccoli-Turkey Casserole (p. 150)
  303 CALORIES
- 3/4 cup Sauteed Corn with Tomatoes & Basil (p. 182)
  85 CALORIES
- 1 big green salad (see Free Foods Chart on p. 53) with 1 tablespoon reduced-fat salad dressing
  FREE FOOD
- 1 cup fat-free milk
  86 CALORIES
- 3/4 cup Vanilla Tapioca Pudding (p. 242)
  133 CALORIES
- Coffee (with sugar substitute and liquid non-dairy creamer if desired)
  FREE FOOD

DINNER TOTAL: 607 CALORIES

SNACKS:

- 3/4 cup air-popped popcorn
  24 CALORIES
- 1 cup fresh raspberries
  60 CALORIES

WEEK 2, DAY 5, TOTAL: 1,403 CALORIES

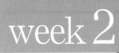

day 6

BREAKFAST:

- 1 serving Caramel Cream Crepes (p. 95)
  206 CALORIES

- 1/2 cup sliced fresh strawberries
  27 CALORIES

- 1 medium plum
  40 CALORIES

- 1 cup fat-free milk
  86 CALORIES

- Coffee (with sugar substitute and liquid non-dairy creamer if desired)
  FREE FOOD

BREAKFAST TOTAL: **359 CALORIES**

LUNCH:

- 1-1/2 cups Italian Sausage Bean Soup (p. 115)
  339 CALORIES

- 1 whole wheat dinner roll
  69 CALORIES

- with 1 teaspoon reduced-fat margarine spread
  FREE FOOD

- 1/3 cup red grapes
  43 CALORIES

- Ice water
  FREE FOOD

LUNCH TOTAL: **451 CALORIES**

DINNER & DESSERT:

- 4 ounces beef tenderloin steak, broiled
  200 CALORIES

- 1 small baked sweet potato
  128 CALORIES

- 1/2 cup Parmesan Roasted Carrots (p. 181)
  82 CALORIES

- Ice water
  FREE FOOD

- 1 cup fat-free milk
  86 CALORIES

- Hot tea (with sugar substitute if desired)
  FREE FOOD

DINNER TOTAL: **496 CALORIES**

SNACKS:

- 9 tiny twist fat-free pretzels served with 1 tablespoon honey mustard for dipping
  50 CALORIES

- 1 cup prepared sugar-free gelatin
  8 CALORIES

- 1 small orange
  45 CALORIES

WEEK 2, DAY 6, TOTAL: 1,409 CALORIES

day 7

BREAKFAST:

- 1-1/2 cup Wheaties
  161 CALORIES

- with 1 cup fat-free milk
  86 CALORIES

- 1 medium grapefruit
  92 CALORIES

- Coffee (with sugar substitute and liquid non-dairy creamer if desired)
  FREE FOOD

BREAKFAST TOTAL: **339 CALORIES**

LUNCH:

- 1 Spinach-Feta Chicken Roll (p. 109)
  272 CALORIES

- 1/2 cup cubed fresh pineapple
  37 CALORIES

- 1 cup fat-free milk
  86 CALORIES

LUNCH TOTAL: **395 CALORIES**

DINNER & DESSERT:

- 1 serving Sirloin Roast with Gravy (p. 227)
  185 CALORIES

- 1 serving Golden Au Gratin Potatoes (p. 196)
  167 CALORIES

- 1 big green salad (see Free Foods Chart on p. 53) with 1 tablespoon reduced-fat salad dressing
  FREE FOOD

- Ice water
  FREE FOOD

- 1 piece Raspberry Pie with Oat Crust (p. 249)
  167 CALORIES

- Hot tea (with sugar substitute if desired)
  FREE FOOD

DINNER TOTAL: **519 CALORIES**

SNACKS:

- 3/4 cup air-popped popcorn
  24 CALORIES

- 1 cup whole fresh strawberries
  54 CALORIES

- 1 medium apple
  72 CALORIES

WEEK 2, DAY 7, TOTAL: 1,403 CALORIES

meal plan | THE COMFORT FOOD DIET

day 1

BREAKFAST:

- 1-1/2 cups Cheerios
  122 CALORIES

- with 1/2 cup fat-free milk
  43 CALORIES

- 1 Frozen Fruit Cup (p. 237)
  48 CALORIES

- 3/4 cup orange juice
  83 CALORIES

- Coffee (with sugar substitute and liquid nondairy creamer if desired)
  FREE FOOD

  BREAKFAST TOTAL: 296 CALORIES

LUNCH:

- 1 piece Focaccia Sandwich (p. 101)
  113 CALORIES

- 3/4 cup Mediterranean Salad (p. 101)
  69 CALORIES

- 1/3 cup red grapes
  43 CALORIES

- 1 cup fat-free milk
  86 CALORIES

- 1/2 cup Colorful Frozen Yogurt (p. 215)
  143 CALORIES

  LUNCH TOTAL: 454 CALORIES

DINNER & DESSERT:

- 1 Turkey Pecan Enchilada (p. 139)
  263 CALORIES

- 3/4 cup Mexican Veggies (p. 178)
  60 CALORIES

- Baby corn
  FREE FOOD

- 1 cup fat-free milk
  86 CALORIES

- 1/3 cup Lemon Sorbet (p. 242)
  138 CALORIES

  DINNER TOTAL: 547 CALORIES

SNACKS:

- 1/2 cup canned sliced peaches in juice
  53 CALORIES

- 1 medium plum
  40 CALORIES

- Baby carrots with 1 tablespoon reduced fat ranch salad dressing
  FREE FOOD

  WEEK 3, DAY 1, TOTAL: 1,390 CALORIES

day 2

BREAKFAST:

- 1 Blueberry Oatmeal Pancake with 1 tablespoon syrup (p. 270)
  141 CALORIES

- 3/4 cup Melon 'n' Grape Medley (p. 239)
  74 CALORIES

- 1 cup fat-free milk
  86 CALORIES

  BREAKFAST TOTAL: 301 CALORIES

LUNCH:

- 1 Chicken Caesar Wrap (p. 115)
  332 CALORIES

- Baby carrots
  FREE FOOD

- 1 dill pickle spear
  FREE FOOD

- 1/2 cup Apple Cranberry Delight (p. 238)
  70 CALORIES

- 1 cup fat-free milk
  86 CALORIES

  LUNCH TOTAL: 488 CALORIES

DINNER & DESSERT:

- 1 serving Asian Orange Beef with 1/2 cup cooked rice (p. 157)
  351 CALORIES

- 1 big green salad (see Free Foods Chart on p. 53) with 1 tablespoon reduced-fat salad dressing
  FREE FOOD

- Steamed fresh broccoli florets
  FREE FOOD

- Carbonated water
  FREE FOOD

- 1 serving Warm Chocolate Melting Cups (p. 212)
  131 CALORIES

- Hot tea (with sugar substitute if desired)
  FREE FOOD

  DINNER TOTAL: 482 CALORIES

SNACKS:

- 1/2 ounce Swiss cheese and 2 butter-flavored crackers
  87 CALORIES

- 1 cup sliced fresh strawberries
  54 CALORIES

  WEEK 3, DAY 2, TOTAL: 1,412 CALORIES

> Store leftover Blueberry Oatmeal Pancakes in the freezer to use on other mornings when time is tight.

day 3

BREAKFAST:

- 2 frozen waffles
  196 CALORIES

- with 1 tablespoon sugar-free syrup
  FREE FOOD

- 1 medium banana
  100 CALORIES

- 1 cup fat-free milk
  86 CALORIES

- Coffee (with sugar substitute and liquid nondairy creamer if desired)
  FREE FOOD

BREAKFAST TOTAL: 382 CALORIES

LUNCH:

- 1 Grilled Fish Sandwich (p. 276)
  241 CALORIES

- 1/3 cup red grapes
  43 CALORIES

- 1 cup cubed watermelon
  40 CALORIES

- Celery sticks with 1 tablespoon fat-free ranch salad dressing
  FREE FOOD

- 1 cup fat-free milk
  86 CALORIES

LUNCH TOTAL: 410 CALORIES

DINNER & DESSERT:

- 1 serving Pork Chop Skillet (p. 162)
  360 CALORIES

- 1 big green salad (see Free Foods Chart on p. 53) with 1 tablespoon reduced-fat salad dressing
  FREE FOOD

- 1 slice Frozen Pistachio Dessert with Raspberry Sauce (p. 220)
  214 CALORIES

- Hot tea (with sugar substitute if desired)
  FREE FOOD

DINNER TOTAL: 574 CALORIES

SNACKS:

- 1 cup air-popped popcorn sprinkled with Italian seasoning
  31 CALORIES

- 1 cup prepared sugar-free gelatin
  8 CALORIES

WEEK 3, DAY 3, TOTAL: 1,405 CALORIES

day 4

BREAKFAST:

- 2 Italian Mini Frittatas (p. 93)
  172 CALORIES

- 1/2 cup Orange Fruit Cup (p. 87)
  80 CALORIES

- 1 cup skinny latte (made with fat-free milk)
  80 CALORIES

BREAKFAST TOTAL: 332 CALORIES

LUNCH:

- 1 cup Southwest Black Bean Soup with 1/4 cup rice and 1 tablespoon sour cream (p. 109)
  273 CALORIES

- 1 medium apple
  72 CALORIES

- 1 cup fat-free milk
  86 CALORIES

LUNCH TOTAL: 431 CALORIES

DINNER & DESSERT:

- 1 serving Turkey with Apple Slices (p. 138)
  263 CALORIES

- 2/3 cup Great Grain Pilaf (p. 194)
  154 CALORIES

- 1 big green salad (see Free Foods Chart on p. 53) with 1 tablespoon reduced-fat salad dressing
  FREE FOOD

- Iced tea (with sugar substitute if desired)
  FREE FOOD

- 1 slice No-Bake Cheesecake Pie (p. 214)
  141 CALORIES

DINNER TOTAL: 558 CALORIES

SNACKS:

- 1 medium plum
  40 CALORIES

- 1/2 cup cheese popcorn
  40 CALORIES

WEEK 3, DAY 4, TOTAL: 1,401 CALORIES

Top off slices of angel food cake with fresh fruit and a dollop of reduced-fat whipped topping or frozen yogurt for a no-fuss dessert that's light, too.

day 5

BREAKFAST:

- 1 Fresh Fruit Parfait (p. 216)
  149 CALORIES

- 1 Cafe Mocha Mini Muffin (p. 266)
  81 CALORIES

- 1 cup fat-free milk
  86 CALORIES

- Coffee (with sugar substitute and liquid nondairy creamer if desired)
  FREE FOOD

BREAKFAST TOTAL: 316 CALORIES

LUNCH:

- 1 Apricot Turkey Sandwich (p. 116)
  338 CALORIES

- Broccoli florets with 2 tablespoons fat-free ranch salad dressing
  FREE FOOD

- 1/2 medium banana
  50 CALORIES

- 1 cup fat-free milk
  86 CALORIES

LUNCH TOTAL: 474 CALORIES

DINNER & DESSERT:

- 3 Italian Cheese-Stuffed Shells with 3/4 cup sauce (p. 158)
  351 CALORIES

- 1 big green salad (see Free Foods Chart on p. 53) with 1 tablespoon reduced-fat salad dressing
  FREE FOOD

- Sugar-free flavored water
  FREE FOOD

- 1 Makeover Oatmeal Bar (p. 211)
  127 CALORIES

- Hot tea (with sugar substitute if desired)
  FREE FOOD

DINNER TOTAL: 478 CALORIES

SNACKS:

- 1/3 cup grapes with 1 tablespoon fat-free whippd topping
  45 CALORIES

- 7 miniature caramel-flavored rice cakes
  60 CALORIES

- 1/2 cup fresh strawberries
  27 CALORIES

WEEK 3, DAY 5, TOTAL: 1,400 CALORIES

day 6

BREAKFAST:

- 2 large scrambled eggs
  202 CALORIES

- 1 slice whole wheat toast
  69 CALORIES

- with 1 teaspoon reduced-fat margarine spread
  FREE FOOD

- 1 cup fat-free milk
  86 CALORIES

- Ice water
  FREE FOOD

BREAKFAST TOTAL: 357 CALORIES

LUNCH:

- 1 cup Chili Con Carne (p. 113)
  299 CALORIES

- 1 cup cubed fresh pineapple
  74 CALORIES

- 1/2 cup cubed watermelon
  20 CALORIES

- Baby carrots
  FREE FOOD

- Diet soft drink
  FREE FOOD

LUNCH TOTAL: 393 CALORIES

DINNER & DESSERT:

- 2 Baked Chicken Fajitas (p.286)
  340 CALORIES

- 3/4 cup Citrus Spinach Salad (p. 173)
  52 CALORIES

- 1 cup fat-free milk
  86 CALORIES

- 2 crisp lady finger cookies
  60 CALORIES

- Coffee (with sugar substitute and liquid nondairy creamer if desired)
  FREE FOOD

DINNER TOTAL: 538 CALORIES

SNACKS:

- 5 medium cooked shrimp with 2 tablespoons cocktail sauce
  77 CALORIES

- 1 clementine
  35 CALORIES

WEEK 3, DAY 6, TOTAL: 1,400 CALORIES

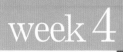

meal plan | THE COMFORT FOOD DIET

day 7

BREAKFAST:

- 1 cup Tropical Fruit Smoothie (p. 87)
  97 CALORIES
- 1 mini bagel
  72 CALORIES
- 1 medium banana
  100 CALORIES
- Coffee (with sugar substitute and liquid nondairy creamer if desired)
  FREE FOOD

BREAKFAST TOTAL: **269 CALORIES**

LUNCH:

- 2 Chive Crab Cakes (p. 256)
  242 calories
- 1 whole wheat dinner roll
  69 CALORIES
- 1 cup cubed fresh pineapple
  74 CALORIES
- 1 cup fat-free milk
  86 CALORIES

LUNCH TOTAL: **471 CALORIES**

DINNER & DESSERT:

- 1 serving Creole Chicken with 2/3 cup sauce and 1/2 cup rice (p. 154)
  320 CALORIES
- 1 big green salad (see Free Foods Chart on p. 53) with 1 tablespoon reduced-fat salad dressing
  FREE FOOD
- 1 cup fat-free milk
  86 CALORIES
- 2/3 cup Rich Peach Ice Cream (p. 213)
  140 CALORIES
- Hot tea (with sugar substitute if desired)
  FREE FOOD

DINNER TOTAL: **546 CALORIES**

SNACKS:

- 2 chocolate kisses
  49 CALORIES
- 1 medium kiwifruit
  46 CALORIES
- Sliced zucchini with 2 tablespoons salsa
  FREE FOOD

WEEK 3, DAY 7, TOTAL: 1,381 CALORIES

day 1

BREAKFAST:

- 3 pancakes from Homemade Pancake Mix (p. 281)
  303 CALORIES
- with 2 tablespoons sugar-free syrup
  FREE FOOD
- 1/3 cup red grapes
  43 CALORIES
- Coffee (with sugar substitute and liquid nondairy creamer if desired)
  FREE FOOD

BREAKFAST TOTAL: **346 CALORIES**

LUNCH:

- 1 Presto Chicken Taco (p. 273)
  206 CALORIES
- with 1 tablespoon taco sauce and 1 tablespoon reduced-fat sour cream
  FREE FOOD
- 1 medium pear
  96 CALORIES
- Steamed broccoli florets
  FREE FOOD
- 1 cup fat-free milk
  86 CALORIES
- Coffee (with sugar substitute and liquid nondairy creamer if desired)
  FREE FOOD

LUNCH TOTAL: **388 CALORIES**

DINNER & DESSERT:

- 1 BBQ Beef Sandwich (p. 233)
  354 CALORIES
- 2/3 cup Home-Style Coleslaw (p. 183)
  88 CALORIES
- 1 cup fat-free milk
  86 CALORIES
- Hot tea (with sugar substitute if desired)
  FREE FOOD

DINNER TOTAL: **528 CALORIES**

SNACKS:

- 1/4 cup pretzel sticks with 1 tablespoon honey mustard
  77 CALORIES
- 1 clementine
  35 CALORIES
- Red and green pepper strips with 1 tablespoon reduced-fat ranch salad dressing
  FREE FOOD

WEEK 4, DAY 1, TOTAL: 1,374 CALORIES

day 2

BREAKFAST:

- 1 piece Monterey Quiche (p. 98)
  265 CALORIES
- 1/3 cup red grapes
  43 CALORIES
- 1 cup fat-free milk
  86 CALORIES
- Hot tea (with sugar substitute if desired)
  FREE FOOD

BREAKFAST TOTAL: **394 CALORIES**

LUNCH:

- 1 whole sandwich made with 2 pieces whole wheat bread and 4 slices deli smoked turkey breast spread with 2 teaspoons fat-free mayonnaise
  178 CALORIES
- 10 baked potato chips
  100 CALORIES
- 1 cup fat-free milk
  86 CALORIES
- 1 Frozen Fruit Cup (p. 237)
  48 CALORIES
- Diet soft drink
  FREE FOOD

LUNCH TOTAL: **412 CALORIES**

DINNER & DESSERT:

- 1 serving Tilapia with Grapefruit Salsa (p. 140)
  264 CALORIES
- 1 big green salad (see Free Foods Chart on p. 53) with 1 tablespoon reduced-fat salad dressing
  FREE FOOD
- 1/2 Grandma's Stuffed Yellow Squash (p. 240)
  103 CALORIES
- Iced tea (with sugar substitute if desired)
  FREE FOOD
- 1 serving Broiled Fruit Dessert (p. 209)
  80 CALORIES
- Hot tea (with sugar substitute if desired)
  FREE FOOD

DINNER TOTAL: **447 CALORIES**

SNACKS:

- 1/2 cup fat-free vanilla frozen yogurt
  95 CALORIES
- 1 cup sliced fresh strawberries
  54 CALORIES

WEEK 4, DAY 2, TOTAL: 1,402 CALORIES

day 3

BREAKFAST:

- 2 frozen waffles
  196 CALORIES
- with 1 tablespoon sugar-free syrup
  FREE FOOD
- 1 cup sliced fresh strawberries
  54 CALORIES
- 1 cup fat-free milk
  86 CALORIES
- 1 cup coffee (with sugar substitute and 1 tablespoon liquid nondairy creamer if desired)
  FREE FOOD

BREAKFAST TOTAL: **336 CALORIES**

LUNCH:

- 1 serving Ratatouille with Polenta (p. 271)
  195 CALORIES
- 1 piece Tropical Meringue Tart (p. 215)
  145 CALORIES
- Ice water
  FREE FOOD

LUNCH TOTAL: **340 CALORIES**

DINNER & DESSERT:

- 1 serving Pork Medallions with Dijon Sauce (p. 284)
  323 CALORIES
- 3/4 cup Herbed Potato Salad (p. 191)
  142 CALORIES
- Shredded cabbage topped with 1 tablespoon reduced-fat salad dressing
  FREE FOOD
- 1 sliced medium apple with cinnamon
  72 CALORIES
- Hot tea (with sugar substitute if desired)
  FREE FOOD

DINNER TOTAL: **537 CALORIES**

SNACKS:

- 1 ice cream cake cone filled with 1/3 cup fat-free strawberry yogurt and 1/4 cup blueberries
  81 CALORIES
- 1 piece string cheese
  80 CALORIES
- 1 clementine
  35 CALORIES

WEEK 4, DAY 3, TOTAL: 1,409 CALORIES

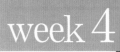

day 4

BREAKFAST:

- 1 Hawaiian Breakfast Cup (p. 242)
  131 CALORIES
- 1 cup orange juice
  110 CALORIES
- 1/2 cup fresh raspberries
  30 CALORIES
- Coffee (with sugar substitute and liquid nondairy creamer if desired)
  FREE FOOD

BREAKFAST TOTAL: 271 CALORIES

LUNCH:

- 1 Garbanzo Bean Pita (1 filled pita half) (p. 105)
  241 CALORIES
- 3/4 cup Mediterranean Salad (p. 101)
  69 CALORIES
- 1 clementine
  35 CALORIES
- 1 cup fat-free milk
  86 CALORIES

LUNCH TOTAL: 431 CALORIES

DINNER & DESSERT:

- 1 serving Burgundy Beef Stew with 1 cup noodles (p. 234)
  388 CALORIES
- Steamed broccoli florets with 1 teaspoon reduced-fat margarine spread
  FREE FOOD
- 1 cup fat-free milk
  86 CALORIES
- 1/2 cup Cappuccino Pudding (p. 210)
  105 CALORIES
- Iced tea (with sugar substitute if desired)
  FREE FOOD

DINNER TOTAL: 579 CALORIES

SNACKS:

- 1 medium kiwifruit
  46 CALORIES
- 1 crisp ladyfinger cookie
  30 CALORIES
- 1/2 cup cheese popcorn
  40 CALORIES

WEEK 4, DAY 4, TOTAL: 1,397 CALORIES

day 5

BREAKFAST:

- 1 serving Baked Blueberry & Peach Oatmeal (p. 99)
  277 CALORIES
- 1 cup fat-free milk
  86 CALORIES
- Hot tea (with sugar substitute if desired)
  FREE FOOD

BREAKFAST TOTAL: 363 CALORIES

LUNCH:

- 1 Grilled Fish Sandwich (p. 276)
  241 CALORIES
- 1 medium peach
  40 CALORIES
- 1 dill pickle spear
  FREE FOOD
- 1/2 cup fat-free milk
  43 CALORIES
- Club soda
  FREE FOOD

LUNCH TOTAL: 324 CALORIES

DINNER & DESSERT:

- 4 ounce salmon fillet, broiled
  184 CALORIES
- 1 whole wheat dinner roll
  69 CALORIES
- with 1 teaspoon reduced-fat margarine spread
  FREE FOOD
- 1/2 cup Peas a la Francais (p. 188)
  112 CALORIES
- 1 big green salad (see Free Foods Chart on p. 53) with 1 tablespoon reduced-fat salad dressing
  FREE FOOD
- Ice water
  FREE FOOD
- 1 serving Coconut Custard Pie (p. 254)
  214 CALORIES
- Coffee (with sugar substitute and liquid nondairy creamer if desired)
  FREE FOOD

DINNER TOTAL: 579 CALORIES

SNACKS:

- 1/2 medium apple with 1/2 ounce sharp cheddar cheese
  93 CALORIES
- 1/2 cup fat-free milk
  43 CALORIES

WEEK 4, DAY 5, TOTAL: 1,402 CALORIES

meal plan | THE COMFORT FOOD DIET

day 6

BREAKFAST:

- 1-1/2 cups Cheerios
  167 CALORIES

- with 1/2 cup fat-free milk
  43 CALORIES

- 1/2 medium banana
  50 CALORIES

- 1/2 cup orange juice
  55 CALORIES

- Coffee (with sugar substitute and liquid nondairy creamer if desired)
  FREE FOOD

BREAKFAST TOTAL: **315 CALORIES**

LUNCH:

- 1-1/3 cup Chicken Caesar Pasta Toss (p. 120)
  363 CALORIES

- 1 whole wheat dinner roll
  76 CALORIES

- with 1 teaspoon reduced-fat margarine spread
  FREE FOOD

- 1/2 cup fat-free milk
  43 CALORIES

LUNCH TOTAL: **482 CALORIES**

DINNER & DESSERT:

- 1 serving Grilled Pork Tenderloin (p. 250)
  171 CALORIES

- 1 serving Coconut-Pecan Sweet Potatoes (p. 229)
  211 CALORIES

- Steamed green beans
  FREE FOOD

- 1 cup cubed watermelon
  40 CALORIES

- 3/4 cup Vanilla Tapioca Pudding (p. 242)
  133 CALORIES

DINNER TOTAL: **555 CALORIES**

SNACKS:

- Baby carrots and celery sticks with 1 tablespoon reduced-fat ranch salad dressing
  FREE FOOD

- 1 cup prepared sugar-free gelatin
  8 CALORIES

- 9 tiny twist fat-free pretzels with 1 tablespoon honey mustard
  50 CALORIES

WEEK 4, DAY 6, TOTAL: 1,410 CALORIES

day 7

BREAKFAST:

- 1-1/2 cups Wheaties
  161 CALORIES

- with 1 cup fat-free milk
  86 CALORIES

- 1/2 cup blueberries
  41 CALORIES

- 1/2 cup sliced fresh strawberries
  27 CALORIES

- Coffee (with sugar substitute and liquid nondairy creamer if desired)
  FREE FOOD

BREAKFAST TOTAL: **315 CALORIES**

LUNCH:

- 1 Super Flatbread Wrap (p. 261)
  348 CALORIES

- Red and green pepper strips with 1 tablespoon reduced-fat ranch sald dressing
  FREE FOOD

- 1 cup fat-free milk
  86 CALORIES

LUNCH TOTAL: **434 CALORIES**

DINNER & DESSERT:

- 1 serving Crunchy Onion Barbecue Chicken (p. 258)
  286 CALORIES

- 2 Mashed Potato Cakes (p. 193)
  147 CALORIES

- 1 big green salad (see Free Foods Chart on p. 53) with 1 tablespoon reduced-fat salad dressing
  FREE FOOD

- Ice water
  FREE FOOD

- 1 serving Sangria Gelatin Dessert (p. 240)
  95 CALORIES

- Hot tea (with sugar substitute if desired)
  FREE FOOD

DINNER TOTAL: **528 CALORIES**

SNACKS:

- 1/3 cup Strawberry-Raspberry Ice (p. 241)
  79 CALORIES

- 7 miniature caramel-flavored rice cakes
  60 CALORIES

WEEK 4, DAY 7, TOTAL: 1,416 CALORIES

day 1

BREAKFAST:

- 1 Zucchini Pancake (p. 88)
  88 CALORIES

- with 2 tablespoons sugar-free syrup
  FREE FOOD

- 1 Turkey Breakfast Sausage (p. 267)
  85 CALORIES

- 1/2 small grapefruit with 1 teaspoon sugar
  48 CALORIES

- 1 cup fat-free milk
  86 CALORIES

BREAKFAST TOTAL: **307 CALORIES**

LUNCH:

- 1 cup Sausage Kale Soup (p. 252)
  194 CALORIES

- 1 half-sandwich made with 1 piece whole wheat bread and 2 slices deli smoked turkey breast spread with 1 teaspoon fat-free mayonnaise
  89 CALORIES

- 1/3 cup red grapes
  43 CALORIES

- Diet soft drink
  FREE FOOD

LUNCH TOTAL: **326 CALORIES**

DINNER & DESSERT:

- 1 serving Homemade Spaghetti Sauce with 1/2 cup cooked spaghetti (p. 133)
  230 CALORIES

- 1 big green salad (see Free Foods Chart on p. 53) with 1 tablespoon reduced-fat salad dressing
  FREE FOOD

- 1 whole wheat roll
  76 CALORIES

- 1 piece Lemon Fluff Dessert (p. 243)
  135 CALORIES

- 1 cup fat-free milk
  86 CALORIES

DINNER TOTAL: **527 CALORIES**

SNACKS:

- 3 cups air-popped popcorn
  94 CALORIES

- 1/2 cup Pretzel Bones (p. 84)
  98 CALORIES

WEEK 5, DAY 1, TOTAL: **1,352 CALORIES**

day 2

BREAKFAST:

- 1 cup Tropical Fruit Smoothie (p. 87)
  97 CALORIES

- 1 mini bagel
  72 CALORIES

- 1/2 small grapefuit with 1 teaspoon sugar
  48 CALORIES

- 1 cup fat-free milk
  86 CALORIES

BREAKFAST TOTAL: **303 CALORIES**

LUNCH:

- 1 serving Spicy Warm Chicken Salad (p. 292)
  417 CALORIES

- 1 kiwifruit
  46 CALORIES

- Baby carrots
  FREE FOOD

- Iced tea (with sugar substitute if desired)
  FREE FOOD

LUNCH TOTAL: **463 CALORIES**

DINNER & DESSERT:

- 1 serving Herbed Beef Tenderloin (3 ounces) (p. 253)
  198 CALORIES

- 3/4 cup Gruyere Mashed Potatoes (p. 197)
  193 CALORIES

- Steamed green beans with 1 teaspoon reduced-fat margarine spread
  FREE FOOD

- 1 cup fat-free milk
  86 CALORIES

- 1 No-Bake Peanut Butter Treat (p. 82)
  70 CALORIES

DINNER TOTAL: **547 CALORIES**

SNACKS:

- 1 cup Parmesan Popcorn (p. 81)
  49 CALORIES

- 13 almonds
  95 CALORIES

WEEK 5, DAY 2, TOTAL: **1,411 CALORIES**

Keep a bag of frozen peas on hand. Toss a handful of peas into soups, sauces, casseroles...even morning omelets. They add a nice burst of color and extra nutrition.

day 3

BREAKFAST:

- 1 serving Baked Eggs with Cheddar & Bacon (p. 267)
  107 CALORIES
- 2 slices whole wheat toast
  138 CALORIES
- with 1 tablespoon no-sugar-added jam
  FREE FOOD
- Coffee (with sugar substitute and liquid nondairy creamer if desired)
  FREE FOOD

BREAKFAST TOTAL: 245 CALORIES

LUNCH:

- 1 Turkey Tortilla Roll-Up (p. 117)
  353 CALORIES
- 2 pineapple rings
  41 CALORIES
- Baby carrots
  FREE FOOD
- Sugar-free flavored water
  FREE FOOD

LUNCH TOTAL: 394 CALORIES

DINNER & DESSERT:

- 1-1/3 cups Cheesy Rigatoni Bake (p. 144)
  274 CALORIES
- 3/4 cup Italian Vegetable Medley (p. 180)
  79 CALORIES
- 1 cup fat-free milk
  86 CALORIES
- 1 piece Tres Leches Cake (p. 224)
  233 CALORIES

DINNER TOTAL: 672 CALORIES

SNACKS:

- 1/3 cup 1% cottage cheese with 2 tablesoons chopped green onion
  58 CALORIES
- 1 cup cubed watermelon
  40 CALORIES

WEEK 5, DAY 3, TOTAL: 1,409 CALORIES

> **Taking time for breakfast has lots of benefits.** You get energy, jump-start your metabolism and are less likely to overeat later. If preparing breakfast becomes too difficult on busy weekday mornings, a little planning can do wonders. Smoothies can be made a day early and many breakfast bakes can be prepared the night before.

day 4

BREAKFAST:

- 1 piece Blueberry-Stuffed French Toast with 1/4 cup sauce (p. 92)
  167 CALORIES
- 1 cup fat-free milk
  86 CALORIES
- 1 small orange
  45 CALORIES

BREAKFAST TOTAL: 298 CALORIES

LUNCH:

- 1 Super-Duper Tuna Sandwich (p. 112)
  291 CALORIES
- 10 baked potato chips
  100 CALORIES
- 1/2 cup sliced fresh strawberries
  27 CALORIES
- Diet soft drink
  FREE FOOD

LUNCH TOTAL: 418 CALORIES

DINNER & DESSERT:

- 2 roasted chicken drumsticks, skin removed
  154 CALORIES
- 1/2 small baked potato with 1 tablespoon fat-free sour cream
  81 CALORIES
- 1 big green salad (see Free Foods Chart on p. 53) with 1 tablespoon reduced-fat salad dressing
  FREE FOOD
- 1 cup fat-free milk
  86 CALORIES
- 1 slice Tart Cherry Pie (p. 251)
  174 CALORIES

DINNER TOTAL: 495 CALORIES

SNACKS:

- 3 pieces snack rye bread topped with 1 tablespoon reduced-fat garden vegetable cream cheese and 6 cucumber slices
  89 CALORIES
- 1/2 medium apple with 1/2 ounce sharp cheddar cheese
  93 CALORIES

WEEK 5, DAY 4, TOTAL: 1,393 CALORIES

day 5

BREAKFAST:

- 1 cup Cheerios
  111 CALORIES
- with 1/2 cup fat-free milk
  43 CALORIES
- 1/2 medium banana with 2 teaspoons reduced-fat creamy peanut butter
  50 CALORIES
- 1 cup orange juice
  110 CALORIES

BREAKFAST TOTAL: 314 CALORIES

LUNCH:

- 1 cup Makeover Curried Chicken Rice Soup (p. 107)
  263 CALORIES
- 1 whole wheat dinner roll
  76 CALORIES
- Broccoli florets with 1 tablespoon fat-free ranch salad dressing
  FREE FOOD
- 1 cup fat-free milk
  86 CALORIES

LUNCH TOTAL: 425 CALORIES

DINNER & DESSERT:

- 1 serving Tuscan Chicken for Two (p. 274)
  217 CALORIES
- 3/4 cup Snow Pea Medley (p. 181)
  83 CALORIES
- 1 whole wheat dinner roll
  76 CALORIES
- Ice water
  FREE FOOD
- 2 Pecan Kisses (p. 256)
  92 CALORIES
- Hot tea (with sugar substitute if desired)
  FREE FOOD

DINNER TOTAL: 468 CALORIES

SNACKS:

- 2 Cheesecake Phyllo Cups (p. 80)
  92 CALORIES
- 1 cup Parmesan Popcorn (p. 81)
  49 CALORIES
- 1/3 cup red grapes
  43 CALORIES

WEEK 5, DAY 5, TOTAL: 1,391 CALORIES

day 6

BREAKFAST:

- 1 wedge Spring Frittata (p. 91)
  163 CALORIES
- 1 Frozen Fruit Cup (p. 237)
  48 CALORIES
- 1 cup fat-free milk
  86 CALORIES

BREAKFAST TOTAL: 297 CALORIES

LUNCH:

- 1 Better Than Egg Salad sandwich (p. 110)
  274 CALORIES
- Baby carrots
  FREE FOOD
- 1 medium plum
  40 CALORIES
- 1 cup fat-free milk
  86 CALORIES

LUNCH TOTAL: 400 CALORIES

DINNER & DESSERT:

- 1 Basil Tuna Steak (p. 130)
  214 CALORIES
- 1/2 cup cooked long-grain brown rice
  108 CALORIES
- Steamed green beans with 1 teaspoon reduced-fat margarine spread
  FREE FOOD
- 1 serving Triple-Berry Cobbler (p. 222)
  235 CALORIES
- Hot tea (with sugar substitute if desired)
  FREE FOOD

DINNER TOTAL: 557 CALORIES

SNACKS:

- 1/2 cup canned sliced peaches in juice
  53 CALORIES
- 1/2 cup fat-free vanilla frozen yogurt
  95 CALORIES

WEEK 5, DAY 6, TOTAL: 1,402 CALORIES

Drinking water has lots of benefits for your body and can keep you from feeling hungry between meals. Here are a few suggestions to help you get into the habit of drinking plenty of it:

- Keep a pitcher of water in your refrigerator so it's handy, well-chilled and inviting.
- Keep a big mug or bottle of water with you at work. You'll find yourself reaching for it automatically.
- Perk up plain water with a squeeze of lemon.

week 5

day 7

BREAKFAST:

- 1 Scrambled Egg Muffin (p. 268)
  133 CALORIES
- 1 cup orange juice
  110 CALORIES
- 1 medium banana
  100 CALORIES
- Coffee (with sugar substitute and liquid nondairy creamer if desired)
  FREE FOOD

BREAKFAST TOTAL: 343 CALORIES

LUNCH:

- 1 cup White Bean Soup (p. 108)
  270 CALORIES
- 1 whole wheat dinner roll
  76 CALORIES
- 1 cup fat-free milk
  86 CALORIES

LUNCH TOTAL: 432 CALORIES

DINNER & DESSERT:

- 1-1/4 cups Weeknight Beef Skillet with 3/4 cup noodles (p. 292)
  389 CALORIES
- 1 big green salad (see the Free Foods Chart on p. 53) with 1 tablespoon reduced-fat salad dressing
  FREE FOOD
- Iced tea (with sugar substitute if desired)
  FREE FOOD
- 1 Quick Crisp Snack Bar (p. 268)
  144 CALORIES

DINNER TOTAL: 533 CALORIES

SNACKS:

- 3/4 cup tomato juice
  31 CALORIES
- 3/4 cup skinny latte (made with fat-free milk)
  60 CALORIES

WEEK 5, DAY 7, TOTAL: 1,399 CALORIES

> When buying fruit juice, remember that words such as "punch," "cocktail," "beverage" or "drink" on the label mean you're likely not getting 100% juice.

week 6

day 1

BREAKFAST:

- 1 piece Baked Peach Pancake (p. 246)
  157 CALORIES
- 1 cup cubed watermelon
  40 CALORIES
- 1 cup fat-free milk
  86 CALORIES

BREAKFAST TOTAL: 283 CALORIES

LUNCH:

- 1 Apricot Turkey Sandwich (p. 116)
  338 CALORIES
- Baby carrots
  FREE FOOD
- 10 baked potato chips
  100 CALORIES
- Ice water
  FREE FOOD
- 1 cup prepared sugar-free gelatin
  8 CALORIES

LUNCH TOTAL: 446 CALORIES

DINNER & DESSERT:

- 1 boneless pork loin chop (4 ounces) broiled
  154 CALORIES
- 1/2 cup cooked egg noodles
  111 CALORIES
- 1 serving Balsamic Asparagus (p. 173)
  45 CALORIES
- 1 piece Banana Split Cheesecake (p. 223)
  247 CALORIES
- Hot tea (with sugar substitute if desired)
  FREE FOOD

DINNER TOTAL: 557 CALORIES

SNACKS:

- 1 piece string cheese
  80 CALORIES
- 1 clementine
  35 CALORIES

WEEK 6, DAY 1, TOTAL: 1,401 CALORIES

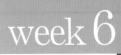

day 2

BREAKFAST:

- 1 piece Potato Egg Bake (p. 98)
  235 CALORIES
- 1 mini bagel
  72 CALORIES
- with 1 tablespoon whipped cream cheese
  35 CALORIES
- 1 medium kiwifruit
  46 CALORIES
- Coffee (with sugar substitute and liquid nondairy creamer if desired)
  FREE FOOD

BREAKFAST TOTAL: **388 CALORIES**

LUNCH:

- 1 Chili Beef Quesadilla (p. 117)
  353 CALORIES
- 1/3 cup red grapes
  43 CALORIES
- 1 cup fat-free milk
  86 CALORIES

LUNCH TOTAL: **482 CALORIES**

DINNER & DESSERT:

- 3/4 cup Garlic Lemon Shrimp (p. 123)
  163 CALORIES
- 1/2 cup cooked long-grain brown rice
  108 CALORIES
- Steamed broccoli with 1 teaspoon reduced-fat margarine spread
  FREE FOOD
- 1 cup fat-free milk
  86 CALORIES
- 1/2 cup Cappuccino Pudding (p. 210)
  105 CALORIES

DINNER TOTAL: **462 CALORIES**

SNACKS:

- 1 cup air-popped popcorn sprinkled with Italian seasoning
  31 CALORIES
- 1 clementine
  35 CALORIES
- Baby carrots
  FREE FOOD

WEEK 6, DAY 2, TOTAL: 1,398 CALORIES

day 3

BREAKFAST:

- 1 serving French Toast with Apple Topping (p. 96)
  219 CALORIES
- 1 medium grapefruit
  92 CALORIES
- 1 cup fat-free milk
  86 CALORIES

BREAKFAST TOTAL: **397 CALORIES**

LUNCH:

- 1 serving Raspberry Chicken Salad (p. 283)
  320 CALORIES
- 1 whole wheat dinner roll
  76 CALORIES
- Ice water
  FREE FOOD

LUNCH TOTAL: **396 CALORIES**

DINNER & DESSERT:

- 2 cups Chicken Artichoke Pasta (p. 289)
  378 CALORIES
- 1 big green salad (see Free Foods Chart on p. 53) with 1 tablespoon reduced-fat salad dressing
  FREE FOOD
- 2 Pecan Kisses (p. 265)
  92 CALORIES
- Hot tea (with sugar substitute if desired)
  FREE FOOD

DINNER TOTAL: **470 CALORIES**

SNACKS:

- 1/2 piece of string cheese
  40 CALORIES
- 1 cup Parmesan Popcorn (p. 81)
  49 CALORIES
- 1/2 cup canned sliced peaches in juice
  53 CALORIES

WEEK 6, DAY 3, TOTAL: 1,405 CALORIES

day 4

BREAKFAST:

- 3/4 cup Three-Fruit Smoothies (p. 97)
  225 CALORIES
- 1 mini bagel
  72 CALORIES
- 1/2 cup orange juice
  55 CALORIES
- Coffee (with sugar substitute and liquid nondairy creamer if desired)
  FREE FOOD

BREAKFAST TOTAL: 352 CALORIES

LUNCH:

- 1 cup Italian Vegetable Soup (p. 103)
  164 CALORIES
- 1 half-sandwich made with 1 piece whole wheat bread and 2 slices deli smoked turkey breast spread with 1 teaspoon fat-free mayonnaise
  89 CALORIES
- 1 medium banana
  100 CALORIES
- 1 cup fat-free milk
  86 CALORIES

LUNCH TOTAL: 439 CALORIES

DINNER & DESSERT:

- 1 serving Skillet Arroz Con Pollo (p. 164)
  373 CALORIES
- 1 big green salad (see Free Foods Chart on p. 53) with 1 tablespoon reduced-fat salad dressing
  FREE FOOD
- Iced tea (with sugar substitute if desired)
  FREE FOOD
- 1 serving Coconut-Cherry Cream Squares (p. 214)
  142 CALORIES

DINNER TOTAL: 515 CALORIES

SNACKS:

- 1 cup Tex-Mex Popcorn (p. 79)
  44 CALORIES
- 1 Mini Polenta Pizza (p. 81)
  57 CALORIES

WEEK 6, DAY 4, TOTAL: 1,407 CALORIES

day 5

BREAKFAST:

- 2 Apple Walnut Pancakes (p. 95)
  208 CALORIES
- with 2 tablespoons sugar-free syrup
  FREE FOOD
- 1 cup cubed watermelon
  40 CALORIES
- 1 cup fat-free milk
  86 CALORIES

BREAKFAST TOTAL: 334 CALORIES

LUNCH:

- 1 Red, White & Blue Pita Pocket (one filled half), (p. 116)
  351 CALORIES
- 1/3 cup red grapes
  43 CALORIES
- 1 cup fat-free milk
  86 CALORIES

LUNCH TOTAL: 480 CALORIES

DINNER & DESSERT:

- 1 serving Italian Hot Dish (p. 166)
  391 CALORIES
- 1 big green salad (see Free Foods Chart on p. 53) with 1 tablespoon reduced-fat salad dressing
  FREE FOOD
- 1 slice Peach-Topped Cake (p. 210)
  121 CALORIES
- Hot tea (with sugar substitute if desired)
  FREE FOOD

DINNER TOTAL: 512 CALORIES

SNACKS:

- 1 medium peach
  40 CALORIES
- 1 cup prepared sugar-free gelatin
  8 CALORIES

WEEK 6, DAY 5, TOTAL: 1,374 CALORIES

Don't forget to clip out the calorie chart on the back flap of this book. Tape it to the inside of a kitchen cabinet to give your family ideas for lower-calorie snacks.

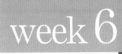

day 6

BREAKFAST:

- 1 large scrambled egg
  101 CALORIES
- 2 slices whole wheat toast
  138 CALORIES
- 1/2 cup orange juice
  55 CALORIES

BREAKFAST TOTAL: 294 CALORIES

LUNCH:

- 1 Colorful Beef Wrap (p. 284)
  325 CALORIES
- 1/2 cup sliced fresh strawberries
  27 CALORIES
- 1 cup fat-free milk
  86 CALORIES

LUNCH TOTAL: 438 CALORIES

DINNER & DESSERT:

- 1 serving Old-Fashioned Swiss Steak (p. 160)
  359 CALORIES
- 1/2 cup cooked egg noodles
  111 CALORIES
- Steamed broccoli with 1 teaspoon reduced-fat margarine spread
  FREE FOOD
- 2 crisp ladyfinger cookies
  60 CALORIES
- Coffee (with sugar substitute and liquid nondairy creamer if desired)
  FREE FOOD

DINNER TOTAL: 530 CALORIES

SNACKS:

- 1/2 cup strawberry-flavored 1% milk
  75 CALORIES
- 2 tablespoons tuna with 3 wheat crackers
  50 CALORIES

WEEK 6, DAY 6, TOTAL: 1,387 CALORIES

day 7

BREAKFAST:

- 1/2 cup Apple-Cinnamon Oatmeal Mix (p. 94)
  176 CALORIES
- 1 medium banana
  100 CALORIES
- 1 cup fat-free milk
  86 CALORIES

BREAKFAST TOTAL: 362 CALORIES

LUNCH:

- 1 Breaded Eggplant Sandwich (p. 111)
  288 CALORIES
- 10 baked potato chips
  100 CALORIES
- 1/2 cup sliced fresh strawberries
  27 CALORIES
- Ice water
  FREE FOOD

LUNCH TOTAL: 415 CALORIES

DINNER & DESSERT:

- 1 Black Bean Chicken Taco (p. 141)
  267 CALORIES
- 1/2 cup canned fat-free refried beans
  90 CALORIES
- 1 big green salad (see Free Foods Chart on p. 53) with 1 tablespoon reduced-fat salad dressing
  FREE FOOD
- Iced tea (with sugar substitute if desired)
  FREE FOOD
- 2/3 cup Rich Peach Ice Cream (p. 213)
  140 CALORIES

DINNER TOTAL: 497 CALORIES

SNACKS:

- 1/2 small apple with 2 tablespoons fat-free caramel ice cream topping
  93 CALORIES
- 1 medium plum
  40 CALORIES

WEEK 6, DAY 7, TOTAL: 1,407 CALORIES

When making a salad, skip the croutons and bacon bits. Try to use romaine lettuce or spinach instead of iceberg.

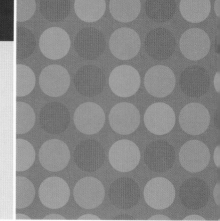

snacks

It's easy to avoid cravings when you indulge in a snack between meals. If you're a woman, enjoy 100 calories worth of snacks per day. Men should eat snacks totaling no more than 200 calories.

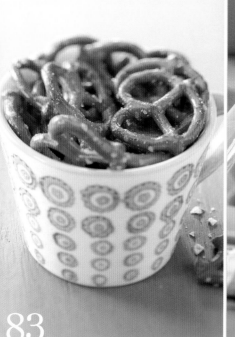

83

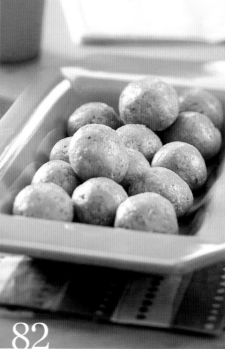

82

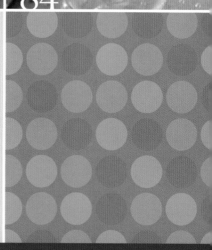

84

See the list at right and on page 78 for effortless snack ideas that are low-calorie yet deliciously satisfying. You'll also find great recipes for snacks and easy appetizers that come in at 100 calories or less on pages 79 through 85. And turn to page 85 for a list of readers' favorite post-workout snacks.

When hunger comes calling, TREAT YOURSELF to a simple bite that's FAST AND EASY but won't pack on the pounds. Each item is an ideal way to satisfy a serious SNACK ATTACK!

50 CALORIES OR LESS

- **3/4 cup tomato juice,** 31 calories

- **1/2 cup blackberries,** 31 calories

- **1 cup air-popped popcorn sprinkled with Italian seasoning,** 31 calories

- **2 apricots,** 34 calories

- **1 clementine,** 35 calories

- **1/2 cinnamon graham cracker,** 35 calories

- **1/3 cup unsweetened applesauce sprinkled with cinnamon,** 35 calories

- **1/2 cup cubed pineapple,** 37 calories

- **1 medium peach,** 40 calories

- **1 medium plum,** 40 calories

- **1 cup cubed watermelon,** 40 calories

- **1/2 cup cheese popcorn,** 40 calories

- **8 sweet cherries,** 41 calories

- **2 pineapple rings,** 41 calories

- **1/2 miniature bagel with 2 teaspoons fat-free cream cheese,** 42 calories

- **1 mini box (.5 ounces) raisins,** 42 calories

- **1/3 cup grapes with 1 tablespoon fat-free whipped topping,** 45 calories

- **1 cup whole strawberries,** 45 calories

- **1 medium kiwifruit,** 46 calories

- **1/2 cup baby carrots with 1 tablespoon hummus,** 48 calories

- **Mixed salad greens with 1 tablespoon crumbled feta cheese and 1 tablespoon fat-free creamy Caesar salad dressing,** 49 calories

- **1 small cucumber, sliced, with 2 tablespoons reduced-fat French onion dip,** 49 calories

- **2 chocolate kisses,** 49 calories

- **2 tablespoons tuna with 3 wheat crackers,** 50 calories

- **1/2 medium banana,** 50 calories

- **1 cup reduced-sodium V8 juice,** 50 calories

- **10 large olives,** 50 calories

51-100 CALORIES

- **1/4 cup dried apples,** 52 calories

- **1/2 cup broccoli florets with 2 tablespoons fat-free ranch salad dressing,** 58 calories

- **1/2 frozen waffle with 1 tablespoon sugar-free syrup,** 58 calories

- **1/2 cup canned peaches (drained),** 58 calories

- **2 crisp lady finger cookies,** 60 calories

- **7 miniature caramel-flavored rice cakes,** 60 calories

- **3/4 cup skinny latte (made with fat-free milk),** 60 calories

- **1 cup raspberries,** 60 calories

- **1 medium orange,** 62 calories

- **1/2 cup red or green grapes,** 65 calories

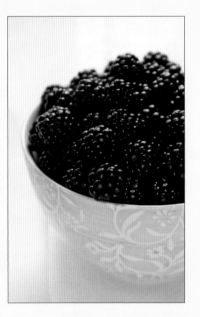

51-100 CALORIES
(CONTINUED)

- **1 fun-size Snickers candy bar,** 71 calories

- **1 medium apple,** 72 calories

- **1/2 cup Honey Nut Cheerios,** 74 calories

- **1/2 cup strawberry-flavored 1% milk,** 75 calories

- **1/2 cup fruit cocktail (drained),** 75 calories

- **2 California roll slices,** 75 calories

- **30 whole grain cheddar Goldfish Crackers,** 76 calories

- **5 medium cooked shrimp with 2 tablespoons cocktail sauce,** 77 calories

- **1/4 cup pretzel sticks with 1 tablespoon honey mustard,** 77 calories

- **10 medium cashews,** 78 calories

- **1 piece of string cheese,** 80 calories

- **1 Hunt's Fat-Free Snack Pack tapioca pudding,** 80 calories

- **4 ounces diced peaches in 100% fruit juice,** 80 calories

- **1/2 cup raspberries with 1 tablespoon chocolate syrup,** 80 calories

- **1 ice cream cake cone filled with 1/3 cup fat-free strawberry yogurt and 1/4 cup blueberries,** 81 calories

- **1/2 cup 1% cottage cheese sprinkled with chives or dill weed,** 81 calories

- **1 ounce deli turkey breast with 3 slices snack rye bread,** 84 calories

- **24 pistachios,** 85 calories

- **1/2 cup 1% chocolate milk,** 85 calories

- **1/2 ounce Swiss cheese and 2 Ritz crackers,** 87 calories

- **8 animal crackers,** 88 calories

- **3 pieces snack rye bread topped with 1 tablespoon reduced-fat garden vegetable cream cheese and 6 cucumber slices,** 89 calories

- **1/3 cup baked beans,** 89 calories

- **1/4 cup miniature marshmallows with 1 tablespoon semisweet chocolate chips,** 90 calories

- **1 crisp rice cereal bar (22 g package),** 90 calories

- **1/2 small pear with 1 tablespoon caramel ice cream topping,** 92 calories

- **3/4 cup sugar-free hot cocoa prepared with fat-free milk,** 92 calories

- **1 cup mandarin orange segments,** 92 calories

- **7 walnut halves,** 93 calories

- **2 tablespoons chocolate-covered raisins,** 93 calories

- **1/2 medium apple with 1/2 ounce sharp cheddar cheese,** 93 calories

- **1/2 small apple with 2 tablespoons caramel ice cream topping,** 93 calories

- **3 cups air-popped popcorn,** 94 calories

- **4 dates,** 94 calories

- **13 almonds,** 95 calories

- **1/2 cup fat-free vanilla frozen yogurt,** 95 calories

- **1 tablespoon peanut butter,** 96 calories

- **6 Ritz Crackers,** 97 calories

- **1/2 cup plain fat-free yogurt with 1/4 cup blueberries,** 98 calories

- **1/2 small banana with 2 teaspoons reduced-fat creamy peanut butter,** 99 calories

- **1/2 cup sugar-free chocolate pudding (prepared with fat-free milk) topped with 1 crushed chocolate wafer,** 99 calories

- **1 container Weight Watchers Berries 'n Cream Yogurt (6 ounces),** 100 calories

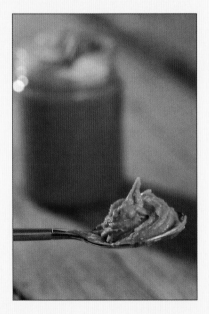

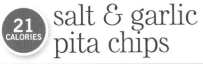

salt & garlic pita chips

21 CALORIES

PREP/TOTAL TIME: 25 minutes

Taste of Home Test Kitchen
With just four ingredients, this recipe is easy to make! The sturdy chips have a satisfying flavor and crunch.

- 1/4 cup olive oil
- 2 garlic cloves, minced
- 6 pita breads (6 inches), split in half
- 3/4 teaspoon kosher salt

- In a bowl, whisk oil and garlic. Brush over rough side of pita halves; sprinkle with salt. Cut each pita half into six wedges. Place rough side up on ungreased baking sheets.

- Bake at 350° for 12-15 minutes or until crisp and golden brown. Cool on wire racks. Store in an airtight container.

YIELD: 6 dozen.

NUTRITION FACTS: 1 chip equals 21 calories, 1 g fat (trace saturated fat), 0 cholesterol, 46 mg sodium, 3 g carbohydrate, trace fiber, trace protein.

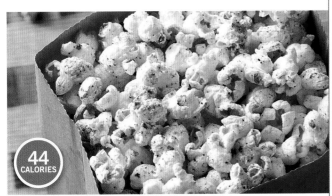

TEX-MEX POPCORN

44 CALORIES

tex-mex popcorn

PREP/TOTAL TIME: 15 minutes

Katie Rose | PEWAUKEE, WISCONSIN
Spicy Southwest seasoning makes this popcorn ideal for any fiesta.

- 1/2 cup popcorn kernels
- 3 tablespoons canola oil
- 1/2 teaspoon cumin seeds
- Refrigerated butter-flavored spray

- 1/4 cup minced fresh cilantro
- 1 teaspoon *each* salt and chili powder
- 1/2 teaspoon garlic powder
- 1/8 teaspoon smoked paprika

- In a Dutch oven over medium heat, heat the popcorn kernels, oil and cumin seeds until oil begins to sizzle. Cover and shake for 2-3 minutes or until popcorn stops popping.

- Transfer to a large bowl; spritz with butter-flavored spray. Add remaining ingredients and toss to coat. Continue spritzing and tossing until popcorn is coated.

YIELD: 4 quarts.

NUTRITION FACTS: 1 cup equals 44 calories, 3 g fat (trace saturated fat), 0 cholesterol, 150 mg sodium, 5 g carbohydrate, 1 g fiber, 1 g protein.

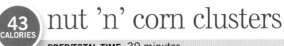

nut 'n' corn clusters

43 CALORIES

PREP/TOTAL TIME: 30 minutes

Maryeileen Jahnke | SOUTH MILWAUKEE, WISCONSIN
My family enjoys munching on these crisp caramel corn clusters.

- 5 quarts popped popcorn
- 2 cups mixed nuts
- 1-1/2 teaspoons butter
- 1 cup sugar
- 1/2 cup *each* honey and corn syrup
- 1 cup peanut butter
- 1 teaspoon *each* vanilla extract and molasses

- Line baking sheets with waxed paper; set aside. Combine popcorn and nuts in a large roasting pan. Bake at 250° for 10-15 minutes or until warm. Meanwhile, grease the sides of a heavy saucepan with 1-1/2 teaspoons butter. Combine sugar, honey and corn syrup in saucepan. Bring to a boil over medium heat, stirring constantly. Boil for 2 minutes without stirring.

- Remove from the heat; stir in peanut butter, vanilla and molasses. Pour over warm popcorn mixture and stir to coat. Working quickly, use buttered hands to form mixture into 1-1/2-in. clusters. Place on prepared baking sheets to dry. Store in an airtight container.

Yield: about 12 dozen.

Editor's Note: If mixture becomes too firm to form into clusters, rewarm in a 250° oven for a few minutes.

NUTRITION FACTS: 1 cluster equals 43 calories, 3 g fat (trace saturated fat), trace cholesterol, 38 mg sodium, 5 g carbohydrate, trace fiber, 1 g protein.

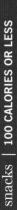
46 CALORIES

CHEESECAKE PHYLLO CUPS

cheesecake phyllo cups

PREP/TOTAL TIME: 25 minutes

Lorraine Chevalier | MERRIMAC, MASSACHUSETTS

I've been making these colorful cheesecake bites for years. Topped with kiwifruit and mandarin oranges, they are just delicious.

> 4 ounces reduced-fat cream cheese
> 1/2 cup reduced-fat sour cream
> Sugar substitute equivalent to 2 tablespoons sugar
> 1 teaspoon vanilla extract
> 2 packages (2.1 ounces *each*) frozen miniature phyllo tart shells, thawed
> 1 can (11 ounces) mandarin orange slices, drained
> 1 kiwifruit, peeled, sliced and cut into quarters

- In a large bowl, beat the cream cheese, sour cream, sugar substitute and vanilla until smooth.

- Pipe or spoon into phyllo shells. Top each with an orange segment and kiwi piece. Refrigerate until serving.

YIELD: 2-1/2 dozen.

EDITOR'S NOTE: This recipe was tested with Splenda sugar blend.

NUTRITION FACTS: 1 cup equals 46 calories, 2 g fat (1 g saturated fat), 4 mg cholesterol, 29 mg sodium, 5 g carbohydrate, trace fiber, 1 g protein.

ham asparagus spirals

PREP: 20 minutes | **BAKE:** 15 minutes

Rosie Huffer | WESTMINSTER, CALIFORNIA

These impressive-looking hors d'ouevres are easy to assemble with only three ingredients. People are always drawn to them because they look so interesting.

> 20 fresh asparagus spears, trimmed
> 20 thin slices deli ham
> 1 package (10.6 ounces) refrigerated Italian breadsticks and garlic spread

- In a large skillet, bring 1/2 in. of water to a boil; add asparagus. Reduce heat; cover and simmer for 2 minutes. Drain and immediately place asparagus in ice water; drain and pat dry.

- Wrap a slice of ham around each asparagus spear. Unroll breadstick dough; spread with garlic spread. Cut each breadstick in half lengthwise. Wrap one piece of dough, garlic spread side out, around each ham-wrapped asparagus spear.

- Place on an ungreased baking sheet. Bake at 375° for 13-15 minutes or until golden brown. Serve immediately.

YIELD: 20 appetizers.

NUTRITION FACTS: 1 spiral equals 49 calories, 2 g fat (trace saturated fat), trace cholesterol, 154 mg sodium, 7 g carbohydrate, trace fiber, 2 g protein.

HAM ASPARAGUS SPIRALS

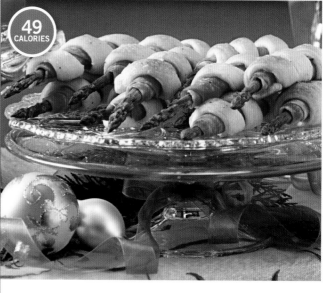

49 CALORIES

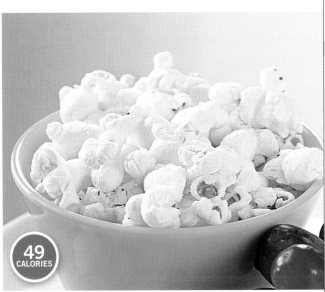

PARMESAN POPCORN

parmesan popcorn

PREP/TOTAL TIME: 10 minutes

Elizabeth King | DULUTH, MINNESOTA

Give popcorn a new twist with this fun and tasty recipe. Kids and adults alike will gobble it up! We enjoy it while watching movies or as an on-the-go snack.

    8 cups air-popped popcorn
    2 tablespoons reduced-fat butter, melted
    2 tablespoons grated Parmesan cheese
  1/4 teaspoon salt
  1/4 teaspoon dried oregano
  1/8 teaspoon garlic salt

- Place popcorn in a large bowl. Drizzle with butter. Combine the remaining ingredients; sprinkle over popcorn and toss to coat.

YIELD: 2 quarts.

NUTRITION FACTS: 1 cup equals 49 calories, 2 g fat (1 g saturated fat), 5 mg cholesterol, 146 mg sodium, 7 g carbohydrate, 1 g fiber, 2 g protein. **DIABETIC EXCHANGE:** 1/2 starch.

mini polenta pizzas

PREP/TOTAL TIME: 30 minutes

Lily Julow | GAINESVILLE, FLORIDA

You can be the talk of the party when you make these delightful appetizers! They're special enough for a fancy gathering, and no one will know they're lighter.

    2 tubes (1 pound *each*) polenta
  1/2 cup grated Parmesan cheese
   12 oil-packed sun-dried tomatoes, halved
  1/4 cup prepared pesto

- Cut polenta into 24 slices; place on ungreased baking sheets. Sprinkle with half of the cheese. Top each with a tomato half and 1/2 teaspoon pesto; sprinkle with remaining cheese.

- Bake at 450° for 7-10 minutes or until the cheese is melted.

YIELD: 2 dozen.

NUTRITION FACTS: 1 mini pizza equals 57 calories, 2 g fat (1 g saturated fat), 2 mg cholesterol, 182 mg sodium, 8 g carbohydrate, 1 g fiber, 2 g protein. **DIABETIC EXCHANGES:** 1/2 starch, 1/2 fat.

MINI POLENTA PIZZAS

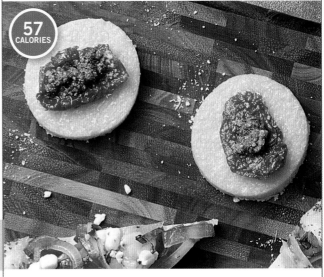

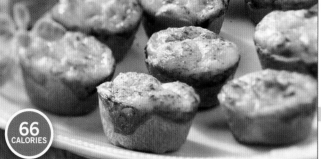

66 CALORIES

MINI SAUSAGE QUICHES

mini sausage quiches

PREP: 25 minutes | **BAKE:** 20 minutes

Jan Mead | MILFORD, CONNECTICUT

These bite-size quiches are loaded with sausage and cheese, and the crescent roll base makes preparation a snap. Serve them for brunch, or keep them on hand for snacking.

- 1/2 **pound bulk hot Italian sausage**
-   2 **tablespoons dried minced onion**
-   2 **tablespoons minced chives**
-   1 **tube (8 ounces) refrigerated crescent rolls**
-   4 **eggs, lightly beaten**
-   2 **cups (8 ounces) shredded Swiss cheese**
-   1 **cup (8 ounces) 4% cottage cheese**
- 1/3 **cup grated Parmesan cheese**

Paprika

- In a large skillet, brown sausage and onion over medium heat for 4-5 minutes or until meat is no longer pink; drain. Stir in chives.

- On a lightly floured surface, unroll crescent dough into one long rectangle; seal seams and perforations. Cut into 48 pieces. Press onto the bottom and up the sides of greased miniature muffin cups.

- Fill each with about 2 teaspoons of sausage mixture. In a large bowl, combine the eggs and cheeses. Spoon 2 teaspoonfuls over sausage mixture. Sprinkle with the paprika.

- Bake at 375° for 20-25 minutes or until a knife inserted in the center comes out clean. Cool for 5 minutes before removing from pans to wire racks. Serve warm. Refrigerate leftovers.

YIELD: 4 dozen.

NUTRITION FACTS: 1 mini quiche equals 66 calories, 5 g fat (2 g saturated fat), 27 mg cholesterol, 116 mg sodium, 2 g carbohydrate, trace fiber, 4 g protein.

no-bake peanut butter treats

PREP/TOTAL TIME: 10 minutes

Sonia Rohda | WAVERLY, NEBRASKA

This quick and tasty dessert is perfect for a road trip or when you're craving something sweet. The treats won't stick to your hands. Keep them in the refrigerator for a guilt-free splurge.

- 1/3 **cup chunky peanut butter**
- 1/4 **cup honey**
- 1/2 **teaspoon vanilla extract**
- 1/3 **cup nonfat dry milk powder**
- 1/3 **cup quick-cooking oats**
-   2 **tablespoons graham cracker crumbs**

- In a small bowl, combine the peanut butter, honey and vanilla. Stir in the milk powder, oats and graham cracker crumbs. Shape into 1-in. balls. Cover and refrigerate until serving.

YIELD: 15 treats.

NUTRITION FACTS: 1 treat equals 70 calories, 3 g fat (1 g saturated fat), 1 mg cholesterol, 46 mg sodium, 9 g carbohydrate, 1 g fiber, 3 g protein. **DIABETIC EXCHANGES:** 1/2 starch, 1/2 fat.

NO-BAKE PEANUT BUTTER TREATS

70 CALORIES

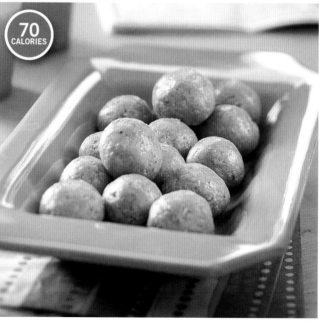

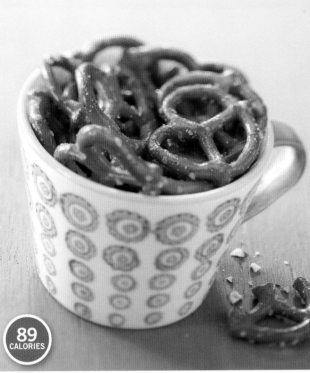

89 CALORIES

PARTY PRETZELS

party pretzels

PREP/TOTAL TIME: 25 minutes

Carrie Shaub I MOUNT JOY, PENNSYLVANIA

Not only are these a perfect midmorning or afternoon snack at work, they're perfect for hungry kids just home from school. Plus, they make for fantastic party food!

- 1 package (16 ounces) fat-free miniature pretzels
- 1/4 cup canola oil
- 3 teaspoons garlic powder
- 1 teaspoon dill weed
- 1/2 teaspoon lemon-pepper seasoning

- Place pretzels in an ungreased 15-in. x 10-in. x 1-in. baking pan. Combine the oil, garlic powder, dill and lemon-pepper; drizzle over pretzels and toss to coat.

- Bake at 350° for 12 minutes, stirring twice. Cool on a wire rack. Store in an airtight container.

YIELD: 12 cups.

NUTRITION FACTS: 1/2 cup equals 89 calories, 2 g fat (trace saturated fat), 0 cholesterol, 290 mg sodium, 16 g carbohydrate, 1 g fiber, 2 g protein. **DIABETIC EXCHANGES:** 1 starch, 1/2 fat.

cheesy pita crisps

PREP/TOTAL TIME: 25 minutes

Christine Mattiko I DALLASTOWN, PENNSYLVANIA

I first made these golden wedges when my college roommates and I wanted garlic bread but only had pitas on hand. My husband likes this "skinny" version even better than the original!

- 4 whole wheat pita pocket halves
- 1/4 cup reduced-fat margarine, melted
- 1/2 teaspoon garlic powder
- 1/2 teaspoon onion powder
- 1/4 teaspoon salt
- 1/4 teaspoon pepper
- 3 tablespoons grated Parmesan cheese
- 1/2 cup shredded part-skim mozzarella cheese

- Split each pita pocket in half. Cut each into two triangles; place rough side up on a baking sheet coated with cooking spray.

- In a bowl, combine the margarine, garlic powder, onion powder, salt and pepper; stir in the Parmesan cheese. Spread over triangles. Sprinkle with mozzarella cheese.

- Bake at 400° for 12-15 minutes or until golden brown.

YIELD: 8 servings.

NUTRITION FACTS: 2 triangles equals 95 calories, 5 g fat (2 g saturated fat), 6 mg cholesterol, 264 mg sodium, 9 g carbohydrate, 1 g fiber, 4 g protein. **DIABETIC EXCHANGES:** 1 fat, 1/2 starch.

CHEESY PITA CRISPS

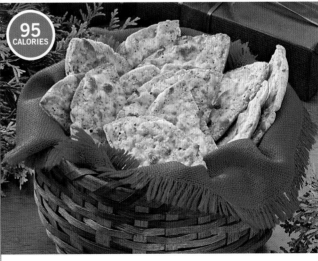

95 CALORIES

> **For a great snack,** I add mild fresh salsa with plenty of cilantro to fat-free cottage cheese. It's perfect when I want something filling and tasty. —**Cathy Hodge Smith**

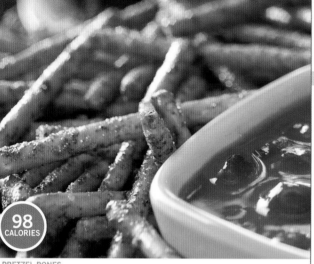

98 CALORIES

PRETZEL BONES

pretzel bones

PREP/TOTAL TIME: 15 minutes

Taste of Home Test Kitchen
Just grab a bag of pretzel sticks, season them and you'll have tasty snack in no time at all! These sweet and savory treats are ideal for munching anytime.

- 1/4 cup honey
- 2-1/2 tablespoons butter
- 2 tablespoons chili powder
- 1 tablespoon onion powder
- 1 package (15 ounces) pretzel sticks

- In a Dutch oven, melt honey and butter; stir in chili powder and onion powder. Add pretzels; toss to coat. Spread in a single layer in 15-in. x 10-in. x 1-in. baking pans coated with cooking spray.

- Bake at 300° for 5 minutes, stirring once. Cool in pans on wire racks. Store in an airtight container.

YIELD: 12 cups.

NUTRITION FACTS: 1/2 cup equals 98 calories, 2 g fat (1 g saturated fat), 3 mg cholesterol, 305 mg sodium, 19 g carbohydrate, 1 g fiber, 2 g protein. **DIABETIC EXCHANGES:** 1 starch.

strawberry mango smoothies for 2

PREP/TOTAL TIME: 10 minutes

Taste of Home Test Kitchen
Have one of these for breakfast, dessert or just as an afternoon snack. They're delicious and creamy, with lots of strawberry and mango flavor.

- 1/2 cup fat-free milk
- 1/4 cup vanilla yogurt
- 3/4 cup halved fresh strawberries
- 1/2 medium mango, peeled and chopped
- 2 to 3 ice cubes

Sugar substitute equivalent to 1-1/2 teaspoons sugar

- In a blender, combine all ingredients; cover and process for 20-30 seconds or until smooth. Stir if necessary. Pour into chilled glasses; serve immediately.

YIELD: 2 servings.

EDITOR'S NOTE: This recipe was tested with Splenda no-calorie sweetener.

NUTRITION FACTS: 1 cup equals 100 calories, 1 g fat (trace saturated fat), 3 mg cholesterol, 47 mg sodium, 21 g carbohydrate, 2 g fiber, 4 g protein. **DIABETIC EXCHANGES:** 1 fruit, 1/2 fat-free milk.

STRAWBERRY MANGO SMOOTHIES FOR 2

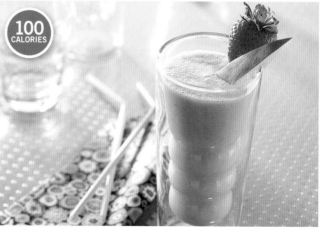

100 CALORIES

SUN-KISSED SMOOTHIES

sun-kissed smoothies

PREP/TOTAL TIME: 10 minutes

Taste of Home Test Kitchen
Grapefruit, banana, pineapple and peaches are a tempting combination in this refreshing sipper. It makes a healthy treat any time of day.

- 3/4 cup ruby red grapefruit juice
- 1 medium ripe banana, cut into chunks and frozen
- 1/2 cup cubed fresh pineapple
- 1/2 cup frozen unsweetened peach slices
- 4 ice cubes
- 1 tablespoon sugar

- In a blender, combine all ingredients; cover and process for 30-45 seconds or until smooth. Pour into chilled glasses; serve immediately.

YIELD: 3 servings.

NUTRITION FACTS: 3/4 cup equals 100 calories, trace fat (trace saturated fat), 0 cholesterol, 2 mg sodium, 25 g carbohydrate, 2 g fiber, 1 g protein. **DIABETIC EXCHANGES:** 1 fruit, 1/2 starch.

Looking for a post-workout snack? Check out these favorites from our readers! For other satisfying ideas, see our list of low-calorie snacks—all have 100 calories or less—on pages 77 and 78, and the Free Foods chart on page 53.

- **100-calorie microwave popcorn. The whole bag is only 100 calories!** Melissa Driver-Algren
- **An apple or a banana...usually an apple, because it takes longer to eat!** Kathy Schaefer
- **Half of a serving of zero-fat Greek yogurt on fresh or frozen fruit.** Mary Oberg Arneson
- **Tomato with fresh mozzarella, basil, olive oil, a little garlic and a sprinkle of balsamic vinegar.** Linda Bolger
- **About 23 M&Ms.** Shannon Davidson
- **Celery with low-fat peanut butter.** John Celestre
- **Fresh cucumbers and tomatoes from the garden.** Barbara Bush
- **Two light string cheese sticks.** Amy Lefavour
- **Cottage cheese with pineapple.** Cindy Johosky
- **A chewy granola bar. It tastes good and takes the edge off my hunger.** Cindy Dupin
- **A package of sweet and salty 100-calorie snack mix.** Brittany Nikolas
- **Sour cream and onion cracker chips.** SuzAnne Holifield
- **Orange creme yogurt.** Michele Lenz
- **Roasted red pepper hummus with veggies.** Cecilia Denny
- **A 100-calorie ice cream sandwich.** Delane Hansen Kempf
- **Four chocolate kisses.** Michele Lenz

breakfasts

Mom told us all along—and she was right. Breakfast is the most important meal of the day. It gets your body going. Try to consume roughly 350 calories in the morning, and you'll have fewer cravings the rest of the day.

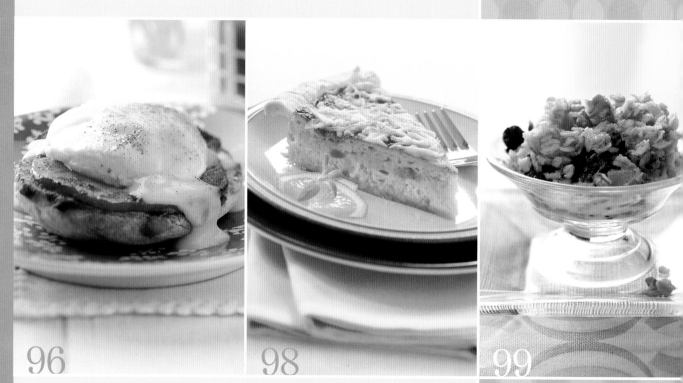

96   98   99

The first section in this chapter has lower-calorie breakfast items. Enjoy them on their own, or pair them with something a bit more substantial. The other two sections are higher-calorie recipes that will surely fill you up as you start your day. See the chart on page 93 for the calorie counts of some typical breakfast foods.

100 Calories or Less 87

101-200 Calories 89

201-300 Calories 95

100 calories or less

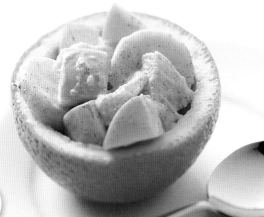

80 CALORIES

ORANGE FRUIT CUPS

orange fruit cups

PREP/TOTAL TIME: 20 minutes

Susan Wiener | **SPRING HILL, FLORIDA**

This is always a favorite with children who come to visit. It's a wonderful treat that's healthy, fast and easy to make.

    2 medium navel oranges, halved
    1 small apple, chopped
    1 small banana, sliced
  1/4 cup plain yogurt
  1/4 teaspoon ground cinnamon
Additional ground cinnamon, optional

- Using a paring or grapefruit knife and spoon, scoop out pulp from oranges, leaving a shell. Separate orange sections and chop; transfer to a small bowl.

- Add the apple, banana, yogurt and cinnamon. Fill orange shells with fruit mixture. Sprinkle with additional cinnamon if desired. Serve immediately.

YIELD: 4 servings.

NUTRITION FACTS: 1/2 cup fruit equals 80 calories, 1 g fat (trace saturated fat), 2 mg cholesterol, 8 mg sodium, 19 g carbohydrate, 3 g fiber, 2 g protein. **DIABETIC EXCHANGE:** 1 fruit.

tropical fruit smoothies

PREP/TOTAL TIME: 10 minutes

Susan Voigt | **PLYMOUTH, MINNESOTA**

Four refreshing fruits go into this frosty smoothie. A bit of honey adds a hint of sweetness.

1-1/2 cups orange juice
    1 can (8 ounces) crushed pineapple, undrained
    1 medium mango, peeled and cut into chunks
    1 cup halved fresh strawberries
    2 medium kiwifruit, peeled and quartered
    1 tablespoon honey
   14 ice cubes
  1/2 cup club soda, chilled

- Place half of the orange juice, pineapple, mango, strawberries, kiwi, honey and ice cubes in a blender; cover and process until blended. Stir in 1/4 cup soda. Pour into chilled glasses; serve immediately. Repeat with remaining ingredients.

YIELD: 7 servings.

NUTRITION FACTS: 1 cup equals 97 calories, trace fat (trace saturated fat), 0 cholesterol, 6 mg sodium, 25 g carbohydrate, 2 g fiber, 1 g protein. **DIABETIC EXCHANGES:** 1 fruit, 1/2 starch

TROPICAL FRUIT SMOOTHIES

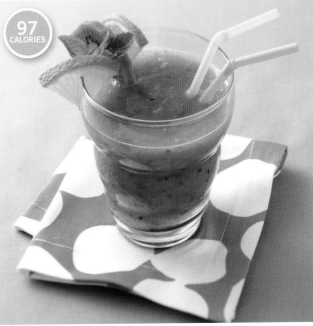

97 CALORIES

I eat egg whites with veggies or oatmeal with fruit and nuts for breakfast. I also have a cup of coffee or green tea every day, since it seems to help increase my metabolism.
—Mary LaJoie, Washington

88 CALORIES

ZUCCHINI PANCAKES

zucchini pancakes

PREP/TOTAL TIME: 20 minutes

Charlotte Goldberg | HONEY GROVE, PENNSYLVANIA
These are a hearty change of pace from ordinary pancakes. Paired with an entree, they're a budget-conscious way to round out a brunch.

- 1-1/2 cups shredded zucchini
- 2 tablespoons biscuit/baking mix
- 3 tablespoons grated Parmesan cheese
Dash pepper
- 1 egg, lightly beaten
- 1 tablespoon canola oil

- In a sieve or colander, drain the zucchini, squeezing to remove excess liquid. Pat dry; set aside. In a small bowl, combine the baking mix, cheese and pepper. Stir in egg until blended. Add the zucchini; toss to coat.

- In a large skillet, heat oil over medium heat; drop 1/4 cupfuls of batter into skillet; press lightly to flatten. Fry for 2 minutes on each side or until golden brown. Drain on paper towels.

YIELD: 4 servings.

NUTRITION FACTS: 1 pancake equals 88 calories, 6 g fat (2 g saturated fat), 56 mg cholesterol, 134 mg sodium, 4 g carbohydrate, 1 g fiber, 4 g protein.

99 CALORIES

banana blueberry smoothies

PREP/TOTAL TIME: 10 minutes

Krista Frank | RHODODENDRON, OREGON
My sons love this smoothie, whether it's served frozen or with a straw. Either way, I feel good serving them this healthy combination of ingredients.

- 1 cup fat-free milk
- 1 cup orange juice
- 1/2 teaspoon vanilla extract
- 2 medium bananas, halved
- 1 cup unsweetened applesauce
- 1 cup frozen unsweetened blueberries

- In a blender, combine all ingredients; cover and process for 30 seconds or until blended. Pour into chilled glasses; serve immediately.

YIELD: 6 servings.

NUTRITION FACTS: 3/4 cup equals 99 calories, trace fat (trace saturated fat), 1 mg cholesterol, 19 mg sodium, 23 g carbohydrate, 2 g fiber, 2 g protein. **DIABETIC EXCHANGE:** 1-1/2 fruit.

granola-to-go bars

PREP: 30 minutes | **BAKE:** 15 minutes + cooling

Sally Haen | MENOMONEE FALLS, WISCONSIN
This grab-and-go goodie makes a great portable breakfast or a hearty snack for a long day out. Chewy and sweet, these fruity oat bars really satisfy!

- 3-1/2 cups quick-cooking oats
- 1 cup chopped almonds
- 1 egg, lightly beaten
- 2/3 cup butter, melted
- 1/2 cup honey
- 1 teaspoon vanilla extract
- 1/2 cup sunflower kernels

101-200 calories

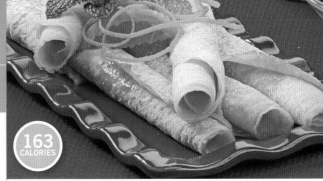

1/2 cup flaked coconut
1/2 cup chopped dried apples
1/2 cup dried cranberries
1/2 cup packed brown sugar
1/2 teaspoon ground cinnamon

- Combine oats and almonds in a 15-in. x 10-in. x 1-in. baking pan coated with cooking spray. Bake at 350° for 15 minutes or until toasted, stirring occasionally.

- In a large bowl, combine egg, butter, honey and vanilla. Stir in sunflower kernels, coconut, apples, cranberries, brown sugar and cinnamon. Stir in oat mixture.

- Press into a 15-in. x 10-in. x 1-in. baking pan coated with cooking spray. Bake at 350° for 13-18 minutes or until set and edges are lightly browned. Cool on a wire rack. Cut into bars. Store in an airtight container.

YIELD: 3 dozen.

NUTRITION FACTS: 1 bar equals 130 calories, 7 g fat (3 g saturated fat), 15 mg cholesterol, 40 mg sodium, 16 g carbohydrate, 2 g fiber, 2 g protein.

GRANOLA-TO-GO BARS

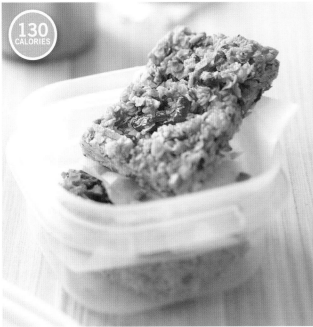

130 CALORIES

FESTIVE FRENCH PANCAKES

163 CALORIES

festive french pancakes

PREP/TOTAL TIME: 15 minutes

Diane Aune | NINE MILE FALLS, WASHINGTON
Not quite as thin as true crepes, these light-as-a-feather pancakes are delightful topped with preserves and a dusting of confectioners' sugar. They're elegant and so easy to make!

2/3 cup milk
  2 eggs
1/3 cup water
1/2 teaspoon vanilla extract
3/4 cup all-purpose flour
  2 tablespoons confectioners' sugar
  1 teaspoon baking powder
1/2 teaspoon salt
Preserves of your choice, optional
Additional confectioners' sugar, optional

- In a blender, combine the milk, eggs, water and vanilla; cover and process until well blended. Combine the flour, confectioners' sugar, baking powder and salt; add to egg mixture. Cover and process until smooth.

- Heat a lightly greased 8-in. nonstick skillet over medium heat; pour 2 tablespoons batter into the center of skillet. Lift and tilt pan to coat bottom evenly. Cook until top appears dry; turn and cook 15-20 seconds longer. Remove to a wire rack.

- Repeat with remaining batter, greasing skillet as needed. Spread preserves over pancakes if desired; roll up. Sprinkle with confectioners' sugar if desired.

YIELD: 8 pancakes.

NUTRITION FACTS: 2 pancakes (calculated without preserves and confectioners' sugar) equals 163 calories, 4 g fat (2 g saturated fat), 112 mg cholesterol, 447 mg sodium, 24 g carbohydrate, 1 g fiber, 7 g protein. **DIABETIC EXCHANGES:** 1-1/2 starch, 1/2 fat.

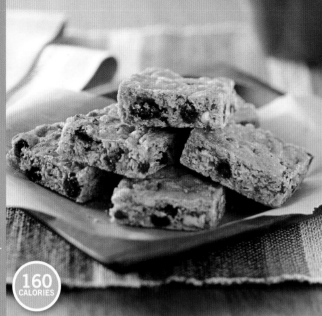

160 CALORIES

CHEWY GRANOLA BARS

chewy granola bars

PREP: 10 minutes | **BAKE:** 25 minutes

Virginia Krites | CRIDERSVILLE, OHIO

For a satisfying breakfast or snack that's both soft and crispy, try this recipe. These bars are a nutritious treat.

    1/2 cup butter, softened
      1 cup packed brown sugar
    1/4 cup sugar
      2 tablespoons honey
    1/2 teaspoon vanilla extract
      1 egg
      1 cup all-purpose flour
      1 teaspoon ground cinnamon
    1/2 teaspoon baking powder
    1/4 teaspoon salt
  1-1/2 cups quick-cooking oats
  1-1/4 cups crisp rice cereal
      1 cup chopped nuts
      1 cup raisins or semisweet chocolate chips,
         optional

- In a large bowl, cream butter and sugars until light and fluffy. Add the honey, vanilla and egg; mix well. Combine the flour, cinnamon, baking powder and salt; gradually add to creamed mixture. Stir in oats, cereal and nuts and raisins or chocolate chips if desired.

- Press into a greased 13-in. x 9-in. baking pan. Bake at 350° for 25-30 minutes or until the top is lightly browned. Cool on a wire rack. Cut into bars.

YIELD: 2 dozen.

NUTRITION FACTS: 1 bar equals 160 calories, 7 g fat (3 g saturated fat), 19 mg cholesterol, 91 mg sodium, 22 g carbohydrate, 1 g fiber, 3 g protein. **DIABETIC EXCHANGES:** 1-1/2 starch, 1-1/2 fat.

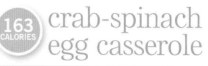

crab-spinach egg casserole

PREP: 10 minutes | **BAKE:** 30 minutes + standing

Steve Heaton | DELTONA, FLORIDA

I came up with this casserole as a special breakfast for our daughter when she was home for a visit. Yum!

      8 eggs
      2 cups half-and-half cream
      2 cans (6 ounces each) crabmeat, drained
      1 package (10 ounces) frozen chopped spinach,
         thawed and squeezed dry
      1 cup dry bread crumbs
      1 cup (4 ounces) shredded Swiss cheese
    1/2 teaspoon salt
    1/4 teaspoon pepper
    1/4 teaspoon ground nutmeg
      2 celery ribs, chopped
    1/2 cup chopped onion
    1/2 cup chopped sweet red pepper
      3 medium fresh mushrooms, chopped
      2 tablespoons butter

- In a large bowl, beat eggs and cream. Stir in the crab, spinach, bread crumbs, cheese, salt, pepper and nutmeg; set aside. In a skillet, saute the celery, onion, red pepper and mushrooms in butter until tender. Add to the spinach mixture.

- Transfer to a greased shallow 2-1/2-qt. baking dish. Bake, uncovered, at 375° for 30-35 minutes or until a thermometer reads 160°. Let stand for 10 minutes before serving.

YIELD: 16 servings.

NUTRITION FACTS: 1 serving equals 163 calories, 9 g fat (5 g saturated fat), 141 mg cholesterol, 265 mg sodium, 8 g carbohydrate, 1 g fiber, 10 g protein.

spring frittata

163 CALORIES

PREP: 35 minutes | **BAKE:** 30 minutes

Diane Higgins | TAMPA, FLORIDA

With roasted veggies, Asiago cheese and plenty of dill, this frittata is packed with great flavors. It looks impressive, but it's really a snap to make.

- 1/2 cup chopped leek (white portion only)
- 1/2 cup cut fresh asparagus (1-inch pieces)
- 2 teaspoons olive oil
- 1/4 teaspoon salt
- 1/4 teaspoon pepper
- 1 cup sliced fresh mushrooms
- 1 cup shredded Asiago cheese
- 4 eggs
- 1 cup egg substitute
- 1/4 cup fat-free milk
- 1 tablespoon snipped fresh dill *or* 1 teaspoon dill weed
- 1 tablespoon minced fresh parsley *or* 1 teaspoon dried parsley flakes

- In small bowl, combine leek and asparagus. Drizzle with oil and sprinkle with salt and pepper; toss to coat.

- Transfer to a baking sheet coated with cooking spray. Bake at 400° for 20-25 minutes or until tender, stirring occasionally. Reduce heat to 350°.

- Place mushrooms on the bottom of a 9-in. deep-dish pie plate coated with cooking spray. Top with roasted vegetables and cheese. In a large bowl, whisk the remaining ingredients; pour over cheese.

- Bake for 30-35 minutes or until a knife inserted near the center comes out clean. Let stand for 5 minutes. Cut into wedges.

YIELD: 6 servings.

NUTRITION FACTS: 1 wedge equals 163 calories, 10 g fat (4 g saturated fat), 158 mg cholesterol, 282 mg sodium, 4 g carbohydrate, 1 g fiber, 14 g protein.

colorful cheese omelet

PREP/TOTAL TIME: 20 minutes

Lynda O'Dell Lynch | PORT HURON, MICHIGAN

When I start my day with this omelet, I know I'm getting valuable nutrients and I'm able to go nonstop.

for 2

- 1 egg
- 2 egg whites
- 2 tablespoons chopped fresh baby spinach
- 1/8 teaspoon hot pepper sauce
- 2 tablespoons chopped sweet red pepper
- 1 green onion, chopped
- 2 tablespoons shredded cheddar cheese

- In a small bowl, whisk the egg, egg whites, spinach and pepper sauce; set aside. In a small nonstick skillet coated with cooking spray, saute red pepper and onion until tender. Reduce heat to medium.

- Add egg mixture to skillet (mixture should set immediately at edges). As eggs set, push cooked edges toward the center, letting uncooked portion flow underneath. When the eggs are set, sprinkle with cheese; fold other side over cheese. Slide omelet onto a plate.

YIELD: 1 serving.

NUTRITION FACTS: 1 omelet equals 167 calories, 9 g fat (5 g saturated fat), 227 mg cholesterol, 276 mg sodium, 4 g carbohydrate, 1 g fiber, 17 g protein. **DIABETIC EXCHANGE:** 2 medium-fat meat.

COLORFUL CHEESE OMELET

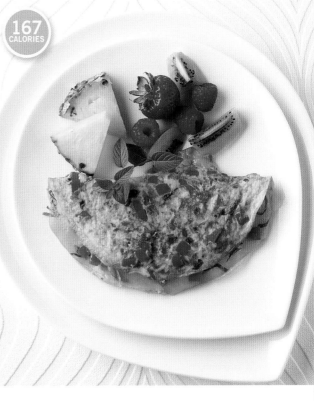

167 CALORIES

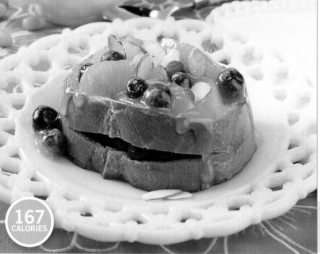

BLUEBERRY-STUFFED FRENCH TOAST

blueberry-stuffed french toast

PREP: 35 minutes | **BAKE:** 15 minutes

Myrna Koldenhoven | SANBORN, IOWA

I came across this recipe several years ago. The fruity French toast is truly company fare.

1-1/2 cups fresh *or* frozen blueberries
3 tablespoons sugar, *divided*
8 slices Italian bread (1-1/4 inches thick)
4 eggs, lightly beaten
1/2 cup orange juice
1 teaspoon grated orange peel
Dash salt

BLUEBERRY ORANGE SAUCE:
3 tablespoons sugar
1 tablespoon cornstarch
1/8 teaspoon salt
1/4 cup orange juice
1/4 cup water
1-1/2 cups orange segments
1 cup fresh *or* frozen blueberries
1/3 cup sliced almonds

- In a small bowl, combine blueberries and 2 tablespoons sugar. Cut a pocket in the side of each slice of bread. Fill each pocket with about 3 tablespoons berry mixture.

- In a shallow bowl, whisk the eggs, orange juice, orange peel, salt and remaining sugar. Carefully dip both sides of bread in egg mixture (do not squeeze out filling). Place in

a greased 15-in. x 10-in. x 1-in. baking pan. Bake at 400° for 7-1/2 minutes on each side, turning gently.

- Meanwhile, in a small saucepan, combine the sugar, cornstarch and salt. Gently whisk in orange juice and water until smooth. Bring to a boil; cook and stir for 1-2 minutes or until thickened. Reduce heat; stir in oranges and blueberries. Cook for 5 minutes or until heated through. Serve with the French toast; sprinkle with almonds.

YIELD: 8 servings.

NUTRITION FACTS: 1 piece with 1/4 cup sauce equals 167 calories, 5 g fat (1 g saturated fat), 106 mg cholesterol, 118 mg sodium, 27 g carbohydrate, 3 g fiber, 5 g protein. **DIABETIC EXCHANGES:** 1-1/2 starch, 1 fat, 1/2 fruit.

italian mini frittatas

PREP: 25 minutes | **BAKE:** 25 minutes

Michelle Anderson | EAGLE, IDAHO

While these individual frittatas contain prosciutto, cheese and butter, the amounts are small so each portion stays slim. They're easy to prepare, simple to serve and fantastic to the final bite.

2 tablespoons chopped sun-dried tomatoes (not packed in oil)
1/2 cup boiling water
2 thin slices prosciutto, finely chopped
1/4 cup chopped shallots
1 teaspoon butter
2 garlic cloves, minced
1/4 cup all-purpose flour
1-1/2 cups fat-free milk
4 egg whites
2 eggs
1 cup (4 ounces) shredded part-skim mozzarella cheese
1/4 cup shredded Asiago cheese
1/2 cup canned water-packed artichoke hearts, rinsed, drained and chopped
2 tablespoons minced fresh basil *or* 2 teaspoons dried basil
3/4 teaspoon salt
1/2 teaspoon white pepper

- Place tomatoes in a small bowl; add boiling water. Cover and let stand for 5 minutes. Drain and set aside.

My motto is 'Eat less and exercise more.' I don't starve. I just always ask myself 'Are you really hungry?' and 'Is this the best food choice you can make?' It completely changes how I look at food, and I learned that food is for when you are hungry. —**A. L. Leslie**

- In a small nonstick skillet, saute prosciutto and shallots in butter until shallots are tender. Add garlic; cook 1 minute longer. Remove from the heat; set aside.

- In a large bowl, whisk flour and milk until smooth; whisk in the egg whites and eggs until blended. Stir in the cheeses, artichokes, basil, salt, pepper, reserved tomatoes and prosciutto mixture.

- Coat 12 muffin cups with cooking spray; fill with egg mixture. Bake at 350° for 25-30 minutes or until a knife inserted near the center comes out clean. Carefully run a knife around edges to loosen; remove from pan. Serve warm.

YIELD: 1 dozen.

NUTRITION FACTS: 2 frittatas equals 172 calories, 7 g fat (4 g saturated fat), 93 mg cholesterol, 642 mg sodium, 11 g carbohydrate, trace fiber, 15 g protein. **DIABETIC EXCHANGES:** 2 lean meat, 1 starch.

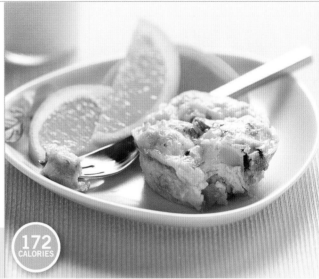

172 CALORIES

ITALIAN MINI FRITTATAS

Here are some typical breakfast foods and the numbers of calories they contain. Use this list as a reference when combining morning mainstays to keep within your goal of a 350-calorie breakfast.

- **1/2 cup fat-free vanilla yogurt topped with 2 tablespoons Wheaties,** 86 calories

- **1/2 cup fat-free plain yogurt topped with 1-1/2 teaspoons honey,** 109 calories

- **1/2 cup fat-free plain yogurt topped with 4 strawberries or 1/4 cup blueberries,** 109 calories

- **6 ounces fat-free fruit-flavored yogurt,** 160 calories

- **1 slice whole wheat toast,** 69 calories

- **1 scrambled egg,** 101 calories

- **1 plain mini bagel,** 72 calories

- **1 tablespoon whipped cream cheese,** 35 calories

- **1/2 toasted whole wheat English muffin with 1 tablespoon peanut butter,** 157 calories

- **1 frozen waffle,** 98 calories

- **1 pancake (6" diameter prepared from dry pancake mix),** 149 calories

- **1 cup Cheerios,** 111 calories

- **1 cup Wheaties,** 107 calories

- **3/4 cup plain oatmeal (made with water),** 109 calories

- **1/3 cup frosted bite-size Shredded Wheat with 1/3 cup fat-free milk,** 89 calories

- **1 cup orange juice,** 110 calories

- **1 cup fat-free milk,** 86 calories

- **1 cup skinny latte (made with fat-free milk),** 80 calories

- **1/2 small grapefruit with 1 teaspoon sugar,** 48 calories

- **1 medium banana,** 100 calories

- **1/2 cup cooked grits,** 76 calories

- **1 medium apple with 1 tablespoon peanut butter,** 161 calories

For additional calorie calculations, check the Nutrition Facts labels on food packages.

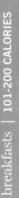

garlic cheese grits

186 CALORIES

PREP/TOTAL TIME: 20 minutes

Rose Tuttle | OVIEDO, FLORIDA

This recipe is the perfect side dish for brunch. The grits are so smooth and creamy and have so much flavor from the cheese and garlic.

for 2

- 1 cup water
- 1/4 cup quick-cooking grits
- 1/2 cup reduced-fat process cheese (Velveeta)
- 1/4 teaspoon garlic powder
- 1/4 cup cornflakes, coarsely crushed
- 1 teaspoon butter, melted

- In a saucepan, bring water to a boil. Slowly stir in grits. Reduce heat; cook and stir for 4-5 minutes or until thickened. Add cheese and garlic powder; stir until cheese is melted. Pour into greased 2-cup baking dish.

- In a small bowl, combine cornflakes and butter; sprinkle over grits. Bake, uncovered, at 350° for 10-15 minutes or until firm and top is lightly toasted.

YIELD: 2 servings.

NUTRITION FACTS: 3/4 cup equals 186 calories, 7 g fat (4 g saturated fat), 20 mg cholesterol, 662 mg sodium, 24 g carbohydrate, 1 g fiber, 9 g protein. **DIABETIC EXCHANGES:** 1-1/2 starch, 1 medium-fat meat, 1/2 fat.

caramel cream crepes

PREP: 20 minutes + chilling | **COOK:** 15 minutes

Taste of Home Test Kitchen

These lovely homemade crepes with a creamy caramel filling are a cinch to whip up. They taste wonderful, too.

- 6 tablespoons fat-free milk
- 6 tablespoons egg substitute
- 1-1/2 teaspoons butter, melted
- 1/2 teaspoon vanilla extract
- 6 tablespoons all-purpose flour
- 6 ounces fat-free cream cheese
- 3 tablespoons plus 6 teaspoons fat-free caramel ice cream topping, *divided*
- 2-1/4 cups reduced-fat whipped topping
- 1-1/2 cups fresh raspberries
- 1/3 cup white wine *or* unsweetened apple juice
- 3 tablespoons sliced almonds, toasted

APPLE-CINNAMON OATMEAL MIX

176 CALORIES

apple-cinnamon oatmeal mix

PREP/TOTAL TIME: 5 minutes

Lynne Van Wagenen | SALT LAKE CITY, UTAH

Oatmeal is a breakfast staple at our house. It's a warm, nutritious start to the day that keeps us going all morning. We used to buy the oatmeal mixes, but we think our homemade version is better! Feel free to substitute raisins or other dried fruit for the apples.

- 6 cups quick-cooking oats
- 1-1/3 cups nonfat dry milk powder
- 1 cup dried apples, diced
- 1/4 cup sugar
- 1/4 cup packed brown sugar
- 1 tablespoon ground cinnamon
- 1 teaspoon salt
- 1/4 teaspoon ground cloves

ADDITIONAL INGREDIENT (FOR EACH SERVING):
- 1/2 cup water

- In a large bowl, combine the first eight ingredients. Store in an airtight container in a cool dry place for up to 6 months. Yield: 8 cups total.

- To prepare oatmeal: Shake mix well. In a small saucepan, bring water to a boil; slowly stir in 1/2 cup mix. Cook and stir over medium heat for 1 minute. Remove from the heat. Cover and let stand for 1 minute or until oatmeal reaches desired consistency.

YIELD: 1 serving.

NUTRITION FACTS: 1/2 cup equals 176 calories, 2 g fat (trace saturated fat), 1 mg cholesterol, 185 mg sodium, 33 g carbohydrate, 4 g fiber, 7 g protein. **DIABETIC EXCHANGE:** 2 starch.

201-300 calories

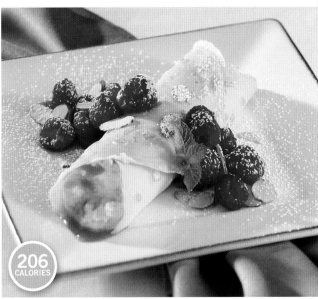

206 CALORIES

CARAMEL CREAM CREPES

- In a blender, combine milk, egg substitute, butter and vanilla; cover and process until blended. Add flour; cover and process until blended. Cover and refrigerate for 1 hour.

- Lightly coat a 6-in. nonstick skillet with cooking spray; heat over medium heat. Pour about 2 tablespoons of batter into center of skillet; lift and tilt pan to evenly coat bottom. Cook until top appears dry and bottom is golden; turn and cook 15-20 seconds longer. Remove to a wire rack. Repeat with remaining batter. Stack cooled crepes with waxed paper or paper towels in between.

- In a small bowl, beat cream cheese and 3 tablespoons caramel topping until smooth. Fold in whipped topping. Spoon down the center of each crepe. Drizzle with remaining caramel topping; roll up.

- In a small microwave-safe bowl, combine the raspberries and wine or juice. Microwave on high for 30-60 seconds or until warm. Using a slotted spoon, place berries over crepes. Sprinkle with almonds.

YIELD: 6 servings.

NUTRITION FACTS: 1 serving equals 206 calories, 6 g fat (4 g saturated fat), 5 mg cholesterol, 227 mg sodium, 25 g carbohydrate, 3 g fiber, 8 g protein. **DIABETIC EXCHANGES:** 1-1/2 starch, 1 lean meat, 1 fat.

apple walnut pancakes

PREP: 15 minutes | **COOK:** 5 minutes/batch

Kerry Blondheim | DENMARK, WISCONSIN

The hearty whole wheat flavor really comes through in these golden pancakes. They're great with a light touch of maple syrup.

- 1 cup all-purpose flour
- 1 cup whole wheat flour
- 1 tablespoon brown sugar
- 2 teaspoons baking powder
- 1 teaspoon salt
- 2 egg whites
- 1 egg, lightly beaten
- 2 cups fat-free milk
- 2 tablespoons canola oil
- 1 medium apple, peeled and chopped
- 1/2 cup chopped walnuts

Maple syrup

- In a large bowl, combine the flours, brown sugar, baking powder and salt. Combine the egg whites, egg, milk and oil; add to dry ingredients just until moistened. Fold in apple and walnuts.

- Pour batter by 1/4 cupfuls onto a hot griddle coated with cooking spray; turn when bubbles form on top. Cook until the second side is golden brown. Serve with syrup.

YIELD: 18 pancakes.

NUTRITION FACTS: 2 pancakes (calculated without syrup) equals 208 calories, 8 g fat (1 g saturated fat), 25 mg cholesterol, 396 mg sodium, 27 g carbohydrate, 3 g fiber, 8 g protein. **DIABETIC EXCHANGES:** 2 starch, 1 fat.

APPLE WALNUT PANCAKES

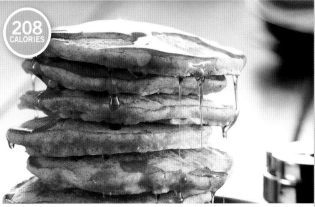

208 CALORIES

By keeping track of the calories I consumed and eating a balanced diet, I lost nearly 85 pounds and went from size 22/24 down to 10/12. I am almost 43 years old, I'm healthier than I was at 25 and I can now fit into my wedding dress from 22 years ago. It is a wonderful feeling! —**Kelly Killian, Wisconsin**

eggs benedict

216 CALORIES

(pictured on page 86)

PREP: 25 minutes | **COOK:** 15 minutes

Rebecca Baird | SALT LAKE CITY, UTAH

The updated hollandaise sauce in this recipe is smooth and creamy and healthier than the regular version.

- 8 slices Canadian bacon
- 8 eggs

HOLLANDAISE SAUCE:

- 2 tablespoons all-purpose flour
- 1/4 teaspoon *each* salt and ground mustard
- 1/8 teaspoon cayenne pepper
- 1/2 cup fat-free milk
- 1/2 cup fat-free evaporated milk
- 1 egg yolk, lightly beaten
- 1 tablespoon butter-flavored sprinkles
- 1 tablespoon lemon juice
- 4 whole wheat English muffins, split and toasted

- In a large nonstick skillet coated with cooking spray, brown bacon on both sides; remove and keep warm.

- Place 2-3 in. of water in a large skillet with high sides. Bring to a boil; reduce heat and simmer gently. Break cold eggs, one at a time, into a custard cup or saucer; holding the cup close to the surface of the water, slip each egg into water. Cook, uncovered, until whites are completely set and yolks begin to thicken but are not hard, about 4 minutes.

- Meanwhile, in a small saucepan, combine flour, salt, mustard and cayenne. Gradually stir in milk and evaporated milk until smooth. Bring to a boil; cook and stir for 1-2 minutes or until thickened. Remove from heat.

- Stir a small amount of sauce into egg yolk; return all to the pan, stirring constantly. Bring to a gentle boil; cook and stir for 2 minutes. Remove from the heat; stir in butter-flavored sprinkles and lemon juice.

- With a slotted spoon, lift each egg out of the water. Top each muffin half with a slice of bacon, an egg and 2 tablespoons sauce. Serve immediately.

YIELD: 8 servings.

EDITOR'S NOTE: This recipe was tested with Molly McButter. Look for it in the spice aisle.

NUTRITION FACTS: 1 serving equals 216 calories, 8 g fat (3 g saturated fat), 252 mg cholesterol, 752 mg sodium, 19 g carbohydrate, 2 g fiber, 17 g protein. **DIABETIC EXCHANGES:** 2 medium-fat meat, 1 starch.

french toast with apple topping

PREP/TOTAL TIME: 20 minutes

Janis Scharnott | FONTANA, WISCONSIN

For breakfast or brunch, you can't top this impressive dish. Warm, sweet apples and a hint of cinnamon make this French toast extra special.

- 1 medium apple, peeled and thinly sliced
- 1 tablespoon brown sugar
- 1/4 teaspoon ground cinnamon
- 2 tablespoons reduced-fat butter, *divided*
- 1 egg
- 1/4 cup 2% milk
- 1 teaspoon vanilla extract
- 4 slices French bread (1/2 inch thick)

Maple syrup, optional

for 2

FRENCH TOAST WITH APPLE TOPPING

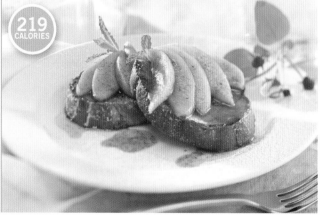

219 CALORIES

- In a large skillet, saute the apple, brown sugar and cinnamon in 1 tablespoon butter until apple is tender.

- In a shallow bowl, whisk the egg, milk and vanilla. Dip both sides of bread in egg mixture.

- In a large skillet, melt remaining butter over medium heat. Cook bread on both sides until golden brown. Serve with apple mixture and maple syrup if desired.

YIELD: 2 servings.

NUTRITION FACTS: 2 slices with 1/4 cup apples equals 219 calories, 10 g fat (5 g saturated fat), 113 mg cholesterol, 279 mg sodium, 29 g carbohydrate, 2 g fiber, 6 g protein. **DIABETIC EXCHANGES:** 1-1/2 starch, 1-1/2 fat, 1/2 fruit.

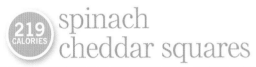

spinach cheddar squares

219 CALORIES

PREP: 15 minutes | **BAKE:** 40 minutes + standing

Elaine Anderson | NEW GALILEE, PENNSYLVANIA
I really enjoy preparing light spinach entrees like this one, which gets many compliments.

- 1 tablespoon dry bread crumbs
- 3/4 cup shredded reduced-fat cheddar cheese, *divided*
- 1 package (10 ounces) frozen chopped spinach, thawed and squeezed dry
- 1/4 cup finely chopped sweet red pepper
- 1-1/2 cups egg substitute
- 3/4 cup fat-free milk
- 2 tablespoons grated Parmesan cheese
- 1/2 teaspoon dried minced onion
- 1/2 teaspoon salt
- 1/4 teaspoon garlic powder
- 1/4 teaspoon pepper

- Sprinkle bread crumbs evenly into an 8-in. square baking dish coated with cooking spray. Top with 1/2 cup cheese, spinach and red pepper. In a small bowl, combine the remaining ingredients; pour over the top.

- Bake, uncovered, at 350° for 35 minutes. Sprinkle with remaining cheese. Bake 2-3 minutes longer or until a knife inserted near the center comes out clean. Let stand for 15 minutes before cutting.

YIELD: 4 servings.

NUTRITION FACTS: 1 piece equals 219 calories, 10 g fat (6 g saturated fat), 31 mg cholesterol, 596 mg sodium, 9 g carbohydrate, 2 g fiber, 26 g protein.

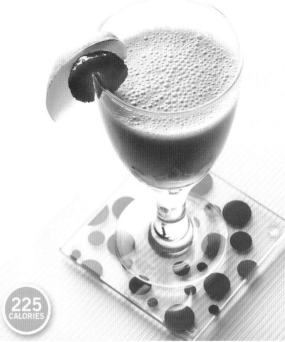

225 CALORIES

THREE-FRUIT SMOOTHIES

three-fruit smoothies

PREP/TOTAL TIME: 10 minutes

Jenny Flake | NEWPORT BEACH, CALIFORNIA
There's nothing more refreshing than a cold, fruit-filled smoothie. I'm thrilled to share this recipe with fellow cooks who enjoy "wowing" guests!

- 1 can (11-1/2 ounces) frozen strawberry breeze juice concentrate, thawed
- 1 cup (8 ounces) vanilla yogurt
- 1/2 cup milk
- 1 tablespoon honey
- 1 teaspoon vanilla extract
- 1 pint fresh strawberries, hulled
- 1 large banana, cut into chunks
- 1 cup chopped peeled fresh peaches *or* frozen unsweetened sliced peaches
- 1 cup crushed ice

- Place half of all ingredients in a blender; cover and process for 15 seconds or until smooth. Pour into chilled glasses. Repeat. Serve immediately.

YIELD: 6 servings.

NUTRITION FACTS: 3/4 cup equals 225 calories, 1 g fat (1 g saturated fat), 4 mg cholesterol, 38 mg sodium, 51 g carbohydrate, 2 g fiber, 4 g protein.

potato egg bake

PREP: 20 minutes | **BAKE:** 35 minutes

Rena Charboneau | GANSEVOORT, NEW YORK

No one will ever guess that this nutritious, mouthwatering breakfast bake is a lighter dish! Potatoes give it a hearty base while cheese and veggies provide color and wonderful flavor.

- 2 pounds Yukon Gold potatoes (about 6 medium), peeled and diced
- 1/2 cup water
- 1 cup frozen chopped broccoli, thawed
- 6 green onions, thinly sliced
- 1 small sweet red pepper, chopped
- 6 eggs
- 8 egg whites
- 1 cup (8 ounces) 1% cottage cheese
- 1 cup (4 ounces) shredded reduced-fat cheddar cheese
- 1/2 cup grated Parmesan cheese
- 1/2 cup fat-free milk
- 2 tablespoons dried parsley flakes
- 1/2 teaspoon salt
- 1/4 teaspoon pepper

- Place potatoes and water in a microwave-safe dish. Cover and microwave on high for 7 minutes or until tender; drain.

- Spread potatoes in a 13-in. x 9-in. baking dish coated with cooking spray. Top with the broccoli, onions and red pepper.

- In a large bowl, whisk the remaining ingredients until blended. Pour over vegetables. Bake, uncovered, at 350° for 35-40 minutes or until center is set.

YIELD: 8 servings.

POTATO EGG BAKE

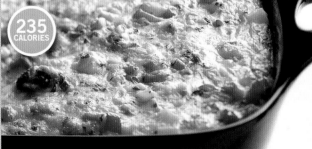

235 CALORIES

NUTRITION FACTS: 1 piece equals 235 calories, 9 g fat (4 g saturated fat), 174 mg cholesterol, 555 mg sodium, 20 g carbohydrate, 2 g fiber, 20 g protein. **DIABETIC EXCHANGES:** 2 medium-fat meat, 1 starch.

265 CALORIES monterey quiche

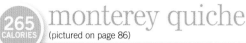

(pictured on page 86)

PREP: 25 minutes | **BAKE:** 45 minutes + standing

Pam Pressly | BEACHWOOD, OHIO

With its creamy goodness and Southwestern flair, this savory specialty is a definite hit with my family. The Taste of Home economists trimmed down the recipe to replicate its original mouthwatering taste with fewer calories. It's perfect for special brunches or lunches with fresh fruit on the side.

- 1/2 cup chopped onion
- 1 tablespoon butter
- 2 garlic cloves, minced
- 8 egg whites, *divided*
- 4 eggs
- 2 cups (16 ounces) 1% small-curd cottage cheese
- 2 cups (8 ounces) shredded reduced-fat Mexican cheese blend *or* Monterey Jack cheese, *divided*
- 2 cans (4 ounces *each*) chopped green chilies
- 1/3 cup all-purpose flour
- 3/4 teaspoon baking powder
- 1/4 teaspoon salt
- 2 unbaked deep-dish pastry shells (9 inches)

- In a small nonstick skillet, cook onion in butter over medium-low heat until tender, stirring occasionally. Add garlic; cook 1 minute longer.

- In a large bowl, combine 6 egg whites, eggs, cottage cheese, 1-1/2 cups shredded cheese, chilies, flour, baking powder, salt and onion mixture. In a large bowl, beat remaining egg whites until stiff peaks form. Fold into cheese mixture. Pour into pastry shells.

- Bake at 400° for 10 minutes. Reduce heat to 350°; bake for 30 minutes. Sprinkle with remaining cheese; bake 5 minutes longer or until a knife inserted near the center comes out clean and cheese is melted. Let stand for 10 minutes before cutting.

YIELD: 2 quiches (6 servings each).

NUTRITION FACTS: 1 piece equals 265 calories, 14 g fat (5 g saturated fat), 88 mg cholesterol, 610 mg sodium, 21 g carbohydrate, 1 g fiber, 16 g protein.

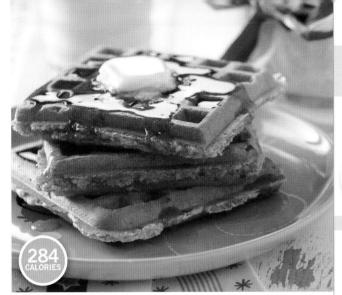

284 CALORIES

WHOLE-GRAIN WAFFLE MIX

whole-grain waffle mix

PREP/TOTAL TIME: 20 minutes

Michelle Sheldon I EDMOND, OKLAHOMA
My mother-in-law shared this recipe, and we love these fluffy waffles. Just add a few ingredients to the mix and you'll be enjoying their homemade goodness in minutes.

  4 cups whole wheat flour
  2 cups all-purpose flour
  1 cup toasted wheat germ
  1 cup toasted oat bran
  1 cup buttermilk blend powder
  3 tablespoons baking powder
  2 teaspoons baking soda
  1 teaspoon salt

ADDITIONAL INGREDIENTS:

  2 eggs
  1 cup water
  2 tablespoons canola oil
  2 tablespoons honey

- In a large bowl, combine the first eight ingredients. Store in an airtight container in the refrigerator for up to 6 months. Yield: 8-1/2 cups mix (about 4 batches).

- To prepare waffles: Place 2 cups waffle mix in a bowl. Combine the eggs, water, oil and honey; stir into waffle mix just until moistened. Bake in a preheated waffle iron according to manufacturer's directions until golden brown.

YIELD: 5 waffles (about 6 inches) per batch.

NUTRITION FACTS: 1 waffle (about 6 inches) equals 284 calories, 9 g fat (2 g saturated fat), 89 mg cholesterol, 482 mg sodium, 43 g carbohydrate, 5 g fiber, 12 g protein. **DIABETIC EXCHANGES:** 3 starch, 1-1/2 fat.

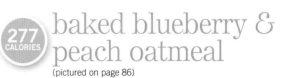

277 CALORIES

baked blueberry & peach oatmeal
(pictured on page 86)

PREP: 20 minutes I **BAKE:** 35 minutes

Rosemarie Weleski I NATRONA HTS., PENNSYLVANIA
This oatmeal bake is a staple in our home. It's very easy to prepare the night before—just keep the dry and wet ingredients separate until ready to bake. I've tried a variety of fruits, but the combination of blueberries and peaches is our favorite.

      3 cups old-fashioned oats
    1/2 cup packed brown sugar
      2 teaspoons baking powder
    1/2 teaspoon salt
      2 egg whites
      1 egg
  1-1/4 cups fat-free milk
    1/4 cup canola oil
      1 teaspoon vanilla extract
      1 can (15 ounces) sliced peaches in juice, drained and chopped
      1 cup fresh *or* frozen blueberries
    1/3 cup chopped walnuts
  Additional fat-free milk, optional

- In a large bowl, combine oats, brown sugar, baking powder and salt. Whisk egg whites, egg, milk, oil and vanilla; add to dry ingredients and stir until blended. Let stand for 5 minutes. Stir in peaches and blueberries.

- Transfer to an 11-in. x 7-in. baking dish coated with cooking spray. Sprinkle with walnuts. Bake, uncovered, at 350° for 35-40 minutes or until top is lightly browned and a thermometer reads 160°. Serve with additional milk if desired.

YIELD: 9 servings.

NUTRITION FACTS: 1 serving (calculated without additional milk) equals 277 calories, 11 g fat (1 g saturated fat), 24 mg cholesterol, 263 mg sodium, 38 g carbohydrate, 3 g fiber, 8 g protein. **DIABETIC EXCHANGES:** 2 starch, 2 fat, 1/2 fruit.

lunches

A good midday meal is essential for keeping up your metabolism and avoiding excessive snacking. Try to stick to 450 calories when planning your lunch. Check out page 103 for a chart with the calorie counts of some brown-bag staples to help round out this important meal.

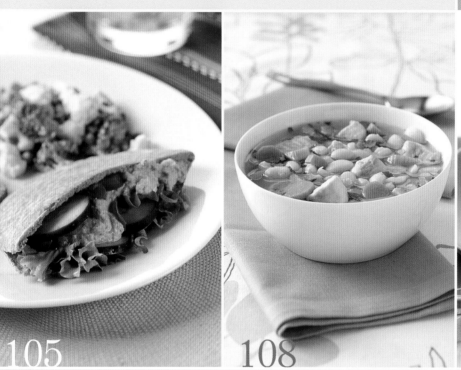

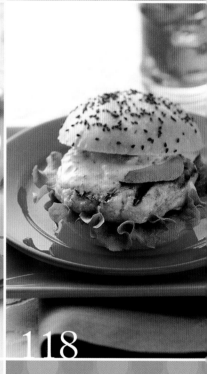

105   108   118

The first section in this chapter has lower-calorie items you might pair with a piece of fruit or a salad. The other sections offer foods that are slightly higher in calories. These satisfying dishes just need a beverage.

250 Calories or Less 101
251-350 Calories 106
351-450 Calories 116

250 calories or less

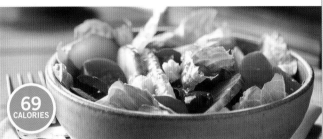

69 CALORIES

MEDITERRANEAN SALAD

mediterranean salad

PREP/TOTAL TIME: 20 minutes

Pat Stevens I GRANBURY, TEXAS

Want to get more veggies in your meals? This big-batch salad also makes a great accompaniment to any grilled main dish. It's our backyard barbecue staple.

- 18 cups torn romaine (about 2 large bunches)
- 1 medium cucumber, sliced
- 1 cup crumbled feta cheese
- 1 cup cherry tomatoes, quartered
- 1 small red onion, thinly sliced
- 1/2 cup julienned roasted sweet red peppers
- 1/2 cup pitted Greek olives, halved

DRESSING:

- 2/3 cup olive oil
- 1/4 cup red wine vinegar
- 1 garlic clove, minced
- 1 teaspoon Italian seasoning
- 1/4 teaspoon salt
- 1/4 teaspoon pepper

- In a very large salad bowl, combine the first seven ingredients. In a jar with a tight-fitting lid, combine the remaining ingredients; shake well. Drizzle over salad and toss to coat. Serve immediately.

YIELD: 28 servings (3/4 cup each).

NUTRITION FACTS: 3/4 cup equals 69 calories, 6 g fat (1 g saturated fat), 2 mg cholesterol, 117 mg sodium, 2 g carbohydrate, 1 g fiber, 1 g protein. **DIABETIC EXCHANGES:** 1 vegetable, 1 fat.

focaccia sandwich

PREP/TOTAL TIME: 15 minutes

Peggy Woodward I EAST TROY, WISCONSIN

Slices of this pretty sandwich are great for any casual get-together. Add or change ingredients to your taste.

- 1/3 cup mayonnaise
- 1 can (4-1/4 ounces) chopped ripe olives, drained
- 1 focaccia bread (about 12 ounces), halved lengthwise
- 4 romaine leaves
- 1/4 pound shaved deli ham
- 1 medium sweet red pepper, thinly sliced into rings
- 1/4 pound shaved deli turkey
- 1 large tomato, thinly sliced
- 1/4 pound thinly sliced hard salami
- 1 jar (7 ounces) roasted sweet red peppers, drained
- 4 to 6 slices provolone cheese

- In a small bowl, combine mayonnaise and olives; spread over the bottom half of bread. Layer with remaining ingredients; replace bread top. Cut into wedges; secure with toothpicks.

YIELD: 24 servings.

NUTRITION FACTS: 1 piece equals 113 calories, 6 g fat (2 g saturated fat), 13 mg cholesterol, 405 mg sodium, 9 g carbohydrate, 1 g fiber, 5 g protein.

FOCACCIA SANDWICH

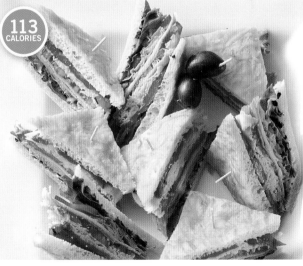

113 CALORIES

I found the most important part of my diet was to eat something I wanted every day, even if it was a teeny piece of chocolate. I needed something to anticipate. In four months, I reached my goal of losing 30 pounds. —**Ashley Latimer, Oregon**

winter harvest vegetable soup

PREP: 25 minutes | **COOK:** 50 minutes

Barbara Marakowski | LOYSVILLE, PENNSYLVANIA
Rich, earthy root vegetables blend with savory spices and the tartness of apples in this wonderful soup.

- 3 medium carrots, halved and thinly sliced
- 3/4 cup chopped celery
- 1 medium onion, chopped
- 2 green onions, thinly sliced
- 1 tablespoon butter
- 1 tablespoon olive oil
- 1 garlic clove, minced
- 7 cups reduced-sodium chicken broth *or* vegetable broth
- 3 cups cubed peeled potatoes
- 2 cups cubed peeled butternut squash
- 2 large tart apples, peeled and chopped

WINTER HARVEST VEGETABLE SOUP

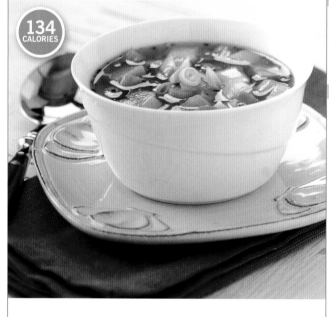

134 CALORIES

- 2 medium turnips, peeled and chopped
- 2 parsnips, peeled and sliced
- 1 bay leaf
- 1/2 teaspoon dried basil
- 1/4 teaspoon dried thyme
- 1/4 teaspoon pepper

Additional thinly sliced green onions, optional

- In a Dutch oven over medium heat, cook and stir the carrots, celery and onions in butter and oil until tender. Add garlic; cook 1 minute longer.

- Add the broth, potatoes, squash, apples, turnips, parsnips and bay leaf. Bring to a boil. Reduce heat; simmer, uncovered, for 20 minutes.

- Stir in the basil, thyme and pepper; simmer 15 minutes longer or until vegetables are tender. Discard bay leaf before serving. Garnish with additional green onions if desired.

YIELD: 12 servings (3 quarts).

NUTRITION FACTS: 1 cup equals 134 calories, 2 g fat (1 g saturated fat), 3 mg cholesterol, 404 mg sodium, 27 g carbohydrate, 5 g fiber, 4 g protein. **DIABETIC EXCHANGES:** 1-1/2 starch, 1 vegetable, 1/2 fat.

italian vegetable soup

PREP: 15 minutes | **COOK:** 25 minutes

Lea Reiter | THOUSAND OAKS, CALIFORNIA
Laced with a splash of white wine, this hearty soup is packed with garden-fresh nutrition and veggies! Leafy escarole adds color and plenty of vitamin A. You could substitute spinach or kale for the escarole if you wish.

- 2 celery ribs, sliced
- 1 medium onion, chopped
- 1 medium carrot, halved and sliced
- 1 tablespoon olive oil
- 2 cups water
- 1 can (15 ounces) white kidney *or* cannellini beans, rinsed and drained

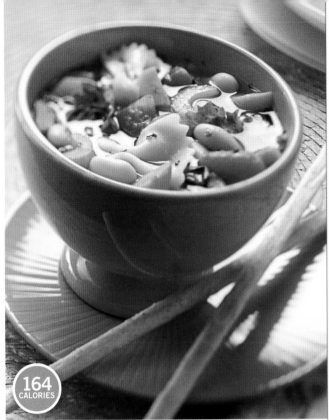

164 CALORIES

ITALIAN VEGETABLE SOUP

1 can (14-1/2 ounces) diced tomatoes, undrained

1 can (14-1/2 ounces) reduced-sodium chicken broth

1/2 cup marsala wine *or* additional reduced-sodium chicken broth

1 teaspoon *each* dried basil, marjoram, oregano and thyme

1/4 teaspoon salt

1/4 teaspoon pepper

1 cup uncooked bow tie pasta

6 cups torn escarole (about 1 small head)

- In a Dutch oven, saute the celery, onion and carrot in oil until tender. Stir in the water, beans, tomatoes, broth, wine and seasonings. Bring to a boil. Stir in pasta.

- Reduce heat; simmer, uncovered, for 13-15 minutes or until pasta is tender, adding escarole during last 3 minutes of cooking.

YIELD: 7 servings.

NUTRITION FACTS: 1 cup equals 164 calories, 3 g fat (trace saturated fat), 0 cholesterol, 426 mg sodium, 26 g carbohydrate, 5 g fiber, 6 g protein. **DIABETIC EXCHANGES:** 1-1/2 starch, 1 vegetable, 1/2 fat.

Below are a few items you might rely on when preparing a basic lunch. When packing a lunch or adding something to your afternoon menu, use this list to make sure you stick to your goal of 450 total calories.

- **1 slice whole wheat bread,** 69 calories
- **1 slice reduced-calorie white bread,** 48 calories
- **1 large pita (6-1/2" diameter),** 165 calories
- **1 flour tortilla (6" diameter),** 90 calories
- **1 corn tortilla (6" diameter),** 58 calories
- **1 whole wheat dinner roll,** 76 calories
- **1 hamburger bun,** 79 calories
- **1 hard roll,** 83 calories
- **1 slice American cheese (1 ounce),** 93 calories
- **1 slice Swiss cheese (1 ounce),** 106 calories
- **1 slice cheddar cheese (1 ounce),** 113 calories
- **1/4 cup diced cheddar cheese,** 113 calories
- **1/2 cup 1% cottage cheese,** 81 calories
- **1 tablespoon shredded Parmesan cheese,** 21 calories
- **1 cup red or green grapes,** 129 calories
- **1 medium orange,** 62 calories
- **1 medium apple,** 72 calories
- **1 cup mandarin orange segments,** 92 calories
- **1/2 cup baked beans,** 134 calories
- **1 cup cubed watermelon,** 40 calories
- **1/2 cup cubed pineapple,** 37 calories
- **1/4 cup cubed avocado,** 60 calories
- **2 tablespoons peanut butter,** 192 calories
- **1 ounce deli ham or turkey,** 22 calories
- **1 beef hot dog,** 147 calories
- **20 baked potato chips,** 200 calories
- **3/4 cup miniature pretzel twists,** 112 calories

For the calorie counts of other typical lunch side dishes, see the Smart Snacks list on pages 77-78. You might also check the Free Foods Chart on page 53.

For calorie calculations of other foods, see the Nutrition Facts labels on food packages.

195 CALORIES

SIMPLE CHICKEN SOUP

simple chicken soup

PREP/TOTAL TIME: 20 minutes

Sue West | ALVORD, TEXAS

I revised a recipe that my family loved so it would be lighter and easier to make. This tasty soup is the result. It's a hearty and healthy meal served with a green salad and fresh bread.

  2 cans (14-1/2 ounces *each*) reduced-sodium chicken broth
  1 tablespoon dried minced onion
  1 package (16 ounces) frozen mixed vegetables
  2 cups cubed cooked chicken breast
  2 cans (10-3/4 ounces *each*) reduced-fat reduced-sodium condensed cream of chicken soup, undiluted

- In a large saucepan, bring the broth and onion to a boil. Reduce heat. Add the vegetables; cover and cook for 6-8 minutes or until crisp-tender. Stir in the chicken and soup; heat through.

YIELD: 6 servings.

NUTRITION FACTS: 1-1/3 cup equals 195 calories, 3 g fat (1 g saturated fat), 44 mg cholesterol, 820 mg sodium, 21 g carbohydrate, 3 g fiber, 19 g protein.

hot swiss chicken sandwiches

PREP/TOTAL TIME: 20 minutes

Edith Tabor | VANCOUVER, WASHINGTON

I've been making these open-faced sandwiches for years, and people always ask for the recipe.

I sometimes serve the filling on slices of sourdough or tucked into pitas.

  1/4 cup reduced-fat mayonnaise
  1/4 teaspoon salt
  1/4 teaspoon lemon juice
1-1/2 cups diced cooked chicken breast
  2/3 cup chopped celery
  1/2 cup shredded reduced-fat Swiss cheese
    4 teaspoons butter, softened
    6 slices Italian bread (about 3/4 inch thick)
    6 slices tomato
  3/4 cup shredded lettuce

- In a large bowl, combine the mayonnaise, salt and lemon juice. Stir in the chicken, celery and cheese. Spread butter on each slice of bread; top each with 1/3 cup chicken mixture.

- Place in a 15-in. x 10-in. x 1-in. baking pan. Broil 4-6 in. from the heat for 3-4 minutes or until heated through. Top with tomato and lettuce.

YIELD: 6 servings.

NUTRITION FACTS: 1 sandwich equals 218 calories, 9 g fat (3 g saturated fat), 44 mg cholesterol, 438 mg sodium, 17 g carbohydrate, 1 g fiber, 17 g protein. **DIABETIC EXCHANGES:** 2 lean meat, 1 starch, 1/2 fat.

HOT SWISS CHICKEN SANDWICHES

218 CALORIES

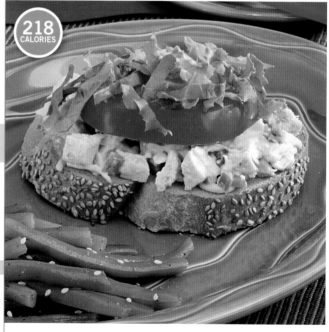

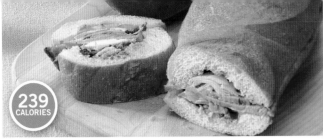

ARTICHOKE-LAMB SANDWICH LOAVES

artichoke-lamb sandwich loaves

PREP: 50 minutes + marinating
BAKE: 1 hour 20 minutes + chilling

Helen Hassler | DENVER, PENNSYLVANIA

These tender sandwiches will surely become the talk of any get-together. I hollow out sourdough baguettes before filling them with cucumber, cheese, marinated lamb and artichokes. Simply delicious, the mouthwatering bites are perfect for a brunch or lunch.

- 1/2 cup lemon juice
- 1/2 cup olive oil
- 6 garlic cloves, minced
- 2 tablespoons minced fresh rosemary
- 1 teaspoon salt
- 1/4 teaspoon cayenne pepper
- 1 boneless leg of lamb (2-1/2 pounds)
- 2 cans (14 ounces *each*) water-packed artichoke hearts, rinsed and drained
- 2/3 cup plus 6 tablespoons reduced-fat balsamic vinaigrette, *divided*
- 2 sourdough baguettes (1 pound *each*)
- 1 medium cucumber, thinly sliced
- 2 medium tomatoes, thinly sliced
- 1 package (5.3 ounces) fresh goat cheese, sliced

- In a large resealable plastic bag, combine the first six ingredients; add lamb. Seal bag and turn to coat. Refrigerate for 8 hours or overnight.

- Drain and discard marinade. Place lamb on a rack in a shallow roasting pan. Bake, uncovered, at 325° for 80-90 minutes or until meat reaches desired doneness (for medium-rare, a meat thermometer should read 145°; medium, 160°; well-done, 170°). Cool to room temperature. Cover and refrigerate for at least 2 hours.

- Place artichokes in a resealable plastic bag; add 2/3 cup vinaigrette. Seal bag and turn to coat; let stand for 10 minutes. Drain and discard marinade.

- Cut lamb into thin slices. Cut each baguette in half horizontally. Carefully hollow out top and bottom, leaving a 3/4-in. shell. Brush the bottom half of each loaf with 2 tablespoons vinaigrette. Layer with cucumber, tomatoes, lamb and artichokes; drizzle with remaining vinaigrette. Top with goat cheese.

- Replace bread tops and press down firmly; wrap tightly in plastic wrap. Refrigerate for at least 2 hours. Cut into slices.

YIELD: 24 servings.

NUTRITION FACTS: 2 slices equals 239 calories, 8 g fat (2 g saturated fat), 33 mg cholesterol, 511 mg sodium, 26 g carbohydrate, 1 g fiber, 15 g protein.

garbanzo bean pitas
(pictured on page 100)

PREP/TOTAL TIME: 20 minutes

Susan Le Brun | SULPHUR, LOUISIANA

This a wonderful meatless recipe for informal dinners and quick lunches alike. I add a little horseradish to my pitas for extra flair.

- 1 can (15 ounces) garbanzo beans *or* chickpeas, rinsed and drained
- 1/2 cup fat-free mayonnaise
- 1 tablespoon water
- 2 tablespoons minced fresh parsley
- 2 tablespoons chopped walnuts
- 1 tablespoon chopped onion
- 1 garlic clove, minced
- 1/8 teaspoon pepper
- 2 whole wheat pita pocket halves
- 4 lettuce leaves
- 1/2 small cucumber, thinly sliced
- 1 small tomato, seeded and chopped
- 1/4 cup fat-free ranch salad dressing, optional

- In a blender, combine the first eight ingredients; cover and process until blended. Spoon 1/3 cup bean mixture into each pita half. Top with lettuce, cucumber and tomato. Serve with ranch dressing if desired.

YIELD: 4 servings.

NUTRITION FACTS: 1 filled pita half equals 241 calories, 6 g fat (trace saturated fat), 3 mg cholesterol, 552 mg sodium, 41 g carbohydrate, 8 g fiber, 9 g protein. **DIABETIC EXCHANGES:** 3 starch, 1 lean meat, 1 fat.

251-350 calories

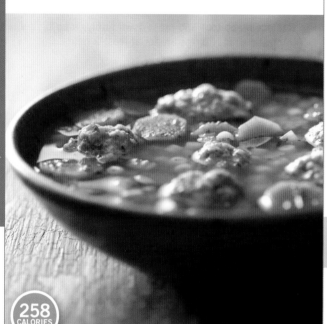

TURKEY MEATBALL SOUP

turkey meatball soup

PREP: 30 minutes | **COOK:** 40 minutes

Christie Ladd | MECHANICSBURG, PENNSYLVANIA
Every Italian-American family I know seems to have their own version of meatball soup. This recipe is based on my family's version.

- 2 egg whites, lightly beaten
- 1/2 cup seasoned bread crumbs
- 1 tablespoon grated Parmesan cheese
- 4 teaspoons Italian seasoning, *divided*
- 1 pound lean ground turkey
- 3 medium carrots, sliced
- 3 celery ribs, finely chopped
- 1 tablespoon olive oil
- 4 garlic cloves, minced
- 3 cans (14-1/2 ounces *each*) reduced-sodium chicken broth

- 1/4 teaspoon pepper
- 1/2 cup ditalini *or* other small pasta

- In a bowl, combine the egg whites, bread crumbs, cheese and 2 teaspoons Italian seasoning. Crumble turkey over mixture and mix well. Shape into 3/4-in. balls.

- Place in a 15-in. x 10-in. x 1-in. baking pan coated with cooking spray. Bake, uncovered, at 350° for 10-15 minutes or until no longer pink.

- Meanwhile, in a Dutch oven, saute carrots and celery in oil until tender. Add garlic; cook 1 minute longer. Add the broth, pepper and remaining Italian seasoning. Bring to a boil. Reduce heat; cover and simmer for 20 minutes.

- Stir in pasta; cook 10-12 minutes longer or until vegetables and pasta are tender. Stir in meatballs; heat through.

YIELD: 6 servings.

NUTRITION FACTS: 1 cup equals 258 calories, 10 g fat (2 g saturated fat), 60 mg cholesterol, 783 mg sodium, 21 g carbohydrate, 2 g fiber, 21 g protein. **DIABETIC EXCHANGES:** 2 lean meat, 1-1/2 starch, 1/2 fat.

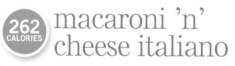

macaroni 'n' cheese italiano

262 CALORIES

PREP: 20 minutes | **BAKE:** 25 minutes + standing

Isabelle Wolters | SCITUATE, MASSACHUSETTS
I've always liked macaroni and cheese, but my husband prefers macaroni with tomato sauce. So I added spaghetti sauce and mozzarella to give my home-style favorite an Italian twist.

- 2 cups uncooked elbow macaroni
- 3/4 cup chopped onion
- 1/4 cup chopped celery
- 1/4 cup chopped green pepper
- 2 teaspoons olive oil
- 1/2 cup meatless spaghetti sauce
- 1/2 teaspoon dried basil
- 1/2 teaspoon dried oregano
- 2 tablespoons all-purpose flour
- 1/2 teaspoon salt
- 1/4 teaspoon ground nutmeg
- 1/8 teaspoon cayenne pepper

> **I am happy to say** that I am 17 pounds lighter than I was five months ago. I have 30 more to lose, and I feel good that my goal is in sight. For me, the magic is a combination of my husband's support, a constantly changing workout routine, online encouragement and minimal cost for all of it. —**Tryna Rhodes, Colorado**

2 cups fat-free milk

1-1/4 cups shredded reduced-fat cheddar cheese

1/2 cup shredded part-skim mozzarella cheese

2 tablespoons grated Parmesan cheese

2 plum tomatoes, seeded and sliced

- Cook pasta according to package directions until cooked but firm. Meanwhile, in a large nonstick skillet, saute the onion, celery and green pepper in oil until tender. Stir in spaghetti sauce, basil and oregano. Bring to a boil. Reduce heat; simmer, uncovered, for 5 minutes. Drain macaroni; stir into sauce. Transfer to a 2-qt. baking dish coated with cooking spray; set aside.

- In a saucepan, combine the flour, salt, nutmeg and cayenne. Gradually stir in milk until smooth. Bring to a boil over medium heat; cook and stir for 2 minutes or until thickened. Reduce heat; stir in cheddar and mozzarella cheeses until melted.

- Pour over macaroni mixture. Top with Parmesan cheese and tomatoes. Bake, uncovered, at 350° for 25-30 minutes or until bubbly and golden brown. Let stand for 5 minutes before serving.

YIELD: 6 servings.

NUTRITION FACTS: 1 serving equals 262 calories, 9 g fat (5 g saturated fat), 25 mg cholesterol, 406 mg sodium, 31 g carbohydrate, 2 g fiber, 16 g protein. **DIABETIC EXCHANGES:** 2 lean meat, 1-1/2 starch, 1 vegetable, 1/2 fat.

makeover curried chicken rice soup

PREP: 15 minutes I **COOK:** 20 minutes

Rebecca Cook I **HELOTES, TEXAS**

This lighter chicken rice soup boasts all the hearty texture, warm comfort and delicious flavor of the original.

1/4 cup butter, cubed

2 large carrots, finely chopped

2 celery ribs, finely chopped

1 small onion, finely chopped

3/4 cup plus 2 tablespoons all-purpose flour

1 teaspoon seasoned salt

1 teaspoon curry powder

2 cans (12 ounces *each*) fat-free evaporated milk

1 cup half-and-half cream

4-1/2 cups reduced-sodium chicken broth

3 cups cubed cooked chicken breast

2 cups cooked brown rice

- In a Dutch oven, melt butter. Add the carrots, celery and onion; saute for 2 minutes. Sprinkle with flour; stir until blended. Stir in seasoned salt and curry. Gradually add milk and cream. Bring to a boil; cook and stir for 2 minutes or until thickened.

- Gradually add broth. Stir in chicken and rice; return to a boil. Reduce heat; simmer, uncovered, for 10 minutes or until vegetables are tender.

YIELD: 11 servings (2-3/4 quarts).

NUTRITION FACTS: 1 cup equals 263 calories, 8 g fat (5 g saturated fat), 54 mg cholesterol, 524 mg sodium, 26 g carbohydrate, 2 g fiber, 20 g protein. **DIABETIC EXCHANGES:** 2 lean meat, 1 starch, 1 fat, 1/2 fat-free milk.

MAKEOVER CURRIED CHICKEN RICE SOUP

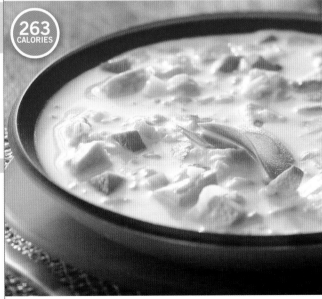

263 CALORIES

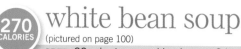

264 CALORIES

BLACK BEAN TACO PIZZA

black bean taco pizza

PREP: 25 minutes | **BAKE:** 10 minutes

Sherie Nelson | DULUTH, MINNESOTA

My husband absolutely loves this pizza. I make it several times a month for family and friends.

- 1 tablespoon cornmeal
- 1 package (6-1/2 ounces) pizza crust mix
- 1 bottle (8 ounces) taco sauce
- 2 medium tomatoes, seeded and chopped
- 3/4 cup canned black beans
- 1/2 cup frozen corn
- 1 can (4 ounces) chopped green chilies
- 2 green onions, chopped
- 1-1/2 cups (6 ounces) shredded reduced-fat Colby-Monterey Jack cheese

Reduced-fat sour cream, optional

- Coat a 12-in. pizza pan with cooking spray; sprinkle with cornmeal. Prepare pizza dough according to package directions. With floured hands, press dough onto prepared pan. Bake at 450° for 7-10 minutes or until lightly browned.

- Spread taco sauce over crust to within 1 in. of edges. Top with tomatoes, beans, corn, chilies, onions and cheese.

- Bake for 10-15 minutes or until cheese is melted and crust is golden brown. Serve with sour cream if desired.

YIELD: 6 servings.

NUTRITION FACTS: 1 slice (calculated without sour cream) equals 264 calories, 6 g fat (4 g saturated fat), 15 mg cholesterol, 783 mg sodium, 38 g carbohydrate, 4 g fiber, 14 g protein. **DIABETIC EXCHANGES:** 2-1/2 starch, 1 medium-fat meat.

270 CALORIES

white bean soup
(pictured on page 100)

PREP: 20 minutes + soaking | **COOK:** 2 hours

Elizabeth Wagner | CLIO, MICHIGAN

I turned to this hearty recipe after my husband had heart surgery. Filled with beans, veggies and chicken, it's chock-full of fiber, and its lean protein fills us up. It makes a big batch and freezes well for fast meals later.

- 1/2 pound dried baby lima beans
- 1/2 pound dried great northern beans
- 2 pounds boneless skinless chicken breasts, cubed
- 1 teaspoon salt, *divided*
- 2 tablespoons canola oil, *divided*
- 1 large onion, chopped
- 3 medium carrots, sliced
- 2 celery ribs, thinly sliced
- 1 garlic clove, minced
- 4 cups reduced-sodium chicken broth
- 2 cups water
- 1/2 teaspoon pepper
- 1/4 cup minced fresh parsley

- Sort beans and rinse with cold water. Place in a Dutch oven; add water to cover by 2 in. Bring to a boil; boil for 2 minutes. Remove from the heat; cover and let stand for 1-4 hours or until beans are softened.

- Drain and rinse beans, discarding liquid; set beans aside. Sprinkle chicken with 1/2 teaspoon salt. In the same pan, saute chicken in 1 tablespoon oil until no longer pink. Drain and set aside. Saute onion in remaining oil until tender. Add the carrots, celery and garlic; saute 1-2 minutes longer.

- Stir in the broth, water, pepper, beans and chicken; bring to a boil. Reduce heat; cover and simmer for 1-3/4 to 2-1/4 hours or until beans are tender. Stir in parsley and remaining salt.

YIELD: 11 servings (1-3/4 quarts).

NUTRITION FACTS: 1 cup equals 270 calories, 5 g fat (1 g saturated fat), 46 mg cholesterol, 499 mg sodium, 30 g carbohydrate, 9 g fiber, 27 g protein. **DIABETIC EXCHANGES:** 3 lean meat, 2 starch, 1/2 fat.

spinach-feta chicken rolls

PREP: 25 minutes | **BAKE:** 45 minutes

Linda Gregg | SPARTANBURG, SOUTH CAROLINA
This dish was inspired by a favorite Greek appetizer. It may take a bit of extra work, but it's well worth it!

- 1/2 cup sun-dried tomatoes (not packed in oil)
- 1 cup boiling water
- 1 package (10 ounces) frozen chopped spinach, thawed and squeezed dry
- 1 cup (4 ounces) crumbled feta cheese
- 4 green onions, thinly sliced
- 1/4 cup Greek olives, chopped
- 1 garlic clove, minced
- 6 boneless skinless chicken breast halves (6 ounces *each*)
- 1/4 teaspoon salt
- 1/4 teaspoon pepper

- Place tomatoes in a small bowl; add boiling water. Let stand for 5 minutes. In another bowl, combine the spinach, feta cheese, onions, olives and garlic. Drain and chop tomatoes; add to spinach mixture.

- Flatten chicken to 1/4-in. thickness; sprinkle with salt and pepper. Spread spinach mixture over chicken. Roll up and secure with toothpicks. Place in a 13-in. x 9-in. baking dish coated with cooking spray.

- Cover and bake at 350° for 30 minutes. Uncover; bake 15-20 minutes longer or until chicken is no longer pink. Discard toothpicks.

YIELD: 6 servings.

NUTRITION FACTS: 1 stuffed chicken breast half equals 272 calories, 9 g fat (3 g saturated fat), 104 mg cholesterol, 583 mg sodium, 7 g carbohydrate, 3 g fiber, 40 g protein. **DIABETIC EXCHANGES:** 5 lean meat, 1 vegetable.

SPINACH-FETA CHICKEN ROLLS

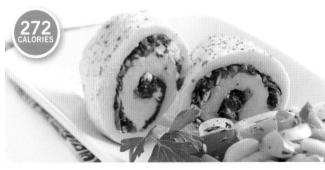

272 CALORIES

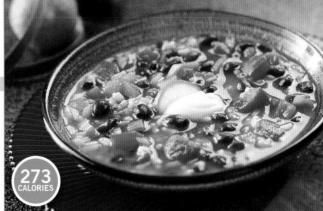

273 CALORIES

SOUTHWEST BLACK BEAN SOUP

southwest black bean soup

PREP: 15 minutes | **COOK:** 35 minutes

Jill Heatwole | PITTSVILLE, MARYLAND
A friend brought this recipe to a gathering, and it has been a hit with my family ever since! I use brown rice for more fiber and whole-grain goodness.

- 1 medium sweet red pepper, chopped
- 2 celery ribs, chopped
- 1 small onion, chopped
- 1 tablespoon canola oil
- 2 cans (15 ounces each) black beans, rinsed and drained
- 1 can (14-1/2 ounces) reduced-sodium chicken broth
- 1 can (14-1/2 ounces) diced tomatoes, undrained
- 1 can (4 ounces) chopped green chilies
- 3/4 teaspoon ground cumin
- 1-1/2 cups cooked instant brown rice
- 6 tablespoons reduced-fat sour cream

- In a nonstick saucepan, saute the pepper, celery and onion in oil until tender. Add the beans, broth, tomatoes, chilies and cumin. Bring to a boil. Reduce heat; simmer, uncovered, for 30 minutes or until thickened.

- Divide rice among six soup bowls; top with soup and sour cream.

YIELD: 6 servings.

NUTRITION FACTS: 1 cup soup with 1/4 cup rice and 1 tablespoon sour cream equals 273 calories, 5 g fat (1 g saturated fat), 5 mg cholesterol, 655 mg sodium, 45 g carbohydrate, 9 g fiber, 12 g protein. **DIABETIC EXCHANGES:** 2-1/2 starch, 1 lean meat, 1 vegetable, 1/2 fat.

I substitute sandwich rounds and tortillas in place of bread or buns, and I drink only water. I swim laps in the community pool and get up hourly at work to walk around.
—Jackie Cobb Woodward

274 CALORIES better than egg salad

PREP/TOTAL TIME: 20 minutes

Lisa Renshaw | KANSAS CITY, MISSOURI
Tofu makes the taste and texture of this "egg" salad unique in this quick-to-fix sandwich.

- 1/4 cup chopped celery
- 2 green onions, chopped
- 1/4 cup reduced-fat mayonnaise
- 2 tablespoons sweet pickle relish
- 1 tablespoon Dijon mustard
- 1/4 teaspoon ground turmeric
- 1/4 teaspoon salt
- 1/8 teaspoon cayenne pepper
- 1 package (12.3 ounces) silken firm tofu, cubed
- 8 slices whole wheat bread
- 4 lettuce leaves

- In a small bowl, combine the first eight ingredients. Gently stir in tofu. Spread over four slices of bread; top with lettuce and remaining bread.

YIELD: 4 servings.

NUTRITION FACTS: 1 sandwich equals 274 calories, 12 g fat (2 g saturated fat), 5 mg cholesterol, 734 mg sodium, 33 g carbohydrate, 5 g fiber, 13 g protein. **DIABETIC EXCHANGES:** 2 starch, 1 lean meat, 1 fat.

turkey enchiladas

PREP: 30 minutes | **BAKE:** 25 minutes

Kimberly Bish | VANDALIA, OHIO
My husband and I hosted a Mexican-themed party, and this was one of the main dishes. It was a huge success! I was thrilled when four of our friends asked for—and left with—a copy of the recipe!

- 1 large onion, chopped
- 1 large green pepper, chopped
- 2 teaspoons canola oil
- 3 tablespoons all-purpose flour
- 1-1/4 teaspoons ground coriander
- 1/4 teaspoon pepper
- 1 can (14-1/2 ounces) reduced-sodium chicken broth
- 1 cup (8 ounces) fat-free sour cream
- 1 cup (4 ounces) shredded reduced-fat cheddar cheese, *divided*
- 3 cups cubed cooked turkey breast
- 3/4 cup salsa
- 8 flour tortillas (6 inches), warmed

- In a large nonstick saucepan coated with cooking spray, cook and stir onion and green pepper in oil until tender. Sprinkle with flour, coriander and pepper; stir until blended. Gradually stir in broth. Bring to a boil; cook and stir for 2 minutes or until thickened. Remove from the heat. Stir in sour cream and 3/4 cup cheese.

- In a bowl, combine the turkey, salsa, and 1 cup cheese mixture. Spoon 1/3 cup turkey mixture down the center of each tortilla. Roll up and place seam side down in a 13-in. x 9-in. baking dish coated with cooking spray. Pour remaining cheese mixture over the top.

- Cover and bake at 350° for 20 minutes. Sprinkle with remaining cheese. Bake, uncovered, 5-10 minutes longer or until heated through and cheese is melted.

YIELD: 8 servings.

NUTRITION FACTS: 1 enchilada equals 284 calories, 8 g fat (2 g saturated fat), 60 mg cholesterol, 610 mg sodium, 26 g carbohydrate, 1 g fiber, 26 g protein. **DIABETIC EXCHANGES:** 3 lean meat, 2 starch.

TURKEY ENCHILADAS

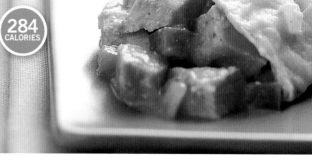

284 CALORIES

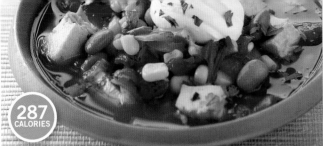

287 CALORIES

HEARTY CHIPOTLE CHICKEN SOUP

hearty chipotle chicken soup

PREP: 15 minutes | **COOK:** 30 minutes

Sonali Ruder | NEW YORK, NEW YORK

Sweet corn and cool sour cream help tame the smoky hot flavor of chipotle pepper in this well-balanced soup that's perfect for chilly days.

- 1 large onion, chopped
- 1 tablespoon canola oil
- 4 garlic cloves, minced
- 4 cups reduced-sodium chicken broth
- 2 cans (15 ounces *each*) pinto beans, rinsed and drained
- 2 cans (14-1/2 ounces *each*) fire-roasted diced tomatoes, undrained
- 3 cups frozen corn
- 2 chipotle peppers in adobo sauce, seeded and minced
- 2 teaspoons adobo sauce
- 1 teaspoon ground cumin
- 1/4 teaspoon pepper
- 2 cups cubed cooked chicken breast
- 1/2 cup fat-free sour cream
- 1/4 cup minced fresh cilantro

- In a Dutch oven, saute onion in oil until tender. Add garlic; cook 1 minute longer. Add the broth, beans, tomatoes, corn, chipotle peppers, adobo sauce, cumin and pepper. Bring to a boil. Reduce heat; simmer, uncovered, for 20 minutes.

- Stir in chicken; heat through. Garnish with sour cream; sprinkle with cilantro.

YIELD: 8 servings (3-1/4 quarts).

NUTRITION FACTS: 1-2/3 cups with 1 tablespoon sour cream equals 287 calories, 4 g fat (1 g saturated fat), 29 mg cholesterol, 790 mg sodium, 42 g carbohydrate, 7 g fiber, 21 g protein. **DIABETIC EXCHANGES:** 2 starch, 2 lean meat, 2 vegetable.

288 CALORIES

breaded eggplant sandwiches

PREP: 30 minutes | **BAKE:** 25 minutes

Holly Gomez | SEABROOK, NEW HAMPSHIRE

Eggplant Parmesan is one of my family's favorite comfort foods. We love this version served open-faced with a salad.

- 1/4 cup minced fresh basil
- 2 teaspoons olive oil
- 1/4 teaspoon dried oregano
- 1/4 teaspoon pepper
- 1/8 teaspoon salt
- 2 egg whites, lightly beaten
- 1 cup seasoned bread crumbs
- 1 medium eggplant
- 2 large tomatoes
- 1-1/2 cups (6 ounces) shredded part-skim mozzarella cheese
- 2 tablespoons grated Parmesan cheese
- 1 garlic clove, peeled
- 12 slices Italian bread (1/2 inch thick), toasted

- Combine the basil, oil, oregano, pepper and salt; set aside. Place egg whites and bread crumbs in separate shallow bowls. Cut eggplant lengthwise into six slices. Dip slices in egg whites, then coat in crumbs.

- Place on a baking sheet coated with cooking spray. Bake at 375° for 20-25 minutes or until tender and golden brown, turning once.

- Cut each tomato into six slices; place two slices on each eggplant slice. Spoon reserved basil mixture over tomatoes and sprinkle with cheeses. Bake for 3-5 minutes or until cheese is melted.

- Meanwhile, rub garlic over one side of each slice of bread; discard garlic. Place each eggplant stack on a slice of bread, garlic side up. Top with remaining bread, garlic side down.

YIELD: 6 servings.

NUTRITION FACTS: 1 sandwich equals 288 calories, 9 g fat (4 g saturated fat), 18 mg cholesterol, 628 mg sodium, 38 g carbohydrate, 5 g fiber, 15 g protein. **DIABETIC EXCHANGES:** 2 starch, 1 lean meat, 1 vegetable, 1 fat.

291
CALORIES

SUPER-DUPER TUNA SANDWICHES

super-duper tuna sandwiches

PREP/TOTAL TIME: 15 minutes

Renee Bartolomeo | INDIANOLA, IOWA
If packing this fantastic sandwich for a brown-bag lunch, keep the bread separate from the salad so it doesn't get soggy. You can also try serving the tuna salad with crackers, as a wrap or on lettuce.

- 2 cans (5 ounces *each*) light water-packed tuna, drained and flaked
- 1/3 cup shredded peeled apple
- 1/3 cup finely shredded cabbage
- 1/3 cup finely shredded carrot
- 3 tablespoons finely chopped celery
- 3 tablespoons finely chopped onion
- 3 tablespoons sweet pickle relish
- 2 tablespoons reduced-fat mayonnaise
- 8 slices whole wheat bread

- In a large bowl, combine the first eight ingredients. Spread 1/2 cup tuna mixture over four slices of bread; top with remaining bread slices.

YIELD: 4 servings.

NUTRITION FACTS: 1 sandwich equals 291 calories, 5 g fat (1 g saturated fat), 28 mg cholesterol, 717 mg sodium, 31 g carbohydrate, 5 g fiber, 29 g protein. **DIABETIC EXCHANGES:** 3 lean meat, 2 starch, 1/2 fat.

293
CALORIES

chicken pesto pizza

PREP: 35 minutes + rising | **BAKE:** 20 minutes

Heather Thompson | WOODLAND HILLS, CALIFORNIA
Keeping the spices simple in this recipe helps the flavor of the chicken and vegetables come through. The pizza tastes great and is good for you, too.

- 2 teaspoons active dry yeast
- 1 cup warm water (110° to 115°)
- 2-3/4 cups bread flour, *divided*
- 1 tablespoon plus 2 teaspoons olive oil, *divided*
- 1 tablespoon sugar
- 1-1/2 teaspoons salt, *divided*
- 1/2 pound boneless skinless chicken breasts, cut into 1/2-inch pieces
- 1 small onion, halved and thinly sliced
- 1/2 *each* small green, sweet red and yellow peppers, julienned
- 1/2 cup sliced fresh mushrooms
- 3 tablespoons prepared pesto
- 1-1/2 cups (6 ounces) shredded part-skim mozzarella cheese
- 1/4 teaspoon pepper

- In a large bowl, dissolve yeast in warm water. Beat in the 1 cup flour, 1 tablespoon oil, sugar and 1 teaspoon salt. Add the remaining flour; beat until combined.

- Turn onto a lightly floured surface; knead until smooth and elastic, about 6-8 minutes. Place in a bowl coated with cooking spray, turning once to coat top. Cover and let rise in a warm place until doubled, about 1 hour.

- In a large nonstick skillet over medium heat, cook the chicken, onion, peppers and mushrooms in remaining oil until chicken is no longer pink and vegetables are tender. Remove from the heat; set aside.

- Punch dough down; roll into a 15-in. circle. Transfer to a 14-in. pizza pan. Build up edges slightly. Spread with pesto. Top with chicken mixture and cheese. Sprinkle with pepper and remaining salt.

- Bake at 400° for 18-20 minutes or until crust and cheese are lightly browned.

YIELD: 8 slices.

NUTRITION FACTS: 1 slice equals 293 calories, 10 g fat (3 g saturated fat), 30 mg cholesterol, 601 mg sodium, 35 g carbohydrate, 2 g fiber, 18 g protein. **DIABETIC EXCHANGES:** 2 starch, 1 lean meat, 1 fat.

299 CALORIES chili con carne

PREP/TOTAL TIME: 20 minutes

Marline Emmal | VANCOUVER, BRITISH COLUMBIA
You'll only need one skillet and 20 minutes to whip up this hearty, slightly spicy Chili Con Carne.

- 1/2 pound lean ground beef (90% lean)
- 1-1/2 cups reduced-sodium tomato juice
- 3/4 cup kidney beans, rinsed and drained
- 2 tablespoons chopped onion
- 1 teaspoon chili powder
- 1/4 teaspoon ground cumin
- 1/4 teaspoon minced garlic
- 2 to 3 drops hot pepper sauce

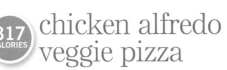

GARNISH:

Thinly sliced green onion, optional

- In a large saucepan, cook beef over medium heat until no longer pink; drain. Stir in the remaining ingredients. Bring to a boil. Reduce heat; simmer, uncovered, for 10 minutes or until slightly thickened, stirring occasionally. Garnish with green onion if desired.

YIELD: 2 servings.

NUTRITION FACTS: 1 cup equals 299 calories, 8 g fat (3 g saturated fat), 56 mg cholesterol, 346 mg sodium, 24 g carbohydrate, 6 g fiber, 30 g protein. **DIABETIC EXCHANGES:** 3 lean meat, 2 vegetable, 1 starch.

317 CALORIES chicken alfredo veggie pizza

PREP: 45 minutes + rising | **BAKE:** 25 minutes

Nancy Lindsay | NEW MARKET, IOWA
I created this pizza myself, and it's become our favorite! The vegetables' bright colors make it very appealing.

- 1 package (1/4 ounce) active dry yeast
- 1 cup warm water (110° to 115°)
- 1 tablespoon canola oil
- 2 teaspoons sugar
- 3/4 teaspoon salt, *divided*
- 1/2 teaspoon garlic-herb seasoning blend
- 1/2 cup whole wheat flour
- 2-1/4 to 2-1/2 cups bread flour
- 1 tablespoon cornmeal
- 1 cup fresh baby spinach
- 4 teaspoons all-purpose flour
- 1-1/4 cups 2% milk
- 1-1/2 cups cubed cooked chicken breast
- 1/3 cup shredded Parmesan cheese

Dash white pepper

- 1 cup sliced fresh mushrooms
- 1 plum tomato, seeded and chopped
- 1 small onion, diced
- 1/2 cup chopped green pepper
- 1/4 cup sliced ripe olives
- 1 cup (4 ounces) shredded part-skim mozzarella cheese
- 1/2 cup shredded Colby-Monterey Jack cheese

- In a bowl, dissolve yeast in warm water. Add the oil, sugar, 1/2 teaspoon salt, seasoning blend, whole wheat flour and 2-1/4 cups bread flour. Beat until smooth. Stir in enough remaining flour to form a stiff dough.

- Turn onto a lightly floured surface; knead until smooth and elastic, about 6-8 minutes. Place in a bowl coated with cooking spray, turning once to coat the top. Cover and let rise for 20 minutes.

- Punch dough down; roll into a 15-in. circle. Sprinkle cornmeal over a 14-in. pizza pan coated with cooking spray. Transfer dough to prepared pan; build up edges slightly. Bake at 425° for 12-14 minutes or until edges are lightly browned.

- Meanwhile, in a large saucepan, bring 1/2 in. of water to a boil. Add spinach; cover and boil for 3-5 minutes or until wilted. Drain and squeeze dry; set aside.

- In a large saucepan, combine flour and milk until smooth. Bring to a boil; cook and stir for 2 minutes or until thickened. Add the chicken, Parmesan cheese, remaining salt, pepper and reserved spinach. Cook and stir over medium heat until cheese is melted.

- Spread sauce over crust; top with remaining ingredients. Bake 10-15 minutes longer or until cheeses are melted.

YIELD: 8 servings.

NUTRITION FACTS: 1 slice equals 317 calories, 9 g fat (4 g saturated fat), 40 mg cholesterol, 476 mg sodium, 38 g carbohydrate, 3 g fiber, 22 g protein. **DIABETIC EXCHANGES:** 2-1/2 starch, 2 lean meat, 1/2 fat.

328 CALORIES · grandma's french tuna salad wraps

PREP/TOTAL TIME: 15 minutes

Jennifer Magrey | STERLING, CONNECTICUT

My French Canadian grandmother always made her tuna salad with chopped egg in it. I tried to recreate her version, added some veggies for complete nutrition and turned it into a wrap. It's a fun lunch or dinner, and we get the memory of my dear grandmother with each savory bite.

for 2

- 1 can (5 ounces) light water-packed tuna, drained and flaked
- 1 celery rib, finely chopped
- 1/4 cup fat-free mayonnaise
- 1/4 teaspoon pepper
- 2 whole wheat tortillas (8 inches), room temperature
- 1/2 cup shredded lettuce
- 1 small carrot, shredded
- 4 slices tomato
- 2 slices red onion, separated into rings
- 1 hard-cooked egg, sliced

- In a small bowl, combine the tuna, celery, mayonnaise and pepper. Spoon tuna mixture down the center of each tortilla. Top with lettuce, carrot, tomato, onion and egg. Roll up tightly; secure with toothpicks.

YIELD: 2 servings.

NUTRITION FACTS: 1 wrap equals 328 calories, 7 g fat (1 g saturated fat), 135 mg cholesterol, 770 mg sodium, 32 g carbohydrate, 4 g fiber, 30 g protein. **DIABETIC EXCHANGES:** 3 lean meat, 2 starch, 1 vegetable.

330 CALORIES · german deli pizza

PREP: 40 minutes + rising | **BAKE:** 15 minutes

Cindy Reams | PHILIPSBURG, PENNSYLVANIA

Take the chill off and serve up great German deli flavor with this savory, cheesy pizza. It has a tender crust and a mild, mustardy bite that people of all ages can appreciate. It's fun to serve a pizza like this that's a little unexpected.

DOUGH:
- 2/3 cup water (70° to 80°)
- 1 tablespoon olive oil
- 1 teaspoon caraway seeds
- 1/4 teaspoon salt
- 1-1/2 cups bread flour
- 1/2 cup rye flour
- 1 teaspoon active dry yeast

SAUCE:
- 1/3 cup chopped red onion
- 1 tablespoon butter
- 1 tablespoon all-purpose flour
- 1 cup fat-free evaporated milk
- 1 tablespoon spicy brown mustard
- 1/4 cup shredded Swiss cheese

TOPPINGS:
- 1/3 cup thinly sliced red onion
- 1 cup cubed fully cooked ham
- 1 cup (4 ounces) shredded Swiss cheese

- In bread machine pan, place dough ingredients in order suggested by manufacturer. Select dough setting (check dough after 5 minutes of mixing; add 1 to 2 tablespoons of water or flour if needed).

- When cycle is completed, turn dough onto a lightly floured surface. Punch dough down; roll into a 13-in. circle. Transfer to a 12-in. pizza pan coated with cooking spray; build up edges slightly. Cover and let rest for 10 minutes.

- Prick dough thoroughly with a fork. Bake at 400° for 6-8 minutes or until edges are lightly browned.

- Meanwhile, for sauce, in a small saucepan, saute chopped onion in butter until tender. Stir in flour until blended; gradually add evaporated milk and mustard. Bring to a boil; cook and stir for 2 minutes or until thickened. Remove from the heat; stir in cheese. Spread over crust. Top with sliced onion, ham and cheese. Bake for 12-15 minutes or until crust and cheese are lightly browned.

YIELD: 6 slices.

NUTRITION FACTS: 1 slice equals 330 calories, 12 g fat (6 g saturated fat), 36 mg cholesterol, 546 mg sodium, 37 g carbohydrate, 3 g fiber, 19 g protein. **DIABETIC EXCHANGES:** 2-1/2 starch, 2 lean meat, 1 fat.

I lost weight by including more fiber and protein in my diet. Choosing the right snacks, like nuts and veggies with hummus, helps keep my hunger at bay between meals and helps me make better choices for lunch and dinner. —**Renee McDaniel**

chicken caesar wraps

PREP/TOTAL TIME: 15 minutes

Nancy Pratt | LONGVIEW, TEXAS

This classic handheld sandwich with tender chicken, Parmesan cheese and chopped Caesar croutons has the perfect amount of dressing for a tasty meal.

- 3/4 cup fat-free creamy Caesar salad dressing
- 1/4 cup grated Parmesan cheese
- 1/2 teaspoon garlic powder
- 1/4 teaspoon pepper
- 3 cups cubed cooked chicken breast
- 2 cups torn romaine
- 3/4 cup Caesar salad croutons, coarsely chopped
- 6 whole wheat tortillas (8 inches)

- In a large bowl, combine the dressing, cheese, garlic powder and pepper. Add the chicken, romaine and croutons. Spoon 2/3 cup chicken mixture down the center of each tortilla; roll up.

YIELD: 6 servings.

NUTRITION FACTS: 1 wrap equals 332 calories, 7 g fat (1 g saturated fat), 57 mg cholesterol, 689 mg sodium, 37 g carbohydrate, 4 g fiber, 27 g protein. **DIABETIC EXCHANGES:** 3 lean meat, 2-1/2 starch, 1/2 fat.

CHICKEN CAESAR WRAPS

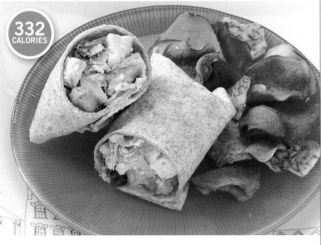

332 CALORIES

339 CALORIES italian sausage bean soup

PREP: 20 minutes | **COOK:** 1-1/2 hours

Glenna Reimer | GIG HARBOR, WASHINGTON

In the colder months, I like to put on a big pot of this comforting soup. It cooks away while I do other things like baking bread, crafting or even cleaning the house.

- 1 pound Italian sausage links, casings removed
- 1 medium onion, finely chopped
- 3 garlic cloves, sliced
- 4 cans (14-1/2 ounces *each*) reduced-sodium chicken broth
- 2 cans (15 ounces *each*) pinto beans, rinsed and drained
- 1 can (14-1/2 ounces) diced tomatoes, undrained
- 1 cup medium pearl barley
- 1 large carrot, sliced
- 1 celery rib, sliced
- 1 teaspoon minced fresh sage
- 1/2 teaspoon minced fresh rosemary *or* 1/8 teaspoon dried rosemary, crushed
- 6 cups chopped fresh kale

- Crumble sausage into a Dutch oven; add onion. Cook over medium heat until meat is no longer pink. Add garlic; cook 1 minute longer. Drain.

- Add the broth, beans, tomatoes, barley, carrot, celery, sage and rosemary. Bring to a boil. Reduce heat; cover and simmer for 45 minutes.

- Stir in kale; return to a boil. Reduce heat; cover and simmer for 25-30 minutes or until vegetables are tender and kale is wilted.

YIELD: 8 servings (3 quarts).

NUTRITION FACTS: 1-1/2 cups equals 339 calories, 9 g fat (3 g saturated fat), 23 mg cholesterol, 1,100 mg sodium, 48 g carbohydrate, 11 g fiber, 19 g protein.

351-450 calories

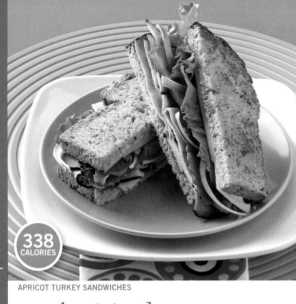

338 CALORIES

APRICOT TURKEY SANDWICHES

apricot turkey sandwiches

PREP/TOTAL TIME: 15 minutes

Charlotte Gehle I BROWNSTOWN, MICHIGAN

Apricot jam adds a hint of sweetness to this savory sandwich that's piled high with thinly sliced peppered turkey, lettuce, tomato, onion and Swiss cheese. It's simple goodness at its best.

for 2

- 2 turkey bacon strips
- 4 pieces multigrain bread, toasted
- 2 tablespoons apricot jam
- 3 ounces thinly sliced deli peppered turkey
- 2 slices tomato
- 2 slices red onion
- 2 pieces leaf lettuce
- 2 slices reduced-fat Swiss cheese
- 4 teaspoons Dijon mustard

- In a small skillet, cook bacon over medium heat until crisp. Remove to paper towels to drain; set aside.

- Spread two toast slices with jam. Layer with turkey, reserved bacon, tomato, onion, lettuce and cheese. Spread remaining toast with mustard; place on top.

YIELD: 2 servings.

NUTRITION FACTS: 1 sandwich equals 338 calories, 10 g fat (3 g saturated fat), 40 mg cholesterol, 1,109 mg sodium, 43 g carbohydrate, 4 g fiber, 23 g protein. **DIABETIC EXCHANGES:** 3 starch, 2 medium-fat meat.

red, white and blue pita pockets

351 CALORIES

PREP: 15 minutes + marinating I **COOK:** 5 minutes

Charlene Chambers I ORMOND BEACH, FLORIDA

Completely packed with delicious fillings, these pockets get their patriotic name from red peppers, white sour cream and tangy blue cheese. But don't wait for the Fourth of July to serve them; they're fantastic any day of the year!

- 2 tablespoons red wine vinegar
- 4 teaspoons olive oil
- 2 garlic cloves, minced
- 1 pound beef top sirloin steak, thinly sliced
- 1/2 cup fat-free sour cream
- 1/3 cup crumbled blue cheese
- 4 whole wheat pita pocket halves
- 2 cups torn red leaf lettuce
- 1/2 cup roasted sweet red peppers, drained and cut into strips
- 1/4 cup sliced red onion

- In a large resealable plastic bag, combine the vinegar, oil and garlic; add the beef. Seal bag and turn to coat; refrigerate for 8 hours or overnight.

- In a small bowl, combine sour cream and blue cheese; set aside. Drain and discard the marinade.

- In a large nonstick skillet or wok coated with cooking spray, stir-fry beef for 2-3 minutes or until no longer pink. Line pita halves with lettuce, red peppers and onion; fill each with 1/3 cup beef. Serve with sour cream mixture.

YIELD: 4 servings.

NUTRITION FACTS: 1 filled pita half equals 351 calories, 12 g fat (4 g saturated fat), 59 mg cholesterol, 522 mg sodium, 26 g carbohydrate, 3 g fiber, 32 g protein. **DIABETIC EXCHANGES:** 4 lean meat, 1-1/2 fat, 1 starch, 1 vegetable.

chili beef quesadillas

PREP: 30 minutes | **BAKE:** 10 minutes

Robyn Larabee | LUCKNOW, ONTARIO
Served in whole wheat tortillas, these scrumptious beef and veggie quesadillas pack a healthy dose of fiber.

- 3/4 pound lean ground beef (90% lean)
- 1 medium onion, chopped
- 3/4 cup finely chopped fresh mushrooms
- 1 medium zucchini, shredded
- 1 medium carrot, shredded
- 2 garlic cloves, minced
- 2 teaspoons chili powder
- 1/4 teaspoon salt
- 1/4 teaspoon hot pepper sauce
- 2 medium tomatoes, seeded and chopped
- 1/4 cup minced fresh cilantro
- 4 whole wheat tortillas (8 inches), warmed

Cooking spray

- 1/2 cup shredded part-skim mozzarella cheese

- In a large nonstick skillet over medium heat, cook beef and onion until meat is no longer pink; drain. Remove and keep warm. In the same skillet, cook and stir the mushrooms, zucchini, carrot, garlic, chili powder, salt and pepper sauce until vegetables are tender. Stir in the tomatoes, cilantro and beef mixture.

- Spritz one side of each tortilla with cooking spray; place plain side up in a 15-in. x 10-in. x 1-in. baking pan coated with cooking spray. Spoon beef mixture over

CHILI BEEF QUESADILLAS

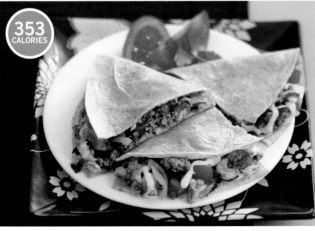

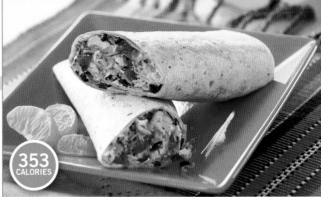

TURKEY TORTILLA ROLL-UPS

half of each tortilla; sprinkle with cheese. Fold tortillas over filling.

- Bake at 400° for 5 minutes. Carefully turn over; bake 5-6 minutes longer or until cheese is melted. Cut into wedges.

YIELD: 4 servings.

NUTRITION FACTS: 1 quesadilla equals 353 calories, 12 g fat (4 g saturated fat), 50 mg cholesterol, 475 mg sodium, 33 g carbohydrate, 5 g fiber, 26 g protein. **DIABETIC EXCHANGES:** 3 lean meat, 2 vegetable, 1-1/2 starch.

turkey tortilla roll-ups

PREP/TOTAL TIME: 10 minutes

Darlene Brenden | SALEM, OREGON
If you're on the run, you won't have to take along a fork and knife to enjoy these tasty, hearty roll-ups.

- 3/4 cup sour cream
- 6 spinach tortillas *or* flour tortillas of your choice (8 inches)
- 1-1/2 cups cubed cooked turkey *or* ready-to-use grilled chicken breast strips
- 1 cup (4 ounces) finely shredded cheddar cheese
- 1 cup shredded lettuce
- 1/2 cup chopped ripe olives
- 1/2 cup chunky salsa

- Spread 2 tablespoons sour cream over each tortilla. Top with turkey, cheese, lettuce, olives and salsa. Roll up each tortilla tightly; wrap in plastic wrap. Refrigerate until serving.

YIELD: 6 servings.

NUTRITION FACTS: 1 roll-up equals 353 calories, 16 g fat (9 g saturated fat), 67 mg cholesterol, 577 mg sodium, 29 g carbohydrate, trace fiber, 20 g protein.

I started choosing healthier food options, and now my body craves them. I drink less soda and allow myself to indulge within limits when a craving hits.
— Jennifer Hughes Winemiller

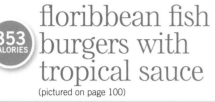

floribbean fish burgers with tropical sauce

(pictured on page 100)

PREP: 35 minutes | **GRILL:** 10 minutes

Virginia Anthony | JACKSONVILLE, FLORIDA
I like to prepare these fish burgers, because they are delicious yet lower in saturated fat and cholesterol than burgers made with beef. Then I figure I can top the sandwiches with some avocado since there's not a lot of other fat in the recipe.

- 1/2 cup fat-free mayonnaise
- 1 tablespoon minced fresh cilantro
- 1 tablespoon minced chives
- 1 tablespoon sweet pickle relish
- 1 tablespoon lime juice
- 1 teaspoon grated lime peel
- 1-1/2 teaspoons Caribbean jerk seasoning
- 1/8 teaspoon hot pepper sauce

BURGERS:
- 1 egg white, lightly beaten
- 4 green onions, chopped
- 1/3 cup soft bread crumbs
- 2 tablespoons minced fresh cilantro
- 2 teaspoons Caribbean jerk seasoning
- 1 garlic clove, minced
- 1/8 teaspoon salt
- 1-1/2 pounds grouper *or* red snapper fillets
- 6 kaiser rolls, split
- 6 lettuce leaves
- 1 medium ripe avocado, peeled and cut into 12 slices

- In a small bowl, combine the first eight ingredients; cover and refrigerate until serving.

- In a large bowl, combine the egg white, onions, bread crumbs, cilantro, jerk seasoning, garlic and salt. Place fish in a food processor; cover and process until finely chopped. Add to egg white mixture and mix well. Shape into six burgers.

- Spray both sides of burgers with cooking spray. Using long-handled tongs, moisten a paper towel with cooking oil and lightly coat the grill rack. Grill burgers, covered, over medium heat or broil 4 in. from the heat for 4-5 minutes on each side or until a meat thermometer reads 160°.

- Serve each on a roll with lettuce, avocado and 5 teaspoons tropical sauce.

YIELD: 6 servings.

NUTRITION FACTS: 1 burger equals 353 calories, 9 g fat (1 g saturated fat), 44 mg cholesterol, 797 mg sodium, 39 g carbohydrate, 4 g fiber, 29 g protein. **DIABETIC EXCHANGES:** 3 lean meat, 2-1/2 starch, 1 fat.

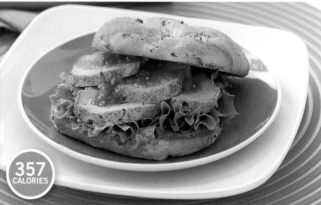

ROAST PORK SANDWICHES WITH PEACH CHUTNEY

roast pork sandwiches with peach chutney

PREP: 15 minutes | **BAKE:** 35 minutes

Lily Julow | GAINESVILLE, FLORIDA
This combination of roast pork with peach chutney used to be a favorite Sunday dinner.

- 1 pork tenderloin (1 pound)
- 2 tablespoons spicy brown mustard

PEACH CHUTNEY:

- 1/4 cup peach preserves
- 3 tablespoons finely chopped onion
- 2 tablespoons red wine vinegar
- 1 small garlic clove, minced
- 1/4 teaspoon mustard seed
- 1/8 teaspoon salt
- 1/8 teaspoon ground ginger
- 1/8 teaspoon ground cinnamon

Dash cayenne pepper

Dash ground cloves

- 1/4 cup fat-free mayonnaise
- 4 onion rolls, split and toasted
- 4 lettuce leaves

- Brush pork with mustard; place on a rack in a shallow roasting pan. Bake at 425° for 35-40 minutes or until a meat thermometer reads 160°. Let stand for 5 minutes before slicing.

- Meanwhile, for chutney, in a small saucepan, combine the preserves, onion, vinegar, garlic and seasonings. Bring to a boil. Reduce heat; simmer, uncovered, for 7-8 minutes or until thickened. Set aside to cool. Spread mayonnaise over roll bottoms. Layer with lettuce, pork slices and chutney. Replace tops.

YIELD: 4 servings.

NUTRITION FACTS: 1 sandwich equals 357 calories, 7 g fat (2 g saturated fat), 65 mg cholesterol, 589 mg sodium, 42 g carbohydrate, 2 g fiber, 29 g protein. **DIABETIC EXCHANGES:** 3 lean meat, 2-1/2 starch.

teriyaki chicken salad with poppy seed dressing

PREP: 30 minutes + marinating | **GRILL:** 10 minutes

Cathleen Leonard | WOODBRIDGE, CALIFORNIA
I've made this salad often and shared it with many people. It's originally from my good friend's daughter, and we always receive compliments on how the wonderful fruit flavors come alive served with the poppy seed dressing.

- 1 cup honey teriyaki marinade
- 1 pound boneless skinless chicken breasts
- 6 cups torn romaine

- 3 medium kiwifruit, peeled and sliced
- 1 can (20 ounces) unsweetened pineapple chunks, drained
- 1 can (11 ounces) mandarin oranges, drained
- 2 celery ribs, chopped
- 1 medium sweet red pepper, chopped
- 1 medium green pepper, chopped
- 1 cup fresh raspberries
- 1 cup sliced fresh strawberries
- 3 green onions, chopped
- 1/2 cup salted cashews
- 1/3 cup reduced-fat poppy seed salad dressing

- Place marinade in a large resealable plastic bag; add the chicken. Seal bag and turn to coat; refrigerate for 8 hours or overnight. Drain and discard marinade.

- Grill chicken, covered, over medium heat or broil 4 in. from the heat for 5-7 minutes on each side or until a meat thermometer reads 170°.

- Slice chicken. Divide the romaine, kiwi, pineapple, oranges, celery, peppers, raspberries and strawberries among six plates; top with chicken. Sprinkle with green onions and cashews. Drizzle with salad dressing.

YIELD: 6 servings.

NUTRITION FACTS: 1 serving equals 361 calories, 11 g fat (2 g saturated fat), 42 mg cholesterol, 761 mg sodium, 49 g carbohydrate, 7 g fiber, 20 g protein. **DIABETIC EXCHANGES:** 2 lean meat, 1-1/2 starch, 1-1/2 fat, 1 vegetable, 1 fruit.

TERIYAKI CHICKEN SALAD WITH POPPY SEED DRESSING

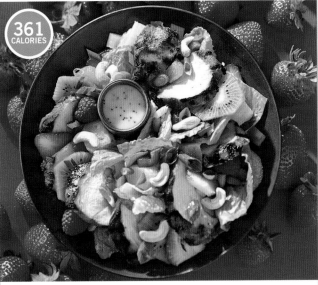

361 CALORIES

363 CALORIES

CHICKEN CAESAR PASTA TOSS

chicken caesar pasta toss

PREP/TOTAL TIME: 30 minutes

Joy Bilbey I HOLT, MICHIGAN

The Taste of Home test kitchen revised my pasta, chicken and asparagus medley flavored with Caesar salad dressing so it's even faster to fix. I created the recipe when looking for a no-hassle dinner to feed my hungry family.

- 3 quarts water
- 2-1/2 cups uncooked tricolor spiral pasta
- 1-1/2 cups cut fresh asparagus (1-inch pieces)
- 1-1/2 pounds boneless skinless chicken breasts, cut into 1-inch pieces
- 2 teaspoons olive oil
- 2 large tomatoes, chopped
- 2/3 cup reduced-fat Caesar vinaigrette
- 3 green onions, chopped
- 3 tablespoons grated Parmesan cheese

- In a Dutch oven, bring water to a boil. Add pasta. Return to a boil; cook for 4 minutes. Add asparagus; cook 6-8 minutes longer or until pasta and asparagus are tender.

- Meanwhile, in a large nonstick skillet, saute chicken in oil until no longer pink. Remove from the heat.

- Drain pasta mixture; return to the pan. Add the chicken, tomatoes and vinaigrette. Cook over low heat until heated through. Sprinkle with onions and Parmesan cheese.

YIELD: 6 servings.

NUTRITION FACTS: 1-1/3 cups equals 363 calories, 10 g fat (2 g saturated fat), 67 mg cholesterol, 609 mg sodium, 35 g carbohydrate, 2 g fiber, 31 g protein. **DIABETIC EXCHANGES:** 3 lean meat, 2 starch, 1 vegetable, 1 fat.

382 CALORIES

chicken fajita pizza

PREP: 25 minutes I **BAKE:** 10 minutes

Rebecca Clark I WARRIOR, ALABAMA

This pizza is packed with flavorful seasonings, but it's the cilantro that gives it the fresh burst of flavor. If you like Southwestern foods, this one is for you!

- 1 tube (13.8 ounces) refrigerated pizza crust
- 1 pound boneless skinless chicken breasts, cubed
- 3 teaspoons canola oil, *divided*
- 1 teaspoon fajita seasoning mix
- 1 medium sweet red pepper, julienned
- 1 medium green pepper, julienned
- 1 medium onion, halved and sliced
- 1 garlic clove, minced
- 1/2 cup salsa
- 1/4 teaspoon pepper
- 1-1/2 cups (6 ounces) shredded reduced-fat Mexican cheese blend
- 2 tablespoons minced fresh cilantro

- Unroll crust into a 15-in. x 10-in. x 1-in. baking pan coated with cooking spray; flatten dough and build up edges slightly. Bake at 425° for 7-10 minutes or until golden brown.

- Meanwhile, in a large nonstick skillet, saute chicken in 2 teaspoons oil until no longer pink. Sprinkle with seasoning mix; cook 30 seconds longer. Remove and keep warm.

- In the same skillet, saute peppers and onion in remaining oil for 3 minutes. Add garlic; cook 1 minute longer or until vegetables are crisp-tender. Remove from the heat; stir in the salsa, pepper and reserved chicken.

- Spoon chicken mixture over crust; sprinkle with cheese. Bake for 6-10 minutes or until cheese is melted. Sprinkle with cilantro.

YIELD: 6 servings.

NUTRITION FACTS: 1 slice equals 382 calories, 12 g fat (4 g saturated fat), 62 mg cholesterol, 807 mg sodium, 38 g carbohydrate, 2 g fiber, 30 g protein. **DIABETIC EXCHANGES:** 3 lean meat, 2 starch, 1 vegetable, 1 fat.

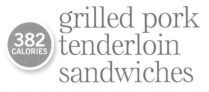

grilled pork tenderloin sandwiches

382 CALORIES

PREP: 15 minutes + marinating | **GRILL:** 25 minutes

Geri Bierschbach | WEIDMAN, MICHIGAN

I got the recipe for these pork sandwiches from a friend at work. I'm always asked for it when I serve this dish.

- 2 tablespoons canola oil
- 2 tablespoons reduced-sodium soy sauce
- 2 tablespoons steak sauce
- 2 garlic cloves, minced
- 1-1/2 teaspoons brown sugar
- 1/2 teaspoon ground mustard
- 1/2 teaspoon minced fresh gingerroot
- 2 pork tenderloins (1 pound *each*)

MUSTARD HORSERADISH SAUCE:

- 1/4 cup fat-free mayonnaise
- 1/4 cup reduced-fat sour cream
- 1-1/2 teaspoons lemon juice
- 1 teaspoon sugar
- 1/2 teaspoon ground mustard
- 1/2 teaspoon Dijon mustard
- 1/2 teaspoon prepared horseradish
- 6 kaiser rolls, split
- 6 lettuce leaves

- In a large resealable plastic bag, combine the first seven ingredients; add pork. Seal bag and turn to coat; refrigerate for 8 hours or overnight.

- Drain and discard marinade. Using long-handled tongs, moisten a paper towel with cooking oil and lightly coat the grill rack. Prepare grill for indirect heat using a drip pan. Place pork over drip pan and grill pork, covered, over indirect medium-hot heat for 25-40 minutes or until a meat thermometer reads 160°. Let stand for 5 minutes before slicing.

- In a small bowl, combine the mayonnaise, sour cream, lemon juice, sugar, ground mustard, Dijon mustard and horseradish. Serve pork on rolls with lettuce and mustard horseradish sauce.

YIELD: 6 servings.

NUTRITION FACTS: 1 sandwich equals 382 calories, 10 g fat (3 g saturated fat), 89 mg cholesterol, 528 mg sodium, 34 g carbohydrate, 2 g fiber, 37 g protein. **DIABETIC EXCHANGES:** 4 lean meat, 2 starch.

one-pot chili

384 CALORIES

PREP: 25 minutes | **COOK:** 15 minutes

Dawn Forsberg | SAINT JOSEPH, MISSOURI

This hearty entree is low in fat and full of flavor. I love that you can cook the dried pasta right in the chili. One less pot to wash! This also reheats in the microwave perfectly.

- 1 pound lean ground turkey
- 1 small onion, chopped
- 1/4 cup chopped green pepper
- 1 teaspoon olive oil
- 2 cups water
- 1 can (15 ounces) pinto beans, rinsed and drained
- 1 can (14-1/2 ounces) reduced-sodium beef broth
- 1 can (14-1/2 ounces) diced tomatoes with mild green chilies, undrained
- 1 can (8 ounces) no-salt-added tomato sauce
- 2 teaspoons chili powder
- 1 teaspoon ground cumin
- 1/2 teaspoon dried oregano
- 2 cups uncooked multigrain penne pasta
- 1/4 cup reduced-fat sour cream
- 1/4 cup minced fresh cilantro

- In a large saucepan coated with cooking spray, cook the turkey, onion and pepper in oil over medium heat until meat is no longer pink; drain.

- Stir in the water, beans, broth, tomatoes, tomato sauce, chili powder, cumin and oregano. Bring to a boil. Add pasta; cook for 15-20 minutes or until tender, stirring occasionally. Serve with sour cream; sprinkle with cilantro.

YIELD: 6 servings (2 quarts).

NUTRITION FACTS: 1-1/3 cups with 2 teaspoons sour cream equals 384 calories, 10 g fat (2 g saturated fat), 64 mg cholesterol, 598 mg sodium, 47 g carbohydrate, 8 g fiber, 25 g protein. **DIABETIC EXCHANGES:** 3 starch, 2 lean meat, 1 vegetable.

dinners

Only the Taste of Home Comfort Food Diet lets you dig into classic fare such as cheesy pizzas, bubbling casseroles and juicy pork chops...and still lose weight! Aim for 500 calories for an entire supper, so when planning your menu, be sure to save a few calories for a side dish and dessert.

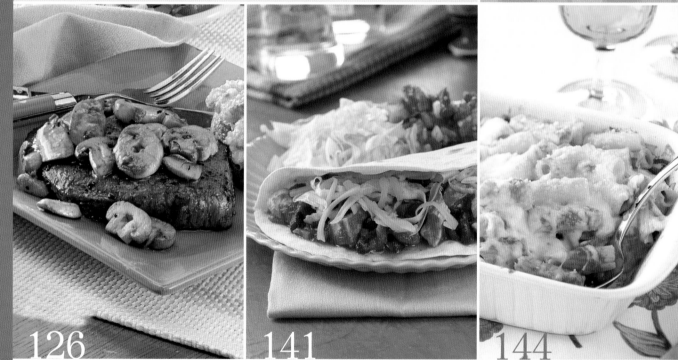

126   141   144

The first section in this chapter has lower-calorie entrees you might pair with side dishes, a green salad, bread, etc. The remaining entree areas are higher-calorie one-dish meals that simply need to be paired with a beverage. See page 127 for calorie counts of some typical dinner foods.

250 Calories or Less 123
251-350 Calories 134
351-450 Calories 157

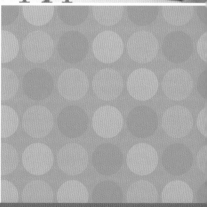

250 calories or less

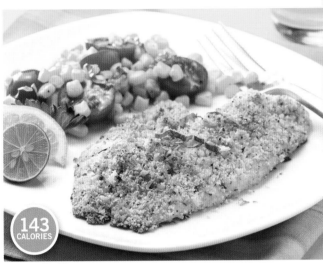

143 CALORIES

BAKED TILAPIA

baked tilapia

PREP/TOTAL TIME: 20 minutes

Brandi Castillo | SANTA MARIA, CALIFORNIA

So much flavor...so few ingredients! A quick and easy crumb coating makes this yummy tilapia recipe ideal for busy weeknights. Try the breading on cod for a change of pace.

- 3/4 cup soft bread crumbs
- 1/3 cup grated Parmesan cheese
- 1 teaspoon garlic salt
- 1 teaspoon dried oregano
- 4 tilapia fillets (5 ounces *each*)

- In a shallow bowl, combine the bread crumbs, cheese, garlic salt and oregano. Coat fillets in crumb mixture. Place on a baking sheet coated with cooking spray.
- Bake at 425° for 8-12 minutes or until fish flakes easily with a fork.

YIELD: 4 servings.

NUTRITION FACTS: 1 fillet equals 143 calories, 2 g fat (1 g saturated fat), 72 mg cholesterol, 356 mg sodium, 2 g carbohydrate, trace fiber, 28 g protein. **DIABETIC EXCHANGE:** 4 lean meat.

garlic lemon shrimp

PREP/TOTAL TIME: 20 minutes

Athena Russell | FLORENCE, SOUTH CAROLINA

You'll be amazed that you can make this simple, elegant pasta in mere minutes. Serve with whole grain bread to soak up all of the garlic lemon sauce.

- 1 pound uncooked large shrimp, peeled and deveined
- 2 tablespoons olive oil
- 3 garlic cloves, sliced
- 1 tablespoon lemon juice
- 1 teaspoon ground cumin
- 1/4 teaspoon salt
- 2 tablespoons minced fresh parsley

Hot cooked pasta *or* rice

- In a large skillet, saute shrimp in oil for 3 minutes. Add the garlic, lemon juice, cumin and salt; cook and stir until shrimp turn pink. Stir in parsley. Serve with pasta or rice.

YIELD: 4 servings.

NUTRITION FACTS: 3/4 cup (calculated without rice or pasta) equals 163 calories, 8 g fat (1 g saturated fat), 138 mg cholesterol, 284 mg sodium, 2 g carbohydrate, trace fiber, 19 g protein. **DIABETIC EXCHANGES:** 3 lean meat, 1-1/2 fat.

GARLIC LEMON SHRIMP

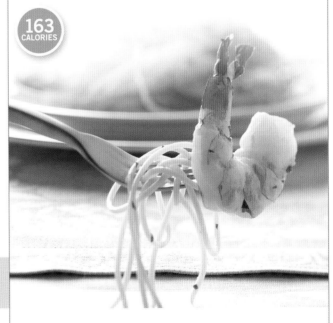

163 CALORIES

In a year and a half, I have lost 65 pounds by prayer, counting calories, better food choices and running. —Jennifer Carr Westmoreland

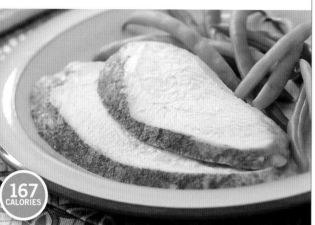

167 CALORIES

PEPPERY GRILLED TURKEY BREAST

peppery grilled turkey breast

PREP: 15 minutes | **GRILL:** 1-1/2 hours + standing

Mary Relyea | CANASTOTA, NEW YORK
This is a combination of several favorite family recipes. People who try it for the first time are amazed to find that it's not only flavorful but healthy as well.

- 2 tablespoons light brown sugar
- 1 tablespoon salt
- 2 teaspoons ground cinnamon
- 1 teaspoon cayenne pepper
- 1/2 teaspoon ground mustard
- 1 bone-in turkey breast (5 pounds)
- 1 cup reduced-sodium chicken broth
- 1/4 cup white vinegar
- 1/4 cup jalapeno pepper jelly
- 2 tablespoons olive oil

- In a small bowl, combine the brown sugar, salt, cinnamon, cayenne and mustard. With fingers, carefully loosen the skin from both sides of turkey breast. Spread half of spice mixture under turkey skin; secure skin to underside of breast with wooden toothpicks. Spread remaining spice mixture over the skin.

- Using long-handled tongs, moisten a paper towel with cooking oil and lightly coat the grill rack. Prepare grill for indirect heat, using a drip pan. Place turkey over drip pan, grill, covered, over indirect medium heat for 30 minutes.

- In a small saucepan, combine the broth, vinegar, jelly and oil. Cook and stir over medium heat for 2 minutes or until jelly is melted. Set aside 1/2 cup. Baste turkey with some of the remaining jelly mixture. Grill 1 to 1-1/2 hours longer or until a meat thermometer reads 170°, basting every 15 minutes.

- Cover and let stand for 10 minutes. Remove and discard turkey skin if desired. Brush with reserved jelly mixture before slicing.

YIELD: 15 servings.

NUTRITION FACTS: 4 ounces cooked turkey (with skin removed) equals 167 calories, 3 g fat (trace saturated fat), 78 mg cholesterol, 565 mg sodium, 6 g carbohydrate, trace fiber, 29 g protein. **DIABETIC EXCHANGES:** 4 lean meat, 1/2 starch, 1/2 fat.

172 CALORIES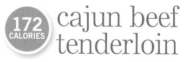

cajun beef tenderloin

PREP: 15 minutes **GRILL:** 50 minutes + standing

Suzanne Dannahower | FORT PIERCE, FLORIDA
This spicy entree really warms up any cold-weather dinner. The dry rub keeps the tenderloin moist.

- 1 beef tenderloin roast (3 pounds)
- 4 teaspoons salt
- 1 tablespoon paprika
- 2-1/4 teaspoons onion powder
- 1-1/2 teaspoons garlic powder
- 1-1/2 teaspoons white pepper
- 1-1/2 teaspoons pepper
- 1 to 3 teaspoons cayenne pepper
- 1 teaspoon dried basil
- 1/2 teaspoon chili powder
- 1/8 teaspoon dried thyme

1/8 teaspoon ground mustard
Dash ground cloves

- Tie tenderloin at 2-in. intervals with kitchen string. Combine the seasonings; rub over beef. Using long-handled tongs, moisten a paper towel with cooking oil and lightly coat the grill rack.

- Prepare grill for indirect heat using a drip pan. Place tenderloin over drip pan and grill, covered, over indirect medium heat for 50-60 minutes, or until meat reaches desired doneness (for medium-rare, a meat thermometer should read 145°; medium, 160°; well-done, 170°), turning occasionally. Let stand for 10 minutes before slicing.

- To roast the tenderloin, bake on a rack in a shallow roasting pan at 425° for 45-60 minutes or until meat reaches desired doneness.

YIELD: 12 servings.

NUTRITION FACTS: 3 ounces cooked beef equals 172 calories, 7 g fat (3 g saturated fat), 50 mg cholesterol, 788 mg sodium, 2 g carbohydrate, 1 g fiber, 25 g protein. DIABETIC EXCHANGE: 3 lean meat.

moroccan beef kabobs

PREP: 25 minutes + marinating | GRILL: 10 minutes

Jennifer Shaw | DORCHESTER, MASSACHUSETTS
My grandma's marinade adds tang to these kabobs. It boosts the flavor without adding lots of calories.

- 1 cup chopped fresh parsley
- 1 cup chopped fresh cilantro
- 1/4 cup grated onion
- 3 tablespoons lemon juice
- 2 tablespoons olive oil
- 1 tablespoon ground cumin
- 1 tablespoon ground coriander
- 1 tablespoon paprika
- 1 tablespoon cider vinegar
- 1 tablespoon ketchup
- 2 garlic cloves, minced
- 1 teaspoon minced fresh gingerroot
- 1 teaspoon Thai red chili paste
- Dash salt and pepper
- 2 pounds beef top sirloin steak, cut into 1-inch pieces

- In a large resealable plastic bag, combine the parsley, cilantro, onion, lemon juice, oil, cumin, coriander, paprika, vinegar, ketchup, garlic, ginger, chili paste, salt and pepper; add beef. Seal bag and turn to coat; refrigerate for 8 hours or overnight.

- Drain and discard marinade. Thread beef cubes onto eight metal or soaked wooden skewers. Using long-handled tongs, moisten a paper towel with cooking oil and lightly coat the grill rack.

- Grill beef, covered, over medium-hot heat or broil 4 in. from the heat for 8-12 minutes or until meat reaches desired doneness, turning occasionally.

YIELD: 8 servings.

NUTRITION FACTS: 1 kabob equals 185 calories, 9 g fat (3 g saturated fat), 63 mg cholesterol, 91 mg sodium, 3 g carbohydrate, 1 g fiber, 22 g protein. DIABETIC EXCHANGES: 3 lean meat, 1/2 fat.

MOROCCAN BEEF KABOBS

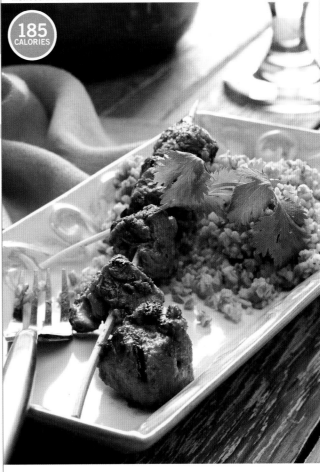

185 CALORIES

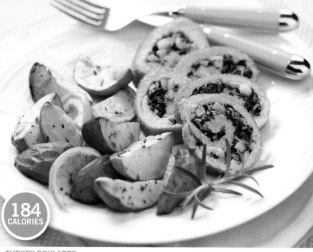

184 CALORIES

TURKEY ROULADES

turkey roulades

PREP: 40 minutes | **BAKE:** 40 minutes

Kari Wheaton | SOUTH BELOIT, ILLINOIS

The filling in this recipe goes so well with turkey. I love the hint of lemon, the savory combo of apples, mushrooms and spinach—and the bread-crumb coating adds a nice crunch.

- 1 cup diced peeled tart apple
- 1 cup diced fresh mushrooms
- 1/2 cup finely chopped onion
- 2 teaspoons olive oil
- 5 ounces frozen chopped spinach, thawed and squeezed dry
- 2 tablespoons lemon juice
- 2 teaspoons grated lemon peel
- 3/4 teaspoon salt, *divided*

Pinch ground nutmeg

- 4 turkey breast tenderloins (8 ounces *each*)
- 1/4 teaspoon pepper
- 1 egg, lightly beaten
- 1/2 cup seasoned bread crumbs

- In a large nonstick skillet coated with cooking spray, saute the apple, mushrooms and onion in oil until tender. Remove from the heat; stir in the spinach, lemon juice, lemon peel, 1/4 teaspoon salt and nutmeg.

- Make a lengthwise slit down the center of each tenderloin to within 1/2 in. of bottom. Open tenderloins so they lie flat; cover with plastic wrap. Flatten to 1/4-in. thickness. Remove plastic; sprinkle turkey with pepper and remaining salt.

- Spread spinach mixture over tenderloins to within 1 in. of edges. Roll up jelly-roll style, starting with a short side; tie with kitchen string. Place egg and bread crumbs in separate shallow bowls. Dip roulades in egg, then roll in crumbs.

- Place in an 11-in. x 7-in. baking pan coated with cooking spray. Bake, uncovered, at 375° for 40-45 minutes or until a meat thermometer reads 170°. Let stand for 5 minutes before slicing.

YIELD: 8 servings.

NUTRITION FACTS: 1/2 roulade equals 184 calories, 4 g fat (1 g saturated fat), 82 mg cholesterol, 405 mg sodium, 9 g carbohydrate, 1 g fiber, 29 g protein. **DIABETIC EXCHANGES:** 3 lean meat, 1/2 starch.

187 CALORIES

broiled sirloin steaks

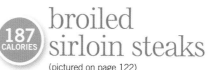

(pictured on page 122)

PREP/TOTAL TIME: 20 minutes

Karol Chandler-Ezell | NACOGDOCHES, TEXAS

A butcher gave me great advice on cooking different types of meat. Marinating and broiling work really well on very lean cuts like this. Let the steaks rest for a couple of minutes before serving to preserve moistness.

- 2 tablespoons lime juice
- 1 teaspoon onion powder
- 1 teaspoon garlic powder
- 1/4 teaspoon ground mustard
- 1/4 teaspoon dried oregano
- 1/4 teaspoon dried thyme
- 4 beef top sirloin steaks (5 ounces *each*)
- 1 cup sliced fresh mushrooms

- In a small bowl, combine the first six ingredients; rub over both sides of steaks.

- Broil 4 in. from the heat for 7 minutes. Turn steaks; top with mushrooms. Broil 7-8 minutes longer or until meat reaches desired doneness (for medium-rare, a meat thermometer should read 145°; medium, 160°; well-done, 170°) and mushrooms are tender.

YIELD: 4 servings.

NUTRITION FACTS: 1 steak with 3 tablespoons mushrooms equals 187 calories, 7 g fat (3 g saturated fat), 80 mg cholesterol, 60 mg sodium, 3 g carbohydrate, trace fiber, 28 g protein. **DIABETIC EXCHANGE:** 4 lean meat.

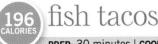

fish tacos

196 CALORIES

PREP: 30 minutes | **COOK:** 20 minutes

Lena Lim | SEATTLE, WASHINGTON

A cool sauce with just a bit of zing tops these crispy, spicy fish tacos. It's great, guilt-free and doesn't break the bank...always a good thing when you're a college kid!

- 3/4 cup fat-free sour cream
- 1 can (4 ounces) chopped green chilies
- 1 tablespoon fresh cilantro leaves
- 1 tablespoon lime juice
- 4 tilapia fillets (4 ounces *each*)
- 1/2 cup all-purpose flour
- 1 egg white, beaten
- 1/2 cup panko (Japanese) bread crumbs
- 1 tablespoon canola oil
- 1/2 teaspoon salt
- 1/2 teaspoon *each* white pepper, cayenne pepper and paprika
- 8 corn tortillas (6 inches), warmed
- 1 large tomato, finely chopped

- Place sour cream, chilies, cilantro and lime juice in a food processor; cover and process until blended. Set aside.

- Cut each tilapia fillet lengthwise into two portions. Place the flour, egg white and bread crumbs in separate shallow bowls. Dip tilapia in flour, then egg white, then crumbs.

- In a large skillet over medium heat, cook tilapia in oil in batches for 4-5 minutes on each side or until fish flakes easily with a fork. Combine the seasonings; sprinkle over fish.

- Place a portion of fish on each tortilla; top with about 2 tablespoons of sour cream mixture. Sprinkle with tomato.

YIELD: 8 servings.

NUTRITION FACTS: 1 taco equals 196 calories, 3 g fat (trace saturated fat), 31 mg cholesterol, 303 mg sodium, 26 g carbohydrate, 2 g fiber, 16 g protein. **DIABETIC EXCHANGES:** 2 lean meat, 1-1/2 starch, 1/2 fat.

dinners | 250 CALORIES OR LESS

Consider these typical dinner foods and their calorie counts to help you stay within a 500-calorie meal.

- **4 oz. ground sirloin beef patty,** 175 calories
- **4 oz. beef tenderloin,** 200 calories
- **2 skinless chicken drumsticks,** 154 calories
- **4 oz. boneless, skinless chicken breast,** 130 calories
- **4 oz. boneless, skinless turkey breast,** 118 calories
- **4 oz. ground turkey (93% lean),** 169 calories
- **4 oz. turkey Italian sausage,** 175 calories
- **4 oz. boneless pork loin chop,** 154 calories
- **4 oz. pork tenderloin,** 136 calories

- **4 oz. ham,** 145 calories
- **4 oz. fresh salmon,** 184 calories
- **4 oz. tilapia,** 134 calories
- **4 oz. cod,** 80 calories
- **4 oz. halibut,** 125 calories
- **4 oz. fresh tuna,** 124 calories
- **4 oz. orange roughy,** 87 calories
- **4 oz. scallops,** 111 calories
- **4 oz. shell-on shrimp,** 90 calories
- **4 oz. imitation crab,** 108 calories
- **4 oz. portobello mushroom cap,** 25 calories
- **1 Morningstar Farms® Garden Veggie Patties™ veggie burger,** 110 calories

- **1/2 cup cooked black beans,** 114 calories
- **1/2 cup cooked pinto beans,** 103 calories
- **1/2 cup cooked kidney beans,** 113 calories
- **1/2 cup spaghetti/marinara sauce,** 111 calories
- **1 cup cooked spaghetti,** 200 calories
- **1 cup cooked whole wheat spaghetti,** 176 calories
- **1/2 cup cooked white rice,** 103 calories
- **1/2 cup cooked brown rice,** 108 calories

Weight given is before cooking. For additional calorie calculations, check the Nutrition Facts labels on food packages.

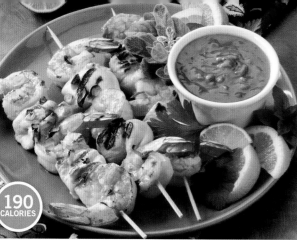

190 CALORIES

CHICKEN AND SHRIMP SATAY

chicken and shrimp satay

PREP: 20 minutes + marinating | **GRILL:** 10 minutes

Hannah Barringer | LOUDON, TENNESSEE

I lightened up a recipe that I found in a cookbook, and these grilled kabobs were the delicious result. The scrumptious dipping sauce is always a hit.

- 3/4 pound uncooked medium shrimp, peeled and deveined
- 3/4 pound chicken tenderloins, cut into 1-inch cubes
- 4 green onions, chopped
- 1 tablespoon butter
- 2 garlic cloves, minced
- 1 tablespoon minced fresh parsley
- 1/2 cup white wine *or* chicken broth
- 1 tablespoon lemon juice
- 1 tablespoon lime juice

SAUCE:
- 1/4 cup chopped onion
- 1 tablespoon butter
- 2/3 cup reduced-sodium chicken broth
- 1/4 cup reduced-fat chunky peanut butter
- 2-1/4 teaspoons brown sugar
- 3/4 teaspoon lemon juice
- 3/4 teaspoon lime juice
- 1/4 teaspoon salt
- 1/4 teaspoon *each* dried basil, thyme and rosemary, crushed
- 1/8 teaspoon cayenne pepper

- Thread shrimp and chicken onto 12 metal or soaked wooden skewers. Place in a large shallow dish; set aside.

- In a small skillet, saute green onions in butter until crisp-tender. Add garlic; cook 1 minute longer. Stir in the parsley, wine, lemon juice and lime juice. Remove from the heat; cool slightly. Pour over skewers and turn to coat. Cover and refrigerate for 4 hours, turning every 30 minutes.

- In a small saucepan, saute onion in butter. Add the remaining sauce ingredients; cook and stir until blended. Remove from the heat; set aside.

- Drain and discard marinade. Using long-handled tongs, moisten a paper towel with cooking oil and lightly coat the grill rack.

- Prepare grill for indirect heat, using a drip pan. Place skewers over drip pan and grill, covered, over indirect medium heat or broil 4 in. from the heat for 7 to 8 minutes, turning often. Brush with 1/4 cup sauce during the last minute of grilling. Serve with remaining sauce.

YIELD: 6 servings.

NUTRITION FACTS: 2 kabobs with 2 tablesspoons sauce equals 190 calories, 7 g fat (3 g saturated fat), 126 mg cholesterol, 339 mg sodium, 7 g carbohydrate, 1 g fiber, 25 g protein. **DIABETIC EXCHANGES:** 3 lean meat, 1 fat, 1/2 starch.

201 CALORIES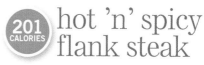

hot 'n' spicy flank steak

PREP: 15 minutes + marinating | **GRILL:** 15 minutes

Julee Wallberg | SALT LAKE CITY, UTAH

With its flavorful marinade, this flank steak makes a succulent meal. I received this recipe from a friend, and it's been a family favorite ever since.

- 3 tablespoons brown sugar
- 3 tablespoons red wine vinegar
- 3 tablespoons sherry *or* reduced-sodium chicken broth
- 3 tablespoons reduced-sodium soy sauce
- 1 tablespoon canola oil
- 1-1/2 teaspoons crushed red pepper flakes
- 1-1/2 teaspoons paprika
- 1-1/2 teaspoons chili powder

I have lost over 100 pounds in the last year and a half by making a lifestyle change! I bake or grill my meat and eat very little red meat. We eat turkey, chicken and salmon burgers. —**Laura Davis**

1-1/2 teaspoons Worcestershire sauce

3/4 teaspoon seasoned salt

3/4 teaspoon garlic powder

3/4 teaspoon dried parsley flakes

1 beef flank steak (1-1/2 pounds)

- In a small bowl, combine the first 12 ingredients. Pour 1/3 cup marinade into a large resealable plastic bag; add steak. Seal bag and turn to coat; refrigerate for 1-3 hours. Cover and refrigerate remaining marinade for basting.

- Using long-handled tongs, moisten a paper towel with cooking oil and lightly coat the grill rack. Grill steak, uncovered, over medium heat or broil 4 in. from the heat for 6-8 minutes on each side or until meat reaches desired doneness (for medium-rare, a meat thermometer should read 145°; medium, 160°; well-done, 170°), basting frequently with remaining marinade. Thinly slice steak across the grain.

YIELD: 6 servings.

NUTRITION FACTS: 3 ounces cooked beef equals 201 calories, 9 g fat (4 g saturated fat), 54 mg cholesterol, 326 mg sodium, 5 g carbohydrate, trace fiber, 22 g protein. **DIABETIC EXCHANGE:** 3 lean meat.

zesty horseradish meat loaf

PREP: 15 minutes I **BAKE:** 45 minutes + standing

Nancy Zimmerman I CAPE MAY COURT HOUSE, NEW JERSEY
This is a tasty, zippy meat loaf. Make sandwiches out of the leftovers and get double duty out of this delicious meat loaf with a kick.

4 slices whole wheat bread, crumbled

1/4 cup fat-free milk

1/2 cup finely chopped celery

1/4 cup finely chopped onion

1/4 cup prepared horseradish

2 tablespoons Dijon mustard

2 tablespoons chili sauce

1 egg, lightly beaten

1-1/2 teaspoons Worcestershire sauce

1/2 teaspoon salt

1/4 teaspoon pepper

1-1/2 pounds lean ground beef (90% lean)

1/2 cup ketchup

- In a large bowl, soak bread in milk for 5 minutes. Drain and discard milk. Stir in the celery, onion, horseradish, mustard, chili sauce, egg, Worcestershire sauce, salt and pepper. Crumble beef over mixture and mix well.

- Shape into a loaf in an 11-in. x 7-in. baking dish coated with cooking spray. Spread top with ketchup. Bake at 350° for 45-55 minutes or until no pink remains and a meat thermometer reads 160°. Let stand for 10 minutes before cutting.

YIELD: 8 servings.

NUTRITION FACTS: 1 slice equals 207 calories, 8 g fat (3 g saturated fat), 79 mg cholesterol, 640 mg sodium, 14 g carbohydrate, 1 g fiber, 19 g protein. **DIABETIC EXCHANGES:** 2 lean meat, 1 starch, 1/2 fat.

ZESTY HORSERADISH MEAT LOAF

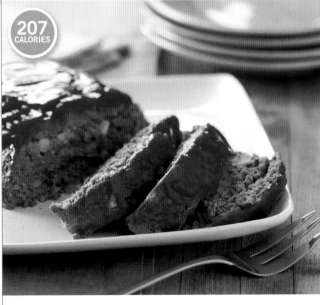

207 CALORIES

214 CALORIES

STUFFED STEAK SPIRALS

stuffed steak spirals

PREP: 35 minutes | **BAKE:** 30 minutes + standing

Margaret Pache | MESA, ARIZONA

When looking for an extra-special entree to serve guests, I rely on this impressive and appealing recipe. Tender and swirled with tangy tomato stuffing, it's a sensational way to showcase flank steak.

- 1/4 cup chopped sun-dried tomatoes (not packed in oil)
- 1/2 cup boiling water
- 1/2 cup grated Parmesan cheese
- 1/4 cup minced fresh parsley
-   1 tablespoon prepared horseradish, drained
-   1 to 1-1/2 teaspoons coarsely ground pepper
-   1 beef flank steak (1-1/2 pounds)
-   2 teaspoons canola oil

- Place tomatoes in a small bowl; add water. Cover and let stand for 5 minutes; drain. Stir in the cheese, parsley, horseradish and pepper; set aside.

- Cut steak horizontally from a long side to within 1/2 in. of opposite side. Open meat so it lies flat; cover with plastic wrap. Flatten to 1/4-in. thickness. Remove plastic; spoon tomato mixture over meat to within 1/2 in. of edges. Roll up tightly jelly-roll style, starting with a long side. Tie with kitchen string.

- Line a shallow roasting pan with heavy-duty foil; coat the foil with cooking spray. In a large nonstick skillet coated with cooking spray, brown meat in oil on all sides. Place in prepared pan.

- Bake, uncovered, at 400° for 30-40 minutes or until meat reaches desired doneness (for medium-rare, a meat thermometer should read 145°; medium, 160°; well-done, 170°). Let stand for 10-15 minutes. Remove string and cut into slices.

YIELD: 6 servings.

NUTRITION FACTS: 3 ounces cooked beef equals 214 calories, 12 g fat (5 g saturated fat), 53 mg cholesterol, 229 mg sodium, 2 g carbohydrate, 1 g fiber, 22 g protein. **DIABETIC EXCHANGES:** 3 lean meat, 1 fat.

basil tuna steaks

PREP/TOTAL TIME: 20 minutes

Linda McLyman | SYRACUSE, NEW YORK

One of my favorite creations is this five-ingredient recipe. Tuna is delicious and can be grilled in no time.

-     6 tuna steaks (6 ounces *each*)
- 4-1/2 teaspoons olive oil
-     3 tablespoons minced fresh basil
-   3/4 teaspoon salt
-   1/4 teaspoon pepper

- Drizzle both sides of tuna steaks with oil. Sprinkle with the basil, salt and pepper.

- Using long-handled tongs, moisten a paper towel with cooking oil and lightly coat the grill rack. Grill tuna, covered, over medium heat or broil 4 in. from the heat for 4-5 minutes on each side for medium-rare or until slightly pink in the center.

YIELD: 6 servings.

NUTRITION FACTS: 1 tuna steak equals 214 calories, 5 g fat (1 g saturated fat), 77 mg cholesterol, 358 mg sodium, trace carbohydrate, trace fiber, 40 g protein. **DIABETIC EXCHANGES:** 5 lean meat, 1 fat.

BASIL TUNA STEAKS

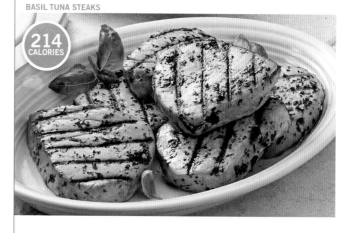

214 CALORIES

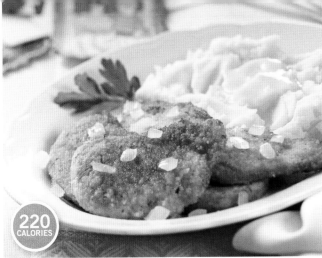

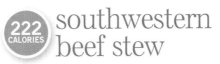

PARMESAN PORK MEDALLIONS

220 CALORIES

parmesan pork medallions

PREP/TOTAL TIME: 20 minutes

Angela Ciocca | SALTSBURG, PENNSYLVANIA

I was so happy to find this recipe. I have served it countless times for family and friends. It takes very little prep time and adapts easily to serve any number.

- 1/2 pound pork tenderloin
- 2 tablespoons seasoned bread crumbs
- 1 tablespoon grated Parmesan cheese
- 1/4 teaspoon salt

Dash pepper

- 2 teaspoons canola oil
- 1/4 cup chopped onion
- 1 garlic clove, minced

- Cut pork into four slices; flatten to 1/4-in. thickness. In a large resealable plastic bag, combine the bread crumbs, cheese, salt and pepper. Add pork, one slice at a time, and shake to coat.

- In a large skillet over medium heat, cook pork in oil for 2-3 minutes on each side or until meat is no longer pink. Remove and keep warm.

- Add onion to the pan; cook and stir until tender. Add garlic, cook 1 minute longer. Serve with pork.

YIELD: 2 servings.

NUTRITION FACTS: 2 medallions equals 220 calories, 9 g fat (2 g saturated fat), 65 mg cholesterol, 487 mg sodium, 8 g carbohydrate, 1 g fiber, 25 g protein. **DIABETIC EXCHANGES:** 3 lean meat, 1 fat, 1/2 starch.

222 CALORIES

southwestern beef stew

PREP: 10 minutes | **COOK:** 1-3/4 hours

Betty Jean Howard | PRINEVILLE, OREGON

This hearty stew is oh-so-tasty, with a good variety of vegetables and a spicy seasoning blend. My husband and I enjoy if often. It's the perfect way to warm up a cool evening. Sometimes I add a can of chopped green chilies for a little more heat.

- 1-1/2 pounds beef top round steak, cut into 1/2-inch cubes
- 1 can (14-1/2 ounces) beef broth
- 1 cup cubed peeled potatoes
- 1 cup sliced carrots
- 1 cup chopped onion
- 1/4 cup chopped sweet red pepepr
- 1 jalapeno pepper, seeded and chopped
- 1 garlic clove, minced
- 1-1/2 teaspoons chili powder
- 1/2 teaspoon salt
- 1 can (14-1/2 ounces) diced tomatoes, undrained
- 2 tablespoons all-purpose flour
- 2 tablespoons water
- 2 tablespoons minced fresh cilantro

- In a Dutch oven coated with cooking spray, brown meat on all sides over medium-high heat. Add the broth, potatoes, carrots, onion, red pepper, jalapeno, garlic, chili powder and salt. Bring to a boil. Reduce heat; cover and simmer for 30 minutes or until potatoes and carrots are tender. Add tomatoes; cover and cook 1 hour longer or until meat is tender.

- Combine flour and water until smooth; stir into pot. Stir in cilantro. Bring to a boil; cook and stir for 2 minutes or until thickened.

YIELD: 6 servings.

EDITOR'S NOTE: We recommend wearing disposable gloves when cutting hot peppers. Avoid touching your face.

NUTRITION FACTS: 1 cup equals 222 calories, 6 g fat (2 g saturated fat), 72 mg cholesterol, 600 mg sodium, 16 g carbohydrate, 3 g fiber, 26 g protein. **DIABETIC EXCHANGES:** 3 lean meat, 2 vegetable, 1/2 starch.

I signed up up for a 90-day fitness boot camp. This step may have saved my life. I started exercising every single day and making even healthier food choices.
— **Tryna Rhodes, Colorado**

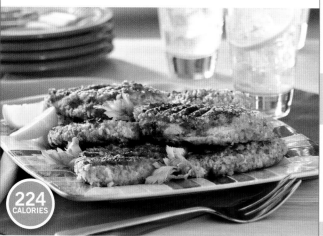

224 CALORIES

GRILLED BREADED CHICKEN

grilled breaded chicken

PREP: 15 minutes + marinating I **GRILL:** 10 minutes

Kristy McClellan I MORGAN, UTAH

When I got married, my husband's aunt gave us all of her favorite recipes. This chicken dish was one of them that we really enjoy.

- 1 cup (8 ounces) reduced-fat sour cream
- 1/4 cup lemon juice
- 4 teaspoons Worcestershire sauce
- 2 teaspoons paprika
- 1 teaspoon celery salt
- 1/8 teaspoon garlic powder
- 8 boneless skinless chicken breast halves (4 ounces *each*)
- 2 cups crushed seasoned stuffing

Refrigerated butter-flavored spray

- In a large resealable plastic bag, combine the first six ingredients; add chicken. Seal bag and turn to coat; refrigerate for up to 4 hours.

- Using long-handled tongs, moisten a paper towel with cooking oil and lightly coat the grill rack. Drain and discard marinade. Coat both sides of chicken with stuffing crumbs; spritz with butter-flavored spray.

- Grill chicken, covered, over medium heat or broil 4 in. from the heat for 4-7 minutes on each side or until a meat thermometer reads 170°.

YIELD: 8 servings.

NUTRITION FACTS: 1 chicken breast half equals 224 calories, 5 g fat (2 g saturated fat), 75 mg cholesterol, 419 mg sodium, 12 g carbohydrate, 0.55 g fiber, 30 g protein. **DIABETIC EXCHANGES:** 3 lean meat, 1 starch.

blue cheese-topped steaks

PREP/TOTAL TIME: 30 minutes

Tiffany Vancil I SAN DIEGO, CALIFORNIA

Steaks are lightly crusted with blue cheese and bread crumbs. They're special enough for holiday dining.

- 2 tablespoons crumbled blue cheese
- 4-1/2 teaspoons dry bread crumbs
- 4-1/2 teaspoons minced fresh parsley
- 4-1/2 teaspoons minced chives

Dash pepper

- 4 beef tenderloin steaks (4 ounces *each*)
- 1-1/2 teaspoons butter
- 1 tablespoon all-purpose flour
- 1/2 cup reduced-sodium beef broth
- 1 tablespoon Madeira wine
- 1/8 teaspoon browning sauce, optional

- In a small bowl, combine the blue cheese, bread crumbs, parsley, chives and pepper. Press onto one side of each steak.

- In a large nonstick skillet coated with cooking spray, cook steaks over medium-high heat for 2 minutes on each side. Transfer to a 15-in. x 10-in. x 1-in. baking pan coated with cooking spray.

- Bake at 350° for 6-8 minutes or until meat reaches desired doneness (for medium-rare, a meat thermometer should read 145°; medium, 160°; well-done, 170°).

- Meanwhile, in a small saucepan, melt butter. Whisk in flour until smooth. Gradually whisk in broth and wine. Bring to a boil; cook and stir for 2 minutes or until thickened. Stir in browning sauce if desired. Serve with steaks.

YIELD: 4 servings.

NUTRITION FACTS: 1 steak equals 228 calories, 11 g fat (5 g saturated fat), 78 mg cholesterol, 197 mg sodium, 4 g carbohydrate, trace fiber, 26 g protein. **DIABETIC EXCHANGE:** 3 lean meat, 1-1/2 fat, 1/2 fat-free milk.

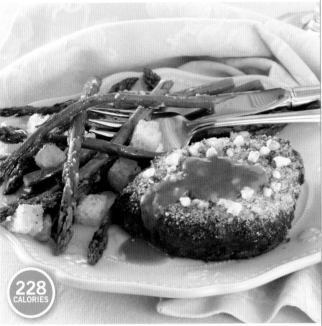

228 CALORIES

BLUE CHEESE-TOPPED STEAKS

homemade spaghetti sauce

PREP: 40 minutes I **COOK:** 50 minutes

Laurinda Johnston I BELCHERTOWN, MASSACHUSETTS
Lean turkey sausage links spice up this hearty sauce that turns pasta into a splendid main dish. I blend a cup of the sauce for my young son, so there are no chunks of vegetables, and he loves it.

- 4 celery ribs, chopped
- 1 large onion, chopped
- 1 large green pepper, chopped
- 2-1/2 cups water, *divided*
- 3 Italian turkey sausage links (4 ounces *each*), casings removed
- 1 can (29 ounces) tomato sauce
- 1 can (28 ounces) diced tomatoes, undrained
- 3 cans (6 ounces *each*) tomato paste
- 1/2 cup minced fresh parsley
- 5 to 6 garlic cloves, minced
- 3 teaspoons Italian seasoning
- 1 teaspoon sugar
- 1/8 teaspoon salt
- 1/8 teaspoon pepper
- 6 cups hot cooked spaghetti

Shredded Parmesan cheese, optional

- In a Dutch oven, combine the celery, onion, green pepper and 1 cup water. Bring to a boil. Reduce heat to medium; cook, uncovered, for 10-12 minutes or until vegetables are tender and water is reduced.

- Crumble sausage over vegetable mixture; cook until meat is no longer pink. Stir in the tomato sauce, tomatoes, tomato paste, parsley, garlic, Italian seasoning, sugar, salt, pepper and remaining water.

- Bring to a boil. Reduce heat; simmer, uncovered, for 45-50 minutes, stirring occasionally. Serve with spaghetti. Garnish with cheese if desired.

YIELD: 12 servings.

NUTRITION FACTS: 1 cup sauce with 1/2 cup spaghetti (calculated without Parmesan cheese) equals 230 calories, 3 g fat (1 g saturated fat), 15 mg cholesterol, 645 mg sodium, 40 g carbohydrate, 6 g fiber, 12 g protein. **DIABETIC EXCHANGE:** 2 starch, 2 vegetable, 1 lean meat.

HOMEMADE SPAGHETTI SAUCE

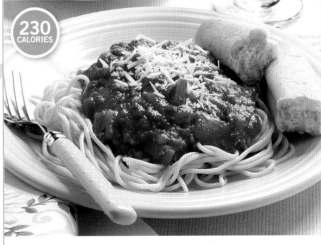

230 CALORIES

251-350 calories

- In the same skillet, saute pepper in oil until crisp-tender. Add garlic; cook 1 minute longer. Stir in the tomatoes, olives, basil, pepper flakes, salt and reserved sausage. Drain pasta. Stir into skillet and heat through. Sprinkle with cheese.

YIELD: 6 servings.

NUTRITION FACTS: 1-3/4 cups equals 249 calories, 9 g fat (2 g saturated fat), 24 mg cholesterol, 480 mg sodium, 32 g carbohydrate, 3 g fiber, 12 g protein. **DIABETIC EXCHANGES:** 2 starch, 1 medium-fat meat, 1/2 fat.

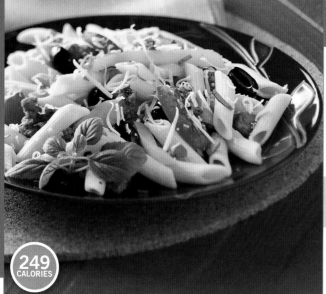

249 CALORIES

TURKEY PASTA TOSS

turkey pasta toss

PREP: 15 minutes I **COOK:** 20 minutes

Heather Savage I CORYDON, INDIANA

This recipe is one of our family's favorites. I served it once for a church supper, and it was a big hit there, too! Make a complete meal by adding salad and some bread. The pasta dish has wonderfully fresh flavor and is so simple to put together.

- 3 cups uncooked penne pasta
- 2 Italian turkey sausage links, casings removed
- 1 large sweet yellow pepper, cut into 1/2-inch strips
- 1 tablespoon olive oil
- 6 garlic cloves, minced
- 4 plum tomatoes, cut into 1-inch chunks
- 20 pitted ripe olives, halved
- 1/4 cup minced fresh basil
- 1/4 teaspoon crushed red pepper flakes
- 1/4 teaspoon salt
- 1/4 cup shredded Romano cheese

- Cook pasta according to package directions. Meanwhile, crumble sausage into a large skillet. Cook over medium heat until meat is no longer pink; drain and keep warm.

252 CALORIES

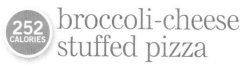

broccoli-cheese stuffed pizza

PREP: 30 minutes + rising I **BAKE:** 20 minutes

Gloria Vallieres I SHORTSVILLE, NEW YORK

I know you'll enjoy this gooey pizza pocket! The filling is very rich and resembles broccoli lasagna. The from-scratch dough gives it irresistible taste that's bound to be popular wherever you serve it.

- 2 packages (1/4 ounce *each*) active dry yeast
- 1-1/2 cups warm water (110° to 115°)
- 5 tablespoons canola oil, *divided*
- 2 teaspoons salt
- 4-1/2 to 5 cups all-purpose flour
- 1 carton (15 ounces) ricotta cheese
- 1/2 teaspoon garlic powder
- 1/2 teaspoon dried oregano
- 2 cups (8 ounces) shredded part-skim mozzarella cheese
- 4 cups frozen broccoli florets, cooked and drained
- 1 jar (4 ounces) sliced mushrooms, drained

- In a large bowl, dissolve yeast in warm water. Add 4 tablespoons oil, salt and enough flour to form a soft dough. Turn onto a floured surface; knead until smooth and elastic, about 6-8 minutes. Place in a greased bowl, turning once to grease top. Cover and let rise in a warm place until doubled, about 1 hour.

- Punch dough down. Turn onto a lightly floured surface, knead for 10 minutes. Divide in half. Roll each portion into a 15-in. x 10-in. rectangle; transfer each to a greased 15-in. x 10-in. x 1-in. baking pan. Cover and let rise until doubled, about 30 minutes.

- Brush one rectangle with remaining oil. Spread with ricotta cheese. Sprinkle with garlic powder and oregano. Layer with mozzarella cheese, broccoli and mushrooms. Invert remaining rectangle over filling; pinch the edges to seal.

- Bake at 400° for 20-30 minutes or until golden brown.

YIELD: 16 servings.

NUTRITION FACTS: 1 piece equals 252 calories, 10 g fat (4 g saturated fat), 22 mg cholesterol, 415 mg sodium, 30 g carbohydrate, 2 g fiber, 10 g protein. **DIABETIC EXCHANGES:** 2 starch, 1 medium-fat meat.

spanish fish

PREP: 10 minutes | **BAKE:** 40 minutes

Pix Stidham | EXETER, CALIFORNIA

These flaky fish fillets get plenty of garden flavor from onions and tomato, plus a little zip from cayenne pepper. This recipe is a particular favorite of my family because the fish doesn't get dry. It stays moist and delicious prepared this way.

1	tablespoon olive oil
1	large onion, thinly sliced
2	tablespoons diced pimientos
6	sea bass *or* halibut fillets (6 ounces *each*)
1-1/4	teaspoons salt
1/4	teaspoon ground mace
1/4	teaspoon cayenne pepper
1/4	teaspoon pepper
6	thick slices tomato
1	cup thinly sliced fresh mushrooms
3	tablespoons chopped green onions
1/4	cup white wine *or* chicken broth
4-1/2	teaspoons butter
1/2	cup dry bread crumbs

- Brush oil onto bottom of a 13-in. x 9-in. baking dish; top with onion and pimientos. Pat fish dry. Combine the salt, mace, cayenne and pepper; sprinkle over both sides of fish.

- Arrange fish over onions and pimientos. Top each fillet with a tomato slice; sprinkle with mushrooms and green onions. Pour wine over fish and vegetables.

- In a nonstick skillet, melt butter; add bread crumbs. Cook and stir over medium heat until lightly browned. Sprinkle over fish.

- Cover and bake at 350° for 20 minutes. Uncover and bake 20-25 minutes longer or until fish flakes easily with a fork.

YIELD: 6 servings.

NUTRITION FACTS: 1 serving equals 251 calories, 9 g fat (3 g saturated fat), 68 mg cholesterol, 700 mg sodium, 11 g carbohydrate, 1 g fiber, 29 g protein. **DIABETIC EXCHANGES:** 4 lean meat, 1 vegetable, 1 fat, 1/2 starch.

SPANISH FISH

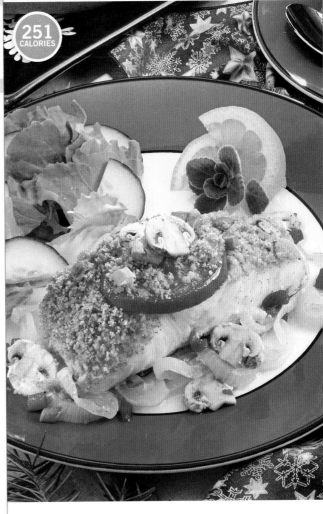

251 CALORIES

254 CALORIES

LITTLE KICK JALAPENO BURGERS

little kick jalapeno burgers

PREP/TOTAL TIME: 20 minutes

Dawn Dhooghe | CONCORD, NORTH CAROLINA
I lightened up one of my husband's favorite burger recipes, and although the original was good, we actually like this sandwich better!

> 2 jalapeno peppers, seeded and finely chopped
> 2 tablespoons minced fresh cilantro
> 2 tablespoons light beer *or* water
> 2 dashes hot pepper sauce
> 2 garlic cloves, minced
> 1/2 teaspoon pepper
> 1/4 teaspoon salt
> 1/4 teaspoon cayenne pepper
> 1 pound extra-lean ground turkey
> 3 slices pepper Jack cheese, cut in half
> 6 dinner rolls, split
> 6 tablespoons salsa
> 6 tablespoons fat-free sour cream
> 6 tablespoons shredded lettuce

- In a large bowl, combine the first eight ingredients. Crumble turkey over mixture and mix well. Shape into six patties.

- Using long-handled tongs, moisten a paper towel with cooking oil and lightly coat the grill rack. Grill burgers, covered, over medium heat or broil 4 in. from the heat for 2-3 minutes on each side or until a meat thermometer reads 165° and juices run clear.

- Top with cheese; cover and grill 1-2 minutes longer or until cheese is melted. Serve on rolls with salsa, sour cream and lettuce.

YIELD: 6 servings.

EDITOR'S NOTE: We recommend wearing disposable gloves when cutting hot peppers. Avoid touching your face.

NUTRITION FACTS: 1 burger equals 254 calories, 7 g fat (2 g saturated fat), 61 mg cholesterol, 471 mg sodium, 23 g carbohydrate, 2 g fiber, 26 g protein. **DIABETIC EXCHANGES:** 3 lean meat, 1-1/2 starch.

braised southwest beef roast

PREP: 20 minutes | **COOK:** 2 hours 25 minutes

Cathy Sestak | FREEBURG, MISSOURI
Seasoned with Southwestern flair, this lean beef roast is fork-tender and gets a little kick from salsa.

> 1-1/2 teaspoons chili powder
> 1 teaspoon ground cumin
> 1/2 teaspoon garlic powder
> 1/2 teaspoon dried oregano
> 1 beef eye of round roast (2 pounds)
> 1 tablespoon canola oil

BRAISED SOUTHWEST BEEF ROAST

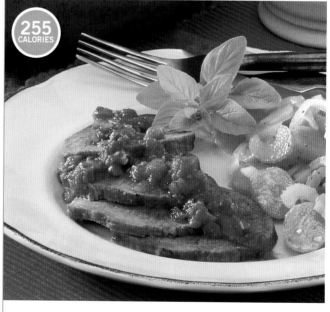

255 CALORIES

> **My son and I** have both lost weight by making simple choices. When we go out to eat, we cut everything in half and then we have a meal for the next day. It works, and we don't feel like we are missing out on anything. —**Sherry Morris**

1 cup reduced-sodium beef broth

1-1/4 cups salsa

1/4 cup water

1 bay leaf

- In a small bowl, combine the chili powder, cumin, garlic powder and oregano; rub over roast. In a Dutch oven, brown meat in oil. Remove from the pan.

- Gradually add broth, stirring to loosen any browned bits from pan. Stir in salsa, water and bay leaf; return meat to pan. Bring to a boil. Reduce heat; cover and simmer for 2-1/4 to 2-1/2 hours or until meat is fork-tender.

- Set meat aside and keep warm. Bring pan juices to a boil. Cook, uncovered, for 10-15 minutes or until sauce is reduced to about 1-1/3 cups; skim fat. Discard bay leaf. Serve sauce with meat.

YIELD: 5 servings.

NUTRITION FACTS: 5 ounces cooked beef with 1/4 cup sauce equals 255 calories, 9 g fat (2 g saturated fat), 84 mg cholesterol, 451 mg sodium, 3 g carbohydrate, 2 g fiber, 35 g protein. **DIABETIC EXCHANGES:** 5 lean meat, 1/2 fat.

pork tenderloin with horseradish sauce

PREP: 15 minutes I **BAKE:** 30 minutes + standing

Ann Berger Osowski I ORANGE CITY, FLORIDA
This delicious pairing receives rave reviews each time I make them, and I've shared the recipe with numerous fans. It's very versatile. The pork can be served hot or cold, and the sauce can also be used as a zesty dip for fresh veggies.

1/2 teaspoon steak seasoning

1/2 teaspoon dried rosemary, crushed

1/2 teaspoon dried thyme

1 pork tenderloin (3/4 pound)

2 garlic cloves, peeled and quartered

1 teaspoon balsamic vinegar

1 teaspoon olive oil

for 2

HORSERADISH SAUCE:

2 tablespoons fat-free mayonnaise

2 tablespoons reduced-fat sour cream

1 teaspoon prepared horseradish

1/8 teaspoon grated lemon peel

Dash salt and pepper

- In a small bowl, combine the steak seasoning, rosemary and thyme; rub over meat. Using the point of a sharp knife, make eight slits in the tenderloin. Insert garlic into slits. Place meat on a rack in a foil-lined shallow roasting pan. Drizzle with vinegar and oil.

- Bake, uncovered, at 350° for 30-40 minutes or until a meat thermometer reads 160°. Let stand for 10 minutes before slicing. Meanwhile, combine the sauce ingredients; chill until serving. Serve with pork.

YIELD: 2 servings.

EDITOR'S NOTE: This recipe was tested with McCormick's Montreal Steak Seasoning. Look for it in the spice aisle.

NUTRITION FACTS: 4 ounces cooked pork with 2 tablespoons sauce equals 258 calories, 10 g fat (3 g saturated fat), 101 mg cholesterol, 450 mg sodium, 5 g carbohydrate, 1 g fiber, 35 g protein. **DIABETIC EXCHANGES:** 5 lean meat, 1 fat.

PORK TENDERLOIN WITH HORSERADISH SAUCE

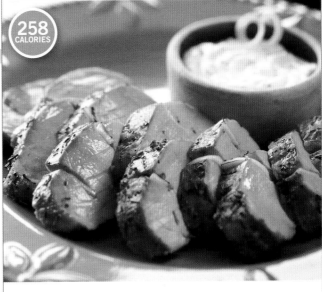

258 CALORIES

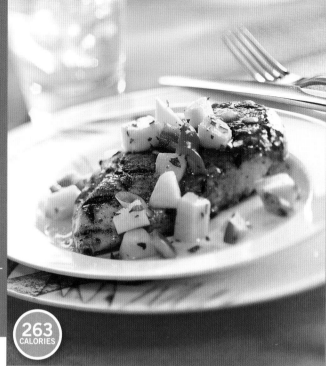

263 CALORIES

SPICY CHICKEN BREASTS WITH PEPPER PEACH RELISH

- Combine the salt, cinnamon, cloves and nutmeg; rub over chicken. In a small bowl, combine the glaze ingredients; set aside. In a small bowl, combine the peaches, peppers, onion, mint and 2 tablespoons glaze; set aside.

- Using long-handled tongs, moisten a paper towel with cooking oil and lightly coat the grill rack. Grill chicken, covered, over medium heat or broil 4 in. from the heat for 6-8 minutes on each side or until a meat thermometer reads 170°, basting frequently with reserved glaze. Serve with reserved relish.

YIELD: 4 servings.

NUTRITION FACTS: 1 chicken breast half with 1/2 cup relish equals 263 calories, 4 g fat (1 g saturated fat), 94 mg cholesterol, 379 mg sodium, 20 g carbohydrate, 2 g fiber, 35 g protein. **DIABETIC EXCHANGES:** 5 lean meat, 1 starch, 1/2 fruit.

spicy chicken breasts with pepper peach relish

PREP: 20 minutes | **GRILL:** 15 minutes

Roxanne Chan | ALBANY, CALIFORNIA

This summery entree is simply packed with the good-for-your-eyes vitamins found in both peaches and peppers.

- 1/2 teaspoon salt
- 1/4 teaspoon *each* ground cinnamon, cloves and nutmeg
- 4 boneless skinless chicken breast halves (6 ounces *each*)

GLAZE:
- 1/4 cup peach preserves
- 2 tablespoons lemon juice
- 1/4 teaspoon crushed red pepper flakes

RELISH:
- 2 medium peaches, peeled and finely chopped
- 1/3 cup finely chopped sweet red pepper
- 1/3 cup finely chopped green pepper
- 1 green onion, finely chopped
- 2 tablespoons minced fresh mint

turkey with apple slices

PREP/TOTAL TIME: 15 minutes

Mary Lou Wayman | SALT LAKE CITY, UTAH

Any day can be "Turkey Day" when you make this smaller-scale main course. The moist tenderloins and tangy apple glaze offer the goodness of turkey without a refrigerator full of leftovers.

- 2 turkey breast tenderloins (about 4 ounces *each*)
- 1 tablespoon butter
- 2 tablespoons maple syrup
- 1 tablespoon cider vinegar
- 1 teaspoon Dijon mustard
- 1/2 teaspoon chicken bouillon granules
- 1 medium tart apple, sliced

for 2

- In a skillet, cook turkey in butter over medium heat for 4-5 minutes on each side or until the juices run clear. Remove from the skillet; cover and keep warm.

- In the same skillet, combine the syrup, vinegar, mustard and bouillon. Add the apple; cook and stir over medium heat for 2-3 minutes or until apple is tender. Serve with turkey.

YIELD: 2 servings.

NUTRITION FACTS: 1 serving equals 263 calories, 7 g fat (4 g saturated fat), 71 mg cholesterol, 374 mg sodium, 24 g carbohydrate, 2 g fiber, 27 g protein. **DIABETIC EXCHANGES:** 3 lean meat, 1-1/2 fat, 1 starch, 1/2 fruit.

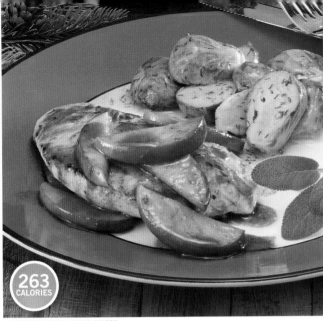

TURKEY WITH APPLE SLICES

- In a large bowl, beat the cream cheese, water, cumin, pepper and salt until smooth. Stir in the onion, turkey and pecans.

- Spoon 1/3 cup turkey mixture down the center of each tortilla. Roll up and place seam side down in a 13-in. x 9-in. baking dish coated with cooking spray. Combine the soup, sour cream, milk and chilies; pour over enchiladas.

- Cover and bake at 350° for 40 minutes. Uncover; sprinkle with cheese. Bake 5 minutes longer or until heated through and cheese is melted. Sprinkle with cilantro.

YIELD: 12 servings.

NUTRITION FACTS: 1 enchilada equals 263 calories, 10 g fat (4 g saturated fat), 59 mg cholesterol, 472 mg sodium, 20 g carbohydrate, 1 g fiber, 22 g protein. **DIABETIC EXCHANGES:** 2 lean meat, 1-1/2 starch, 1/2 fat.

TURKEY PECAN ENCHILADAS

turkey pecan enchiladas

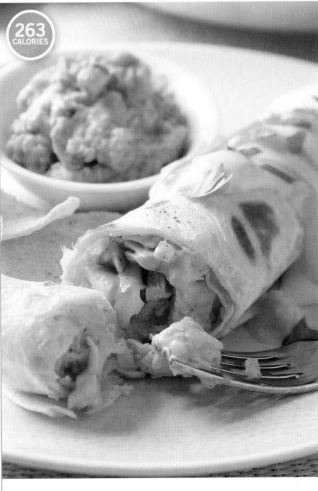

PREP: 25 minutes I **BAKE:** 45 minutes

Cathy Huppe I GEORGETOWN, MASSACHUSETTS
I got this recipe from a friend, and I've often served it at church potlucks. I always go home with an empty dish! It's nice because it's creamy, just a little spicy and unusual.

- 1 medium onion, chopped
- 4 ounces reduced-fat cream cheese
- 1 tablespoon water
- 1 teaspoon ground cumin
- 1/4 teaspoon pepper
- 1/8 teaspoon salt
- 4 cups cubed cooked turkey breast
- 1/4 cup chopped pecans, toasted
- 12 flour tortillas (6 inches), warmed
- 1 can (10-3/4 ounces) reduced-fat reduced-sodium condensed cream of chicken soup, undiluted
- 1 cup (8 ounces) reduced-fat sour cream
- 1 cup fat-free milk
- 2 tablespoons canned chopped green chilies
- 1/2 cup shredded reduced-fat cheddar cheese
- 2 tablespoons minced fresh cilantro

- In a nonstick skillet coated with cooking spray, cook and stir onion over medium heat until tender. Set aside.

> **By eating real and natural foods** and cutting out fake food products, my weight has been steadily going down while still eating lots of meals and snacks.
> —Wendy Steele Nichols

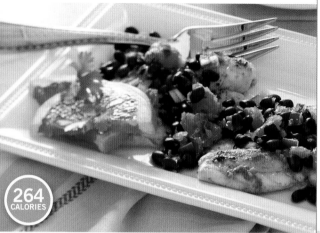

264 CALORIES

TILAPIA WITH GRAPEFRUIT SALSA

tilapia with grapefruit salsa

PREP: 25 minutes + marinating | **COOK:** 10 minutes

Emily Seefeldt | RED WING, MINNESOTA

Not only is tilapia a mild and attractive fish, but it's a snap to find these fillets in single-serving sizes. This satisfying favorite is draped in a spicy grapefruit and black bean salsa.

for 2

- 1/3 cup unsweetened grapefruit juice
- 1/2 teaspoon ground cumin
- 1 garlic clove, minced
- 1/4 teaspoon grated grapefruit peel
- 1/8 teaspoon salt
- 1/8 teaspoon pepper
- Dash to 1/8 teaspoon cayenne pepper
- 2 tilapia fillets (6 ounces *each*)
- 1/2 cup canned black beans, rinsed and drained
- 1/3 cup chopped pink grapefruit sections
- 1/4 cup chopped red onion
- 1 tablespoon minced fresh cilantro
- 1 to 2 teaspoons chopped jalapeno pepper
- 2 teaspoons butter

- For marinade, in a small bowl, combine the first seven ingredients. Set aside 1 tablespoon. Place tilapia in a large resealable plastic bag; add remaining marinade. Seal bag and turn to coat. Refrigerate for 1 hour.

- For the salsa, in a small bowl, combine the beans, grapefruit sections, onion, cilantro, jalapeno and reserved marinade. Cover and refrigerate until serving.

- Drain and discard marinade. In a small skillet over medium heat, cook tilapia in butter for 4-5 minutes on each side or until fish flakes easily with a fork. Serve with salsa.

YIELD: 2 servings.

EDITOR'S NOTE: We recommend wearing disposable gloves when cutting hot peppers. Avoid touching your face.

NUTRITION FACTS: 1 fillet with 1/2 cup salsa equals 264 calories, 6 g fat (3 g saturated fat), 93 mg cholesterol, 369 mg sodium, 18 g carbohydrate, 4 g fiber, 36 g protein. **DIABETIC EXCHANGES:** 5 lean meat, 1 starch, 1 fat.

mexican meat loaf

PREP: 20 minutes | **BAKE:** 45 minutes

Connie Staal | GREENBRIER, ARKANSAS

This great-tasting meat loaf is sure to be requested often by your family. It's moist, tender and chock-full of green pepper, onion and zesty tomato flavor! Why not make two? Tuck one in the oven for supper, the other in the freezer for another night.

- 1 large onion, chopped
- 1 medium green pepper, chopped
- 2 teaspoons olive oil
- 2 garlic cloves, minced
- 3/4 cup dry bread crumbs
- 3/4 cup shredded reduced-fat cheddar cheese
- 1/2 cup tomato sauce
- 1/4 cup fat-free plain yogurt
- 2 tablespoons minced fresh parsley
- 2 teaspoons Worcestershire sauce
- 1 teaspoon chili powder

3/4   pound lean ground turkey
1/4   pound lean ground beef (90% lean)
TOPPING:
1/4   cup tomato sauce
1   teaspoon Worcestershire sauce
1/2   teaspoon chili powder
1/4   cup shredded reduced-fat cheddar cheese

- In a large nonstick skillet, saute onion and green pepper in oil until tender. Add the garlic; cook 1 minute longer.

- Transfer to a large bowl. Stir in the bread crumbs, cheese, tomato sauce, yogurt, parsley, Worcestershire sauce and chili powder. Crumble turkey and beef over mixture and mix well.

- Shape into a loaf. Place in an 11-in. x 7-in. baking dish coated with cooking spray. Bake, uncovered, at 350° for 25 minutes; drain.

- Combine the tomato sauce, Worcestershire sauce and chili powder; spread over meat loaf. Bake for 15 minutes or until no pink remains and a meat thermometer reads 165°. Sprinkle with cheese; bake 2-3 minutes longer or until cheese is melted.

YIELD: 6 servings.

NUTRITION FACTS: 1 slice equals 266 calories, 13 g fat (5 g saturated fat), 70 mg cholesterol, 480 mg sodium, 17 g carbohydrate, 2 g fiber, 21 g protein. **DIABETIC EXCHANGES:** 3 lean meat, 1 starch, 1/2 fat.

MEXICAN MEAT LOAF

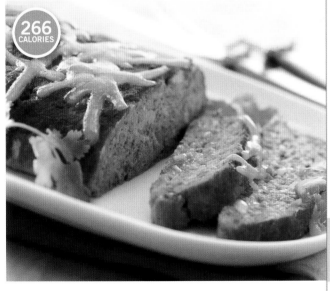

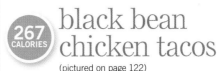

black bean chicken tacos

267 CALORIES

(pictured on page 122)

PREP: 30 minutes | **COOK:** 15 minutes

Teresa Obsnuk | BERWYN, ILLINOIS
Friends and family are delighted when I present my homemade tortillas so they can assemble these tasty tacos.

2   cups all-purpose flour
1   teaspoon baking powder
1-1/2   teaspoons ground cumin, *divided*
2   tablespoons shortening
1/2   cup plus 1 tablespoon warm water
1   pound boneless skinless chicken breast, cubed
2   cups salsa
1   can (15 ounces) black beans, rinsed and drained
1   teaspoon onion powder
1/2   teaspoon chili powder

Shredded lettuce, shredded cheddar cheese, chopped ripe olives, sour cream and additional salsa, optional

- In a large bowl, combine the flour, baking powder and 1/2 teaspoon cumin. Cut in shortening until crumbly. Stir in enough water for mixture to form a ball. Knead on a floured surface for 1 minute. Cover and let rest for 20 minutes.

- Meanwhile, in a large skillet, combine the chicken, salsa, beans, onion powder, chili powder and remaining cumin. Cover and simmer for 15-20 minutes or until chicken juices run clear.

- For tortillas, divide dough into eight balls; roll each ball into an 8-in. circle. In an ungreased skillet, cook tortillas, one at a time, until lightly browned, about 30 seconds on each side.

- Layer between pieces of waxed paper or paper towel; keep warm. Spoon chicken mixture over half of each tortilla and fold over. Serve with lettuce, cheese, olives, sour cream and salsa if desired.

YIELD: 8 servings.

NUTRITION FACTS: 1 taco (calculated without optional toppings) equals 267 calories, 5 g fat (1 g saturated fat), 31 mg cholesterol, 421 mg sodium, 36 g carbohydrate, 3 g fiber, 17 g protein. **DIABETIC EXCHANGES:** 2 starch, 2 lean meat, 1 vegetable, 1 fat.

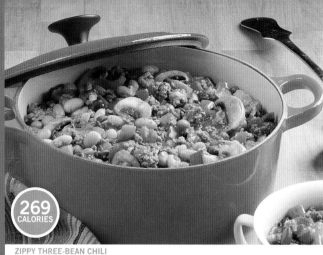

269 CALORIES

ZIPPY THREE-BEAN CHILI

zippy three-bean chili

PREP: 10 minutes I **COOK:** 1 hour 20 minutes

Agnes Hamilton I SCOTT DEPOT, WEST VIRGINIA

I use convenient canned pinto, black and great northern beans to speed up preparation of my hearty chili. This one-dish meal has a stew-like consistency and a peppy Tex-Mex flavor.

- 1 pound lean ground beef (90% lean)
- 1/2 cup chopped onion
- 1 cup chopped fresh mushrooms
- 1/2 cup chopped green pepper
- 1/2 cup chopped sweet red pepper
- 1 garlic clove, minced
- 2 cups water
- 1 can (14-1/2 ounces) diced tomatoes and green chilies, undrained
- 1 envelope reduced-sodium taco seasoning
- 1 can (15-1/2 ounces) great northern beans, rinsed and drained
- 1 can (15 ounces) black beans, rinsed and drained
- 1 can (15 ounces) pinto beans, rinsed and drained
- 8 tablespoons shredded reduced-fat cheddar cheese, *divided*

- In a large saucepan, cook beef and onion over medium heat until meat is no longer pink; drain. Add mushrooms and peppers; cook and stir 3 minutes longer or until vegetables are almost tender. Add garlic; cook 1 minute longer. Stir in the water, tomatoes and taco seasoning.

- Bring to boil. Reduce heat; simmer, uncovered, for 30 minutes. Add beans; simmer 30 minutes longer. Sprinkle each serving with 1 tablespoon cheese.

YIELD: 8 servings (2 quarts).

NUTRITION FACTS: 1 cup equals 269 calories, 6 g fat (3 g saturated fat), 33 mg cholesterol, 738 mg sodium, 32 g carbohydrate, 8 g fiber, 21 g protein. **DIABETIC EXCHANGES:** 2 lean meat, 1-1/2 starch, 1 vegetable.

irish stew

PREP: 15 minutes I **COOK:** 1-1/2 hours

Taste of Home Test Kitchen

Lamb is a great source of protein and adds a delicious flavor to this classic stew. If you can't find it at your grocery store, try using beef stew meat instead.

- 1/3 cup plus 1 tablespoon all-purpose flour, *divided*
- 1-1/2 pounds lamb stew meat, cut into 1-inch cubes
- 3 tablespoons olive oil, *divided*
- 3 medium onions, chopped
- 3 garlic cloves, minced
- 4 cups reduced-sodium beef broth
- 2 medium potatoes, peeled and cubed
- 4 medium carrots, cut into 1-inch pieces
- 1 cup frozen peas
- 1 teaspoon salt
- 1 teaspoon dried thyme
- 1/2 teaspoon pepper
- 1/2 teaspoon Worcestershire sauce
- 2 tablespoons water

- Place 1/3 cup flour in a large resealable plastic bag. Add lamb, a few pieces at a time, and shake to coat.

- In a Dutch oven, brown lamb in batches in 2 tablespoons oil. Remove and set aside. In the same pan, saute onions in remaining oil until tender. Add garlic; cook 1 minute longer.

- Add broth, stirring to loosen browned bits from pan. Return lamb to the pan. Bring to a boil. Reduce heat; cover and simmer for 1 hour or until meat is tender.

- Add potatoes and carrots; cover and cook for 20 minutes. Stir in peas; cook until vegetables are tender.

- Add seasonings and Worcestershire sauce. Combine remaining flour with water until smooth; stir into the stew. Bring to a boil; cook and stir for 2 minutes or until thickened.

YIELD: 8 servings (2-1/2 quarts).

NUTRITION FACTS: 1-1/4 cup equals 271 calories, 10 g fat (2 g saturated fat), 58 mg cholesterol, 618 mg sodium, 24 g carbohydrate, 4 g fiber, 22 g protein. **DIABETIC EXCHANGES:** 2 lean meat, 1 starch, 1 vegetable, 1 fat.

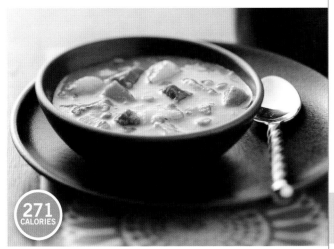

(271 CALORIES)

IRISH STEW

zucchini lasagna

PREP: 45 minutes I **BAKE:** 30 minutes + standing

Ruth Vaught I TEMPE, ARIZONA

Give this meatless lasagna a try. It's chock-full of healthful zucchini and delicious cheeses. You'll be surprised a good serving comes in under 300 calories!

- 6 lasagna noodles
- 1 medium onion, chopped
- 2 teaspoons olive oil
- 2 garlic cloves, minced
- 2 cups water
- 2 cans (6 ounces *each*) tomato paste
- 2-1/2 teaspoons *each* dried thyme, basil and oregano
- 3/4 teaspoon salt
- 3 medium zucchini, thinly sliced
- 1 egg, lightly beaten
- 1 carton (15 ounces) part-skim ricotta cheese
- 2 cups (8 ounces) shredded part-skim mozzarella cheese
- 1/4 cup grated Parmesan cheese

- Cook noodles according to package directions. Meanwhile, in a large nonstick skillet, saute onion in oil until tender. Add garlic; cook 1 minute longer. Stir in the water, tomato paste and seasonings. Bring to a boil. Reduce heat; cover and simmer for 10 minutes.

- Place zucchini in a large saucepan; add 1/2 in. water. Bring to a boil. Reduce heat; cover and cook for 5 minutes. Drain and set aside. In a small bowl, combine egg and ricotta cheese.

- Drain noodles. Place 1/2 cup tomato sauce in a 13-in. x 9-in. baking dish coated with cooking spray; top with three noodles. Layer with half of the ricotta mixture and zucchini. Top with half of the remaining tomato sauce and 1 cup mozzarella cheese. Repeat layers.

- Cover and bake at 375° for 25 minutes. Uncover; sprinkle with Parmesan cheese. Bake 5-10 minutes longer or until bubbly. Let stand for 10 minutes before cutting.

YIELD: 9 servings.

NUTRITION FACTS: 1 piece equals 272 calories, 10 g fat (6 g saturated fat), 55 mg cholesterol, 454 mg sodium, 28 g carbohydrate, 4 g fiber, 18 g protein. **DIABETIC EXCHANGES:** 2 medium-fat meat, 2 vegetable, 1 starch.

ZUCCHINI LASAGNA

(272 CALORIES)

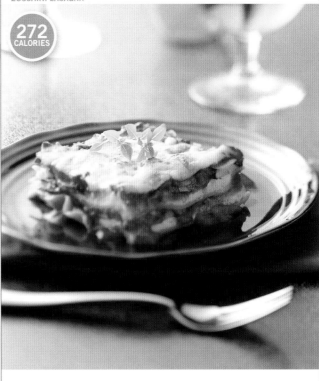

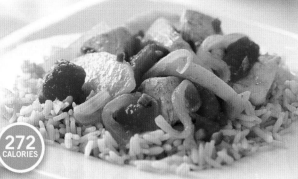

272 CALORIES

CURRIED CHICKEN WITH APPLES

curried chicken with apples

PREP: 20 minutes | **COOK:** 30 minutes

Janice Fakhoury | RALEIGH, NORTH CAROLINA

I got this flavorful recipe from an Indian neighbor who even showed me how to prepare it. This entree is one that people remember.

- 1 pound boneless skinless chicken breasts, cut into 1-inch cubes
- 1 large sweet onion, halved and sliced
- 2 tablespoons canola oil
- 3 garlic cloves, minced
- 2 medium tart apples, peeled and sliced
- 1/2 cup water
- 1 teaspoon salt
- 1 teaspoon ground coriander
- 1 teaspoon minced fresh gingerroot
- 1/2 teaspoon ground turmeric
- 1/4 teaspoon cayenne pepper
- 1 can (14-1/2 ounces) diced tomatoes, drained
- 1 jalapeno pepper, seeded and chopped
- 2 tablespoons minced fresh cilantro

Hot cooked rice

- In a large skillet or wok, stir-fry chicken and onion in oil until onion is tender. Add garlic; cook 1 minute longer. Stir in the apples, water and seasonings.

- Bring to a boil. Reduce heat; simmer, uncovered, for 12-15 minutes or until chicken is no longer pink, stirring occasionally. Stir in the tomatoes, jalapeno and cilantro; heat through. Serve with rice.

YIELD: 4 servings.

EDITOR'S NOTE: We recommend wearing disposable gloves when cutting hot peppers. Avoid touching your face.

NUTRITION FACTS: 1-1/2 cups (calculated without rice) equals 272 calories, 10 g fat (2 g saturated fat), 63 mg cholesterol, 779 mg sodium, 22 g carbohydrate, 4 g fiber, 25 g protein. **DIABETIC EXCHANGES:** 3 lean meat, 1-1/2 fat, 1 starch, 1/2 fruit.

274 CALORIES

cheesy rigatoni bake

(pictured on page 122)

PREP: 20 minutes | **BAKE:** 30 minutes

Nancy Urbine | LANCASTER, OHIO

This is a family favorite. One of our four children always asks for it as a birthday dinner.

- 1 package (16 ounces) rigatoni *or* large tube pasta
- 2 tablespoons butter
- 1/4 cup all-purpose flour
- 1/2 teaspoon salt
- 2 cups milk
- 1/4 cup water
- 4 eggs, lightly beaten
- 2 cans (8 ounces *each*) tomato sauce
- 2 cups (8 ounces) shredded part-skim mozzarella cheese, *divided*
- 1/4 cup grated Parmesan cheese, *divided*

- Cook pasta according to package directions. Meanwhile, in a small saucepan, melt butter. Stir in flour and salt until smooth; gradually add milk and water. Bring to a boil; cook and stir for 2 minutes or until thickened.

- Drain pasta; place in a large bowl. Add eggs. Spoon into two greased 8-in. square baking dishes. Layer each with one can of tomato sauce, half the mozzarella cheese and half the white sauce. Sprinkle each with half the Parmesan cheese.

- Cover and freeze one casserole for up to 3 months. Bake second casserole, uncovered, at 375° for 30-35 minutes or until a meat thermometer reads 160°.

- To use frozen casserole: Thaw in the refrigerator overnight. Cover and bake at 375° for 40 minutes. Uncover; bake 7-10 minutes longer or until a meat thermometer reads 160°.

YIELD: 2 casseroles (6 servings each).

NUTRITION FACTS: 1-1/3 cups equals 274 calories, 9 g fat (5 g saturated fat), 92 mg cholesterol, 440 mg sodium, 34 g carbohydrate, 2 g fiber, 15 g protein. **DIABETIC EXCHANGES:** 2 starch, 1 medium-fat meat, 1/2 fat.

Using a food journal actually helped me to start losing weight. I was completely honest while logging my foods, so it was easy to see when I first started why I wasn't losing any weight. I love to eat out, and the ice cream or extra piece of bread really adds up. —Airus Copeland

277 CALORIES | french cheeseburger loaf

PREP: 25 minutes | **BAKE:** 25 minutes

Nancy Daugherty | CORTLAND, OHIO

Once you prepare this impressive-looking sandwich, you'll never look at refrigerated bread dough the same.

- 3/4 pound lean ground beef (90% lean)
- 1/2 cup chopped sweet onion
- 1 small green pepper, chopped
- 2 garlic cloves, minced
- 2 tablespoons all-purpose flour
- 2 tablespoons Dijon mustard
- 1 tablespoon ketchup
- 1 tube (11 ounces) refrigerated crusty French loaf
- 4 slices reduced-fat process American cheese product
- 1 egg white, lightly beaten
- 3 tablespoons shredded Parmesan cheese

- In a large skillet, cook the beef, onion and pepper over medium heat until meat is no longer pink. Add garlic; cook 1 minute longer. Stir in the flour, mustard and ketchup; set aside.

- Unroll dough starting at the seam. Pat into a 14-in. x 12-in. rectangle. Spoon meat mixture lengthwise down the center of the dough; top with cheese slices. Bring long sides of dough to the center over filling; pinch seams to seal.

- Place seam side down on a baking sheet coated with cooking spray. Brush with egg white. Sprinkle with Parmesan cheese.

- With a sharp knife, cut diagonal slits in top of loaf. Bake at 350° for 25-30 minutes or until golden. Serve warm.

YIELD: 6 servings.

NUTRITION FACTS: 1 slice equals 277 calories, 7 g fat (3 g saturated fat), 33 mg cholesterol, 697 mg sodium, 30 g carbohydrate, 1 g fiber, 21 g protein. **DIABETIC EXCHANGES:** 2 starch, 2 lean meat.

282 CALORIES | enchilada lasagna

PREP: 25 minutes | **BAKE:** 20 minutes + standing

Julie Cackler | WEST DES MOINES, IOWA

Everyone who tries this dish tells me they love the familiar Southwestern taste.

- 1 pound lean ground turkey
- 1 large onion, chopped
- 1 large green pepper, chopped
- 1 small sweet red pepper, chopped
- 1 package (8 ounces) fat-free cream cheese
- 1 teaspoon chili powder
- 1 can (10 ounces) enchilada sauce
- 6 whole wheat flour tortillas (8 inches)
- 1 cup (4 ounces) shredded reduced-fat Mexican cheese blend

Salsa and sour cream, optional

- In a large skillet, cook the turkey, onion and peppers over medium heat until meat is no longer pink; drain. Stir in cream cheese and chili powder.

- Pour enchilada sauce in a shallow bowl. Dip tortillas in sauce to coat. Place two tortillas in a 13-in. x 9-in. baking dish coated with cooking spray; spread with half of the turkey mixture. Sprinkle with 1/3 cup cheese. Repeat layers. Top with remaining tortillas and cheese.

- Cover and freeze for up to 3 months or bake, uncovered, at 400° for 20-25 minutes or until heated through and cheese is melted. Let stand for 10 minutes before serving. Serve with salsa and sour cream if desired.

- To use frozen lasagna: Thaw in the refrigerator overnight. Remove from the refrigerator 30 minutes before baking. Bake as directed.

YIELD: 8 servings.

NUTRITION FACTS: 1 piece (calculated without salsa and sour cream) equals 282 calories, 11 g fat (3 g saturated fat), 57 mg cholesterol, 697 mg sodium, 27 g carbohydrate, 2 g fiber, 22 g protein. **DIABETIC EXCHANGES:** 2 lean meat, 1-1/2 starch, 1 fat.

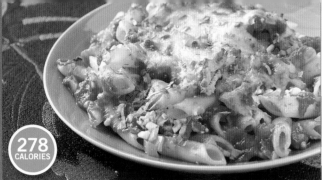

278 CALORIES

BAKED MOSTACCIOLI

baked mostaccioli

PREP: 35 minutes | **BAKE:** 30 minutes

Donna Ebert | RICHFIELD, WISCONSIN
I often serve this for dinner parties and always get tons of compliments.

8	ounces uncooked mostaccioli
1/2	pound lean ground turkey
1	small onion, chopped
1	can (14-1/2 ounces) diced tomatoes, undrained
1	can (6 ounces) tomato paste
1/3	cup water
1	teaspoon dried oregano
1/2	teaspoon salt
1/8	teaspoon pepper
2	cups (16 ounces) fat-free cottage cheese
1	teaspoon dried marjoram
1-1/2	cups (6 ounces) shredded part-skim mozzarella cheese
1/4	cup grated Parmesan cheese

- Cook mostaccioli according to package directions. Meanwhile, in a large saucepan, cook turkey and onion over medium heat until meat is no longer pink; drain.

- Stir in the tomatoes, tomato paste, water, oregano, salt and pepper. Bring to a boil. Reduce heat; cover and simmer for 15 minutes.

- In a small bowl, combine cottage cheese and marjoram; set aside. Drain mostaccioli.

- Spread 1/2 cup meat sauce into an 11-in. x 7-in. baking dish coated with cooking spray. Layer with half of the mostaccioli, meat sauce and mozzarella cheese. Top with cottage cheese mixture. Layer with remaining mostaccioli, meat sauce and mozzarella cheese. Sprinkle with Parmesan cheese (dish will be full).

- Bake, uncovered, at 350° for 30-40 minutes or until bubbly and heated through.

YIELD: 6 servings.

NUTRITION FACTS: 1-1/3 cups equals 278 calories, 7 g fat (3 g saturated fat), 39 mg cholesterol, 607 mg sodium, 32 g carbohydrate, 3 g fiber, 23 g protein. **DIABETIC EXCHANGES:** 3 medium-fat meat, 2 vegetable, 1-1/2 starch.

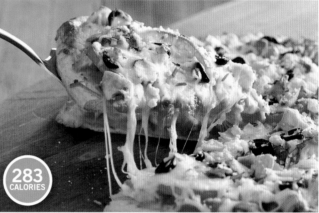

283 CALORIES

GRILLED ARTICHOKE-MUSHROOM PIZZA

grilled artichoke-mushroom pizza

PREP: 20 minutes | **GRILL:** 15 minutes

Brenda Waters | CLARKESVILLE, GEORGIA
This is one of our favorite summer meals because we're always looking for something new to grill.

1	prebaked 12-inch pizza crust
1/2	teaspoon olive oil
2/3	cup tomato and basil spaghetti sauce
2	plum tomatoes, sliced
1/4	cup sliced fresh mushrooms
1/4	cup water-packed artichoke hearts, rinsed, drained and chopped
2	tablespoons sliced ripe olives, optional
1	cup (4 ounces) shredded part-skim mozzarella cheese
1/2	cup crumbled tomato and basil feta cheese
1-1/2	teaspoons minced fresh basil *or* 1/2 teaspoon dried basil
1-1/2	teaspoons minced fresh rosemary *or* 1/2 teaspoon dried rosemary, crushed
1-1/2	teaspoons minced chives

- Brush crust with oil. Spread spaghetti sauce over crust to within 1 in. of edges. Top with tomatoes, mushrooms, artichokes and olives if desired. Sprinkle with cheeses.

- Prepare grill for indirect heat. Grill, covered, over medium indirect heat for 12-15 minutes or until cheese is melted and crust is lightly browned. Sprinkle with herbs during the last 5 minutes of cooking. Let stand for 5 minutes before slicing.

YIELD: 6 servings.

NUTRITION FACTS: 1 slice (calculated without olives) equals 283 calories, 10 g fat (3 g saturated fat), 17 mg cholesterol, 712 mg sodium, 34 g carbohydrate, 1 g fiber, 14 g protein. **DIABETIC EXCHANGES:** 2 starch, 1-1/2 fat, 1 lean meat.

- Drain and discard marinade from tenderloin. Place tenderloin over vegetables. Bake, uncovered, for 30-45 minutes or until meat reaches desired doneness (for medium-rare, a meat thermometer should read 145°; medium, 160°; well-done, 170°).

- Remove beef and let stand for 15 minutes. Check vegetables for doneness. If additional roasting is needed, cover with foil and bake for 10-15 minutes or until tender. Slice beef and serve with vegetables.

YIELD: 8-10 servings.

NUTRITION FACTS: 1 serving equals 283 calories, 8 g fat (3 g saturated fat), 60 mg cholesterol, 627 mg sodium, 16 g carbohydrate, 3 g fiber, 33 g protein. **DIABETIC EXCHANGES:** 4 lean meat, 1 vegetable, 1/2 starch.

BEEF TENDERLOIN WITH ROASTED VEGETABLES

beef tenderloin with roasted vegetables

PREP: 20 minutes + marinating I **BAKE:** 1 hour + standing

Janet Singleton I BELLEVUE, OHIO
I like this recipe because it includes a side dish of roasted potatoes, brussels sprouts and carrots. I make this entree for celebrations throughout the year.

1	beef tenderloin roast (3 pounds)
3/4	cup dry white wine *or* beef broth
3/4	cup reduced-sodium soy sauce
4	teaspoons minced fresh rosemary
4	teaspoons Dijon mustard
1-1/2	teaspoons ground mustard
3	garlic cloves, peeled and sliced
1	pound Yukon Gold potatoes, cut into 1-inch wedges
1	pound brussels sprouts, halved
1	pound fresh baby carrots

- Place tenderloin in a large resealable plastic bag. Combine the wine, soy sauce, rosemary, Dijon mustard, ground mustard and garlic. Pour half of the marinade over tenderloin; seal bag and turn to coat. Refrigerate for 4-12 hours, turning several times. Cover and refrigerate remaining marinade.

- Place the potatoes, brussels sprouts and carrots in a greased 13-in. x 9-in. baking dish; add reserved marinade and toss to coat. Cover and bake at 425° for 30 minutes; stir.

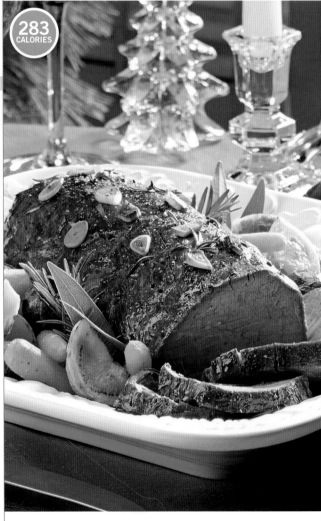

283 CALORIES

I lost 100 pounds in one year by cutting out all sugar, eating smaller portions and switching to whole grains. —Darcie MacLachlan

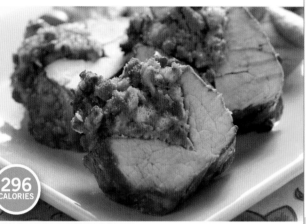

296 CALORIES

GRILLED STUFFED PORK TENDERLOIN

grilled stuffed pork tenderloin

PREP: 20 minutes + marinating | **GRILL:** 25 minutes

Bobbie Carr | LAKE OSWEGO, OREGON

We serve this stuffed tenderloin with a salad and a glass of wine. It's so good and easy you won't believe it.

- 2 pork tenderloins (3/4 pound *each*)
- 3/4 cup dry red wine *or* reduced-sodium beef broth
- 1/3 cup packed brown sugar
- 1/4 cup ketchup
- 2 tablespoons reduced-sodium soy sauce
- 2 garlic cloves, minced
- 1 teaspoon curry powder
- 1/2 teaspoon minced fresh gingerroot
- 1/4 teaspoon pepper
- 1-1/4 cups water
- 2 tablespoons butter
- 1 package (6 ounces) stuffing mix

- Cut a lengthwise slit down the center of each tenderloin to within 1/2 in. of bottom. In a large resealable plastic bag, combine the wine or broth, brown sugar, ketchup, soy sauce, garlic, curry, ginger and pepper; add pork. Seal bag and turn to coat; refrigerate for 2-3 hours.

- In a small saucepan, bring water and butter to a boil. Stir in stuffing mix. Remove from the heat; cover and let stand for 5 minutes. Cool.

- Drain and discard marinade. Open tenderloins so they lie flat; spread stuffing down the center of each. Close tenderloins; tie at 1-1/2-in. intervals with kitchen string.

- Using long-handled tongs, moisten a paper towel with cooking oil and lightly coat the grill rack. Prepare grill for indirect heat using a drip pan. Place pork over drip pan; grill pork, covered, over indirect medium-hot heat for 25-40 minutes or until a meat thermometer reads 160°. Let stand for 5 minutes before slicing.

YIELD: 6 servings.

NUTRITION FACTS: 1 serving equals 296 calories, 9 g fat (4 g saturated fat), 73 mg cholesterol, 678 mg sodium, 24 g carbohydrate, 1 g fiber, 27 g protein. **DIABETIC EXCHANGES:** 3 lean meat, 1-1/2 starch, 1 fat.

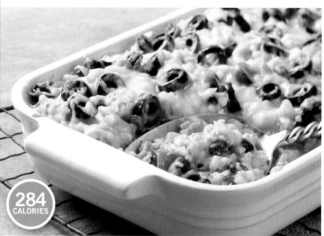

284 CALORIES

SOUTHWEST VEGETARIAN BAKE

southwest vegetarian bake

PREP: 40 minutes | **BAKE:** 35 minutes + standing

Patricia (Trish) Gale | MONTICELLO, ILLINOIS

Creamy and comforting, this hearty Southwestern specialty is perfect for chilly nights.

3/4 cup uncooked brown rice

1-1/2 cups water

1 can (15 ounces) black beans, rinsed and drained

1 can (11 ounces) Mexicorn, drained

1 can (10 ounces) diced tomatoes and green chilies

1 cup salsa

1 cup (8 ounces) reduced-fat sour cream

1 cup (4 ounces) shredded reduced-fat cheddar cheese

1/4 teaspoon pepper

1/2 cup chopped red onion

1 can (2-1/4 ounces) sliced ripe olives, drained

1 cup (4 ounces) shredded reduced-fat Mexican cheese blend

- In a large saucepan, bring rice and water to a boil. Reduce heat; cover and simmer for 35-40 minutes or until tender.

- In a bowl, combine the beans, Mexicorn, tomatoes, salsa, sour cream, cheddar cheese, pepper and rice. Transfer to a shallow 2-1/2-qt. baking dish coated with cooking spray. Sprinkle with onion and olives.

- Bake, uncovered, at 350° for 30 minutes. Sprinkle with Mexican cheese. Bake 5-10 minutes longer or until heated through and cheese is melted. Let stand for 10 minutes before serving.

YIELD: 8 servings.

NUTRITION FACTS: 1 cup equals 284 calories, 10 g fat (6 g saturated fat), 30 mg cholesterol, 879 mg sodium, 35 g carbohydrate, 6 g fiber, 15 g protein. **DIABETIC EXCHANGES:** 2 starch, 1 lean meat, 1 fat.

sirloin strips over rice

PREP: 15 minutes I **COOK:** 30 minutes

Karen Dunn I KANSAS CITY, MISSOURI

I found this recipe in a magazine some 20 years ago. Its great flavor and the fact that leftovers just get better have made it a family favorite!

1-1/2 pounds beef top sirloin steak, cut into thin strips

1 teaspoon salt

1/4 teaspoon pepper

2 teaspoons olive oil, *divided*

2 medium onions, thinly sliced

1 garlic clove, minced

1 can (14-1/2 ounces) diced tomatoes, undrained

1/2 cup reduced-sodium beef broth

1/3 cup dry red wine *or* additional reduced-sodium beef broth

1 bay leaf

1/2 teaspoon dried basil

1/2 teaspoon dried thyme

3 cups hot cooked rice

- Sprinkle beef strips with salt and pepper. In a large nonstick skillet coated with cooking spray, brown beef in 1 teaspoon oil. Remove and keep warm.

- In the same skillet, saute onions in remaining oil until tender. Add garlic; cook 1 minute longer. Stir in the tomatoes, broth, wine, bay leaf, basil and thyme. Bring to a boil. Reduce heat; simmer, uncovered, for 10 minutes.

- Return beef to the pan; cook for 2-4 minutes or until tender and mixture is heated through. Discard bay leaf. Serve with rice.

YIELD: 6 servings.

NUTRITION FACTS: 2/3 cup beef mixture with 1/2 cup rice equals 299 calories, 7 g fat (2 g saturated fat), 63 mg cholesterol, 567 mg sodium, 31 g carbohydrate, 3 g fiber, 25 g protein. **DIABETIC EXCHANGES:** 3 lean meat, 1-1/2 starch, 1 vegetable, 1/2 fat.

SIRLOIN STRIPS OVER RICE

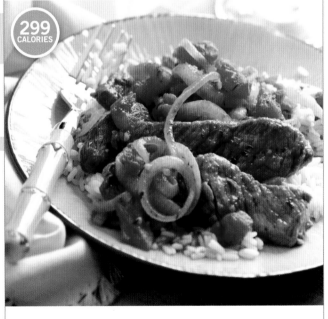

299 CALORIES

303 CALORIES

BROCCOLI-TURKEY CASSEROLE

broccoli-turkey casserole

PREP: 20 minutes I **BAKE:** 45 minutes

Kellie Mulleavy I LAMBERTVILLE, MICHIGAN

I have a lot of company at Thanksgiving, and I enjoy making new things for them. I came up with this recipe as a great way to use up the leftover turkey. Don't have any turkey leftovers? No problem; cooked chicken works well, too.

1-1/2 cups fat-free milk
   1 can (10-3/4 ounces) reduced-fat reduced-sodium condensed cream of chicken soup, undiluted
   1 carton (8 ounces) egg substitute
1/4 cup reduced-fat sour cream
1/2 teaspoon pepper
1/4 teaspoon poultry seasoning
1/8 teaspoon salt
2-1/2 cups cubed cooked turkey breast
   1 package (16 ounces) frozen chopped broccoli, thawed and drained
   2 cups seasoned stuffing cubes
   1 cup (4 ounces) shredded reduced-fat cheddar cheese, *divided*

- In a large bowl, combine the milk, soup, egg substitute, sour cream, pepper, poultry seasoning and salt. Stir in the turkey, broccoli, stuffing cubes and 3/4 cup cheese. Transfer to a 13-in. x 9-in. baking dish coated with cooking spray.

- Bake, uncovered, at 350° for 40 minutes. Sprinkle with remaining cheese. Bake 5-10 minutes longer or until

a knife inserted near the center comes out clean. Let stand for 5 minutes before serving.

YIELD: 6 servings.

NUTRITION FACTS: 1 serving equals 303 calories, 7 g fat (4 g saturated fat), 72 mg cholesterol, 762 mg sodium, 26 g carbohydrate, 3 g fiber, 33 g protein. **DIABETIC EXCHANGES:** 3 lean meat, 1-1/2 starch, 1 vegetable, 1 fat.

light chicken cordon bleu

PREP: 20 minutes I **BAKE:** 25 minutes

Shannon Strate I SALT LAKE CITY, UTAH

I love chicken cordon bleu, but since I watch my cholesterol, I can't afford to indulge in it often. Then I trimmed down a recipe that I received in my high school home economics class years ago, and now I'm satisfied. The creamy sauce makes it extra special.

   8 boneless skinless chicken breast halves (4 ounces *each*)
1/2 teaspoon pepper
   8 slices deli ham (1 ounce *each*)
1-1/2 cups (6 ounces) shredded part-skim mozzarella cheese
2/3 cup fat-free milk
   1 cup crushed cornflakes
   1 teaspoon paprika
1/2 teaspoon garlic powder
1/4 teaspoon salt
SAUCE:
   1 can (10-3/4 ounces) reduced-fat reduced-sodium condensed cream of chicken soup, undiluted
1/2 cup fat-free sour cream
   1 teaspoon lemon juice

- Flatten chicken to 1/4-in. thickness. Sprinkle with pepper; place a ham slice and 3 tablespoons of cheese down the center of each piece. Roll up and tuck in ends; secure with toothpicks. Pour milk into a shallow bowl. In another bowl, combine the cornflakes, paprika, garlic powder and salt. Dip chicken in milk, then roll in crumbs.

- Place in a 13-in. x 9-in. baking dish coated with cooking spray. Bake, uncovered, at 350° for 25-30 minutes or until meat is no longer pink. Meanwhile, in a small saucepan, whisk the soup, sour cream and lemon juice until blended; heat through. Discard toothpicks from chicken; serve with sauce.

YIELD: 8 servings.

NUTRITION FACTS: 1 chicken breast half with 2 tablespoons sauce equals 306 calories, 7 g fat (3 g saturated fat), 91 mg cholesterol, 990 mg sodium, 16 g carbohydrate, trace fiber, 41 g protein.

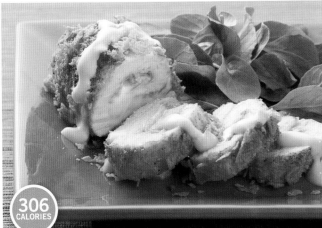

306 CALORIES

LIGHT CHICKEN CORDON BLEU

hungarian goulash

PREP: 15 minutes I **COOK:** 1 hour

Mary Smith I AURORA, NEW YORK

I enjoy preparing this traditional dish, featuring saucy round steak pieces, for a satisfying supper. My mother came to this country from Hungary and brought the recipe with her. I eat it with a lettuce salad full of cucumbers and tomatoes.

2	tablespoons all-purpose flour
1/8	teaspoon salt
1/8	teaspoon pepper
3/4	pound beef top round steak, cut into 1-inch cubes
1/2	cup coarsely chopped onion
1	teaspoon butter
1	teaspoon canola oil
1/2	cup reduced-sodium beef broth
1	tablespoon tomato paste
1	garlic clove, minced

for 2

1	teaspoon paprika
1/8	teaspoon dried marjoram
1/8	teaspoon caraway seeds
1/8	teaspoon lemon juice

Hot cooked noodles, optional

- In a large resealable plastic bag, combine the flour, salt and pepper. Add beef cubes and shake to coat.

- In a large skillet, cook beef and onion in butter and oil until onion is tender. Stir in broth, tomato paste, garlic, paprika, marjoram, caraway seeds and lemon juice. Bring to a boil. Reduce heat; cover and simmer for 1 to 1-1/2 hours or until meat is very tender.

- Serve over noodles if desired.

YIELD: 2 servings.

NUTRITION FACTS: 1 cup equals 310 calories, 10 g fat (3 g saturated fat), 102 mg cholesterol, 333 mg sodium, 13 g carbohydrate, 2 g fiber, 41 g protein. **DIABETIC EXCHANGES:** 5 lean meat, 1 starch, 1 fat.

HUNGARIAN GOULASH

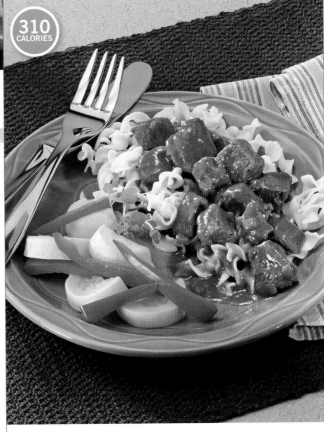

310 CALORIES

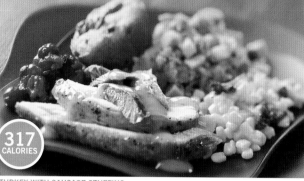

TURKEY WITH SAUSAGE STUFFING

turkey with sausage stuffing

PREP: 30 minutes | **BAKE:** 3 hours + standing

Alma Winberry | GREAT FALLS, MONTANA

My family is addicted to this stuffing and will have no other! It always turns out deliciously, so your guests are sure to be satisfied.

  2 pounds Italian turkey sausage links, casings removed
  6 cups chopped cabbage
  3 medium carrots, shredded
  2 celery ribs, chopped
1/3 cup chopped onion
  3 cups stuffing mix
  3 cups seasoned stuffing cubes
  1 cup reduced-sodium chicken broth
  6 tablespoons egg substitute
1/4 cup half-and-half cream
1/2 teaspoon poultry seasoning
1/2 teaspoon pepper
1/8 teaspoon salt
  1 turkey (12 pounds)

- In a large nonstick skillet coated with cooking spray, cook the sausage, cabbage, carrots, celery and onion over medium heat until meat is no longer pink and vegetables are tender.

- Transfer to a large bowl; stir in the stuffing mix, stuffing cubes, broth, egg substitute, cream, poultry seasoning, pepper and salt.

- Just before baking, loosely stuff turkey with 4 cups of stuffing. Place remaining stuffing in a 13-in. x 9-in. baking dish coated with cooking spray; refrigerate until ready to bake. Skewer turkey openings; tie drumsticks together.

- Place breast side up on a rack in a roasting pan. Bake, uncovered, at 325° for 3 to 3-1/2 hours or until a meat thermometer inserted in the thigh reads 180° for the turkey and 165° for the stuffing, basting occasionally with pan drippings. Cover loosely with foil if turkey browns too quickly.

- Cover and bake additional stuffing for 25-30 minutes. Uncover; bake 10 minutes longer or until lightly browned. Cover turkey and let stand for 20 minutes before removing stuffing and carving turkey.

YIELD: 24 servings (12 cups stuffing).

NUTRITION FACTS: 4 ounces cooked turkey (calculated without skin) with 1/2 cup stuffing equals 317 calories, 10 g fat (3 g saturated fat), 109 mg cholesterol, 568 mg sodium, 12 g carbohydrate, 1 g fiber, 41 g protein. **DIABETIC EXCHANGES:** 5 lean meat, 1 starch.

colorful beef stir-fry

PREP: 35 minutes + marinating | **COOK:** 15 minutes

Deb Blendermann | BOULDER, COLORADO

I really like the easy sesame-ginger marinade and the vibrant mix of vegetables.

1/4 cup reduced-sodium soy sauce
  1 tablespoon honey
  2 teaspoons sesame oil
  3 garlic cloves, minced
1/8 teaspoon ground ginger
1/2 pound boneless beef sirloin steak, thinly sliced
4-1/2 teaspoons cornstarch
1/2 cup reduced-sodium beef broth
1-1/2 teaspoons canola oil, *divided*
  1 small green pepper, cut into chunks
  1 small onion, cut into chunks
  1 medium carrot, julienned
1/4 cup sliced celery
  1 small zucchini, julienned
1/2 cup fresh snow peas
1/2 cup canned bean sprouts, rinsed and drained
Hot cooked rice *or* linguine, optional

- In a bowl, combine the first five ingredients. Place beef in a large resealable plastic bag; add half of the marinade. Seal bag and turn to coat; refrigerate for at least 2 hours. Cover and refrigerate remaining marinade.

- In a small bowl, combine cornstarch and broth until smooth. Stir in reserved marinade; set aside. Drain and discard marinade from beef. In a large nonstick skillet or wok coated with cooking spray, cook beef in 1 teaspoon oil until no longer pink; drain. Remove and keep warm.

- In the same pan, stir-fry green pepper and onion in remaining oil for 2 minutes. Add carrot and celery; stir-fry for 2-3 minutes. Add zucchini and snow peas; stir-fry for 1 minute. Add bean sprouts; cook 1 minute longer.

- Stir broth mixture and stir into vegetable mixture. Bring to a boil; cook and stir for 1-2 minutes or until thickened. Return beef to the pan; heat through. Serve over rice or linguine if desired.

YIELD: 4 cups.

NUTRITION FACTS: 1 cup (calculated without rice) equals 318 calories, 8 g fat (2 g saturated fat), 43 mg cholesterol, 542 mg sodium, 41 g carbohydrate, 4 g fiber, 21 g protein. **DIABETIC EXCHANGES:** 2 lean meat, 1 starch, 1/2 fat.

COLORFUL BEEF STIR-FRY

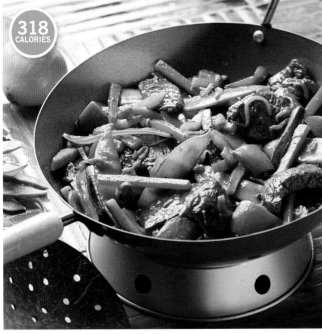

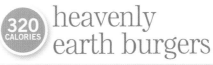 heavenly earth burgers

PREP: 25 minutes | **COOK:** 10 minutes

Wendy McGowan | FONTANA, CALIFORNIA
Packed with nutrition, these rice-and-bean patties make a fun and filling handheld entree. Fresh parsley and carrots add flecks of color, and sunflower kernels provide a touch of crunchiness.

- 1-1/2 cups cooked brown rice
- 1/2 cup finely chopped onion
- 1/4 cup sunflower kernels
- 1/4 cup seasoned bread crumbs
- 1/2 cup shredded carrot
- 3 tablespoons minced fresh parsley
- 2 tablespoons reduced-sodium soy sauce
- 1/2 teaspoon dried thyme
- 1 egg
- 1 egg white
- 1 cup garbanzo beans *or* chickpeas, rinsed and drained
- 1-1/2 teaspoons canola oil
- 6 whole wheat hamburger buns, split
- 6 lettuce leaves
- 6 slices tomato
- 6 slices onion

- In a large bowl, combine the first eight ingredients. In a food processor, combine the egg, egg white and garbanzo beans; cover and process until smooth. Stir into rice mixture. Shape into six patties.

- In a nonstick skillet coated with cooking spray, cook patties in oil for 5-6 minutes on each side or until lightly browned and crisp. Serve on buns with lettuce, tomato and onion.

YIELD: 6 servings.

NUTRITION FACTS: 1 burger equals 320 calories, 9 g fat (1 g saturated fat), 35 mg cholesterol, 634 mg sodium, 49 g carbohydrate, 6 g fiber, 11 g protein. **DIABETIC EXCHANGES:** 3 starch, 1 fat.

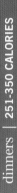

veggie cheese ravioli

PREP/TOTAL TIME: 20 minutes

Gertrudis Miller | EVANSVILLE, INDIANA
Have the best of both worlds with this easy weeknight dish. It tastes really light and refreshing, but the ravioli makes it hearty and filling.

- 1 package (9 ounces) refrigerated cheese ravioli
- 2 small zucchini, julienned
- 1 medium onion, chopped
- 1 can (14-1/2 ounces) diced tomatoes, undrained
- 2 tablespoons chopped ripe olives
- 3/4 teaspoon Italian seasoning
- 3 tablespoons shredded Parmesan cheese

- Cook ravioli according to package directions. Meanwhile, in a large nonstick skillet coated with cooking spray, cook and stir zucchini and onion until tender. Stir in the tomatoes, olives and Italian seasoning. Bring to a boil. Reduce heat; simmer, uncovered, for 5 minutes.

- Drain ravioli and add to the pan; stir gently to combine. Sprinkle with cheese.

YIELD: 3 servings.

NUTRITION FACTS: 1-1/2 cups equals 322 calories, 8 g fat (4 g saturated fat), 37 mg cholesterol, 649 mg sodium, 48 g carbohydrate, 6 g fiber, 17 g protein. **DIABETIC EXCHANGES:** 2 starch, 2 vegetable, 1 lean meat, 1 fat.

VEGGIE CHEESE RAVIOLI

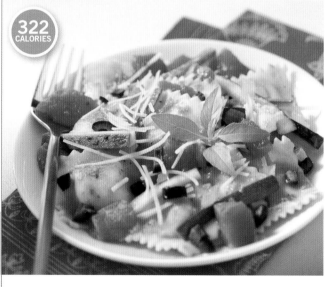

322 CALORIES

CREOLE CHICKEN

320 CALORIES

creole chicken

PREP: 15 minutes | **COOK:** 25 minutes

Susan Shields | ENGLEWOOD, FLORIDA
Chili powder lends just a hint of heat to this full-flavored and oh-so-easy chicken entree.

- 2 boneless skinless chicken breast halves (4 ounces *each*)
- 1 teaspoon canola oil
- 1 can (14-1/2 ounces) stewed tomatoes, cut up
- 1/3 cup julienned green pepper
- 1/4 cup chopped celery
- 1/4 cup sliced onion
- 1/2 to 1 teaspoon chili powder
- 1/2 teaspoon dried thyme
- 1/8 teaspoon pepper
- 1 cup hot cooked rice

for 2

- In a small nonstick skillet coated with cooking spray, cook chicken in oil over medium heat for 5-6 minutes on each side or a meat thermometer reads 170°. Remove and keep warm.

- In the same skillet, combine the tomatoes, green pepper, celery, onion, chili powder, thyme and pepper. Bring to a boil. Reduce heat; cover and simmer for 10 minutes or until vegetables are crisp-tender. Return chicken to pan; heat through. Serve with rice.

YIELD: 2 servings.

NUTRITION FACTS: 1 chicken breast half with 2/3 cup sauce and 1/2 cup rice equals 320 calories, 5 g fat (1 g saturated fat), 63 mg cholesterol, 447 mg sodium, 41 g carbohydrate, 3 g fiber, 27 g protein. **DIABETIC EXCHANGES:** 3 lean meat, 3 starch, 1/2 fat.

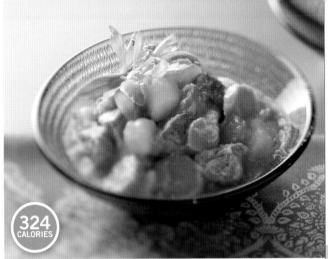

ALL-AMERICAN BEEF STEW

all-american beef stew

PREP: 40 minutes | **COOK:** 1-3/4 hours

Frances Aldal | ANTELOPE, CALIFORNIA
My mother was born and raised in Japan, so she wasn't familiar with many American dishes when she married my father and moved to the States. My paternal grandmother gave her this yummy recipe.

- 3/4 cup all-purpose flour, *divided*
- 1/2 teaspoon seasoned salt
- 1/2 teaspoon pepper, *divided*
- 2 pounds beef stew meat, cut into 1-inch cubes
- 1 tablespoon olive oil
- 4-1/2 cups water, *divided*
- 1 large onion, halved and sliced
- 2 tablespoons Worcestershire sauce
- 1 tablespoon lemon juice
- 2 garlic cloves, minced
- 1 teaspoon sugar
- 1/2 teaspoon salt
- 1/2 teaspoon paprika
- 1/8 teaspoon ground allspice
- 1 bay leaf
- 4 medium potatoes, cubed
- 6 medium carrots, sliced

- Place 1/2 cup flour, seasoned salt and 1/4 teaspoon pepper in a large resealable plastic bag. Add beef, a few pieces at a time, and shake to coat.

- In a Dutch oven, brown meat in oil in batches. Remove and set aside. Add 4 cups water to the pan, stirring to loosen browned bits. Add the onion, Worcestershire sauce, lemon juice, garlic, sugar, salt, paprika, allspice, bay leaf and remaining pepper. Return beef to the pan. Bring to a boil. Reduce heat; cover and simmer for 1 hour.

- Stir in potatoes and carrots. Bring to a boil. Reduce heat; cover and simmer for 30-35 minutes or until meat and vegetables are tender.

- Combine remaining flour and water until smooth; stir into the pan. Bring to a boil; cook and stir for 2 minutes or until thickened. Discard bay leaf.

YIELD: 8 servings (2-1/2 quarts).

NUTRITION FACTS: 1-1/4 cups equals 324 calories, 10 g fat (3 g saturated fat), 70 mg cholesterol, 322 mg sodium, 33 g carbohydrate, 4 g fiber, 25 g protein. **DIABETIC EXCHANGES:** 3 lean meat, 2 starch, 1 vegetable.

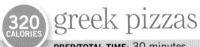

greek pizzas

PREP/TOTAL TIME: 30 minutes

Doris Allers | PORTAGE, MICHIGAN
Pita breads make crispy crusts for these individual pizzas. Topped with feta and ricotta cheese as well as spinach, tomatoes and basil, the fast pizzas are a hit with everyone who tries them.

- 4 pita breads (6 inches)
- 1 cup reduced-fat ricotta cheese
- 1/2 teaspoon garlic powder
- 1 package (10 ounces) frozen chopped spinach, thawed and squeezed dry
- 3 medium tomatoes, sliced
- 3/4 cup crumbled feta cheese
- 3/4 teaspoon dried basil

- Place pita breads on a baking sheet. Combine the ricotta cheese and garlic powder; spread over pitas. Top with spinach, tomatoes, feta cheese and basil.

- Bake at 400° for 12-15 minutes or until bread is lightly browned.

YIELD: 4 servings.

NUTRITION FACTS: 1 pizza equals 320 calories, 7 g fat (4 g saturated fat), 26 mg cholesterol, 642 mg sodium, 46 g carbohydrate, 6 g fiber, 17 g protein. **DIABETIC EXCHANGES:** 2 starch, 2 vegetable, 1 lean meat, 1 fat.

makeover turkey biscuit bake

PREP: 30 minutes | **BAKE:** 15 minutes

Taste of Home Test Kitchen

We lightened up a recipe that had 40 grams of fat per serving. The results are a better-for-you bake that's just as satisfying.

- 1 cup baby carrots, halved lengthwise
- 1 cup julienned parsnips
- 1 tablespoon water
- 2 cups sliced fresh mushrooms
- 2 tablespoons butter
- 1/2 cup all-purpose flour
- 1/2 teaspoon salt
- 1/8 teaspoon white pepper
- 4 cups fat-free milk
- 3 cups diced cooked turkey breast
- 1/2 cup frozen peas, thawed

BISCUITS:

- 1 cup all-purpose flour
- 1/2 cup cake flour
- 3/4 teaspoon baking powder
- 1/2 teaspoon salt
- 1/8 teaspoon baking soda
- 1 egg
- 1/2 cup buttermilk
- 2 tablespoons butter, melted

- In a microwave-safe bowl, combine the carrots, parsnips and water; cover and microwave on high for 4-5 minutes or until tender. Drain and set aside.

- In a large nonstick skillet, saute mushrooms in butter until tender. Combine the flour, salt, white pepper and milk until smooth; stir into mushrooms. Bring to a boil; cook and stir for 1-2 minutes or until thickened. Stir in the carrots, parsnips, turkey and peas. Transfer to a 13-in. x 9-in. baking dish coated with cooking spray.

- For biscuits, in a bowl, combine the flours, baking powder, salt and baking soda. Combine the egg, buttermilk and butter; stir into dry ingredients until a soft dough forms. Drop dough into nine mounds onto turkey mixture.

- Bake at 425° for 15-18 minutes or until a toothpick inserted in biscuits comes out clean and biscuits are golden brown.

YIELD: 9 servings.

EDITOR'S NOTE: This recipe was tested in a 1,100-watt microwave.

NUTRITION FACTS: 2/3 cup turkey mixture with 1 biscuit equals 290 calories, 7 g fat (4 g saturated fat), 82 mg cholesterol, 494 mg sodium, 32 g carbohydrate, 2 g fiber, 24 g protein. **DIABETIC EXCHANGES:** 2 starch, 2 lean meat, 1 vegetable, 1 fat.

MAKEOVER TURKEY BISCUIT BAKE

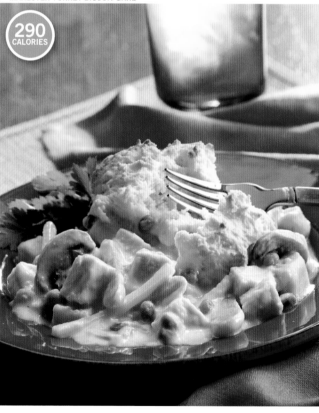

290 CALORIES

351-450 calories

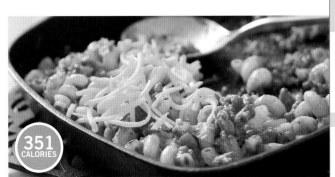

MACARONI SCRAMBLE

macaroni scramble

PREP/TOTAL TIME: 25 minutes

Patricia Kile | NOKOMIS, FLORIDA

This quick and easy dinner has all the pasta, cheese, meat and sweet tomato sauce that make for a family-pleasing classic. Serve with a green salad and crusty bread for a surefire hit.

- 1 cup uncooked cellentani (spiral pasta) *or* elbow macaroni
- 1/2 pound lean ground beef (90% lean)
- 1 small onion, chopped
- 1 celery rib, chopped
- 1 small green pepper, chopped
- 1 garlic clove, minced
- 1 can (10-3/4 ounces) reduced-sodium condensed tomato soup, undiluted
- 1 tablespoon minced fresh parsley *or* 1 teaspoon dried parsley flakes
- 1 teaspoon dried oregano
- 1/4 teaspoon salt
- 1/4 teaspoon pepper
- 1/2 cup shredded reduced-fat cheddar cheese

- Cook pasta according to package directions. Meanwhile, in a large skillet, cook the beef, onion, celery and green pepper over medium heat until meat is no longer pink. Add garlic; cook 1 minute longer. Drain.

- Drain pasta; add to beef mixture. Stir in the soup, parsley, oregano, salt and pepper. Bring to a boil.

Reduce heat; simmer, uncovered, for 4-5 minutes or until heated through. Sprinkle with cheese.

YIELD: 3 servings.

NUTRITION FACTS: 1-1/3 cups equals 351 calories, 11 g fat 5 g saturated fat), 50 mg cholesterol, 758 mg sodium, 38 g carbohydrate, 3 g fiber, 24 g protein. **DIABETIC EXCHANGES:** 3 lean meat, 2 starch, 1 vegetable, 1 fat.

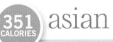 ## asian orange beef

PREP: 20 minutes I **COOK:** 20 minutes

Nancy Bellomo I ST. CHARLES, MISSOURI

Here is the fastest stir-fry ever! Fresh ginger is a must for this recipe and really sparks it up. Everyone just raves about the splash of orange flavor.

- 3 large navel oranges
- 1 bunch green onions
- 3 tablespoons sugar
- 2 tablespoons cornstarch
- 3 tablespoons reduced-sodium soy sauce
- 3 garlic cloves, minced
- 1 tablespoon minced fresh gingerroot
- 1-1/2 pounds beef sirloin steak, cut into 1/2-inch cubes
- 1 tablespoon canola oil
- 3 cups hot cooked rice

- Finely grate the peel from two oranges; set aside. Cut thin strips of orange peel from the remaining orange for garnish; set aside. Squeeze juice from all oranges. Cut onions to separate the white and green parts. Thinly slice white parts; cut green parts into 1-in. lengths for garnish.

- For sauce, in a small bowl, combine sugar and cornstarch; stir in orange juice until smooth. Stir in the soy sauce, garlic, ginger, grated orange peel and white parts of onions; set aside.

- In a large nonstick skillet or wok coated with cooking spray, stir-fry beef in oil until no longer pink. Stir the sauce and add to the pan. Bring to a boil; cook and stir for 2 minutes or until thickened. Serve with rice. Garnish with orange peel strips and remaining onions.

YIELD: 6 servings.

NUTRITION FACTS: 2/3 cup beef mixture with 1/2 cup rice equals 351 calories, 8 g fat (2 g saturated fat), 64 mg cholesterol, 352 mg sodium, 44 g carbohydrate, 3 g fiber, 25 g protein. **DIABETIC EXCHANGES:** 3 lean meat, 2 starch, 1 fruit, 1/2 fat.

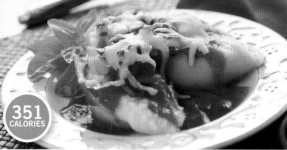

ITALIAN CHEESE-STUFFED SHELLS

italian cheese-stuffed shells

PREP: 1 hour | **BAKE:** 50 minutes

Patty Tappendorf | GALESVILLE, WISCONSIN

I found this recipe in a church cookbook and thought it was a great twist on traditional lasagna. I omitted the meat and added Italian stewed tomatoes.

- 1 medium onion, chopped
- 1/2 cup chopped green pepper
- 1/2 cup chopped sweet red pepper
- 1/2 pound sliced fresh mushrooms
- 2 garlic cloves, minced
- 1-1/2 cups water
- 1 can (14-1/2 ounces) Italian stewed tomatoes
- 1 can (6 ounces) tomato paste
- 1-1/2 teaspoons Italian seasoning
- 2 eggs, lightly beaten
- 1 carton (15 ounces) reduced-fat ricotta cheese
- 2 cups (8 ounces) shredded part-skim mozzarella cheese, *divided*
- 1/2 cup grated Parmesan cheese
- 21 jumbo pasta shells, cooked and drained

- In a nonstick skillet coated with cooking spray, cook onion and peppers over medium heat for 2 minutes. Add mushrooms; cook 4-5 minutes until tender. Add garlic; cook 1 minute longer. Stir in the water, tomatoes, tomato paste and Italian seasoning. Bring to a boil. Reduce heat; cover and simmer for 30 minutes.

- Meanwhile, in a small bowl, combine the eggs, ricotta, 1/2 cup mozzarella and Parmesan cheeses. Stuff into shells. Spread 1 cup vegetable sauce in a 13-in. x 9-in. baking dish coated with cooking spray. Arrange shells over sauce; top with remaining sauce.

- Cover and bake at 350° for 45 minutes. Uncover; sprinkle with remaining mozzarella. Bake 5-10 minutes

longer or until bubbly and cheese is melted. Let stand for 5 minutes before serving.

YIELD: 7 servings.

NUTRITION FACTS: 3 stuffed shells with 3/4 cup sauce equals 351 calories, 11 g fat (6 g saturated fat), 99 mg cholesterol, 457 mg sodium, 39 g carbohydrate, 4 g fiber, 23 g protein. **DIABETIC EXCHANGES:** 2 medium-fat meat, 2 vegetable, 1-1/2 starch.

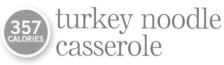

turkey noodle casserole

PREP: 25 minutes | **BAKE:** 45 minutes

Ramona Fish | COLUMBUS, INDIANA

In this hearty supper, I blend spinach with turkey breast, cottage cheese and mozzarella. Yum!

- 2-1/2 cups uncooked yolk-free noodles
- 2 cups cubed cooked turkey breast
- 1 can (10-3/4 ounces) reduced-fat reduced-sodium condensed cream of chicken soup, undiluted
- 1/8 teaspoon garlic salt
- 1/8 teaspoon dried rosemary, crushed

Dash pepper

- 1 package (10 ounces) frozen chopped spinach, thawed and squeezed dry
- 1 cup (8 ounces) fat-free cottage cheese
- 3/4 cup shredded part-skim mozzarella cheese, *divided*
- 1/8 teaspoon paprika

- Cook noodles according to package directions. Meanwhile, in a bowl, combine the turkey, soup, garlic salt, rosemary and pepper. In a bowl, combine the spinach, cottage cheese and 1/2 cup mozzarella cheese.

- Drain noodles. Place half of the noodles in a 2-qt. baking dish coated with cooking spray; layer with half of the turkey and cottage cheese mixtures. Repeat layers.

- Cover and bake at 350° for 35 minutes. Uncover; sprinkle with remaining mozzarella. Bake 10-15 minutes longer until edges are lightly browned. Sprinkle with paprika. Let stand for 5 minutes before serving.

YIELD: 4 servings.

NUTRITION FACTS: 1-1/2 cups equals 357 calories, 6 g fat (3 g saturated fat), 81 mg cholesterol, 746 mg sodium, 32 g carbohydrate, 4 g fiber, 40 g protein. **DIABETIC EXCHANGES:** 5 lean meat, 1-1/2 starch, 1 vegetable, 1/2 fat.

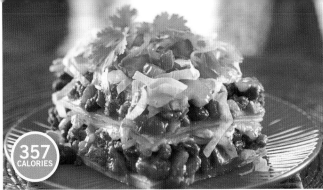

ENCHILADA CASSER-OLÉ!

357 CALORIES

enchilada casser-olé!

PREP: 25 minutes | **BAKE:** 30 minutes

Marsha Wills | HOMOSASSA, FLORIDA

My husband loves this casserole, but it never lasts too long around our house! Packed with black beans, cheese, tomatoes and Southwest flair, it's an impressive-looking entree that's as simple to make as it is simply delicious!

- 1 pound lean ground beef (90% lean)
- 1 large onion, chopped
- 2 cups salsa
- 1 can (15 ounces) black beans, rinsed and drained
- 1/4 cup reduced-fat Italian salad dressing
- 2 tablespoons reduced-sodium taco seasoning
- 1/4 teaspoon ground cumin
- 6 flour tortillas (8 inches)
- 3/4 cup reduced-fat sour cream
- 1 cup (4 ounces) shredded reduced-fat Mexican cheese blend
- 1 cup shredded lettuce
- 1 medium tomato, chopped
- 1/4 cup minced fresh cilantro

- In a large skillet, cook beef and onion over medium heat until meat is no longer pink; drain. Stir in the salsa, beans, dressing, taco seasoning and cumin. Place three tortillas in a 2-qt. baking dish coated with cooking spray. Layer with half of the meat mixture, sour cream and cheese. Repeat layers.

- Cover and bake at 400° for 25 minutes. Uncover; bake 5-10 minutes longer or until heated through. Let stand for 5 minutes before topping with lettuce, tomato and cilantro.

YIELD: 8 servings.

NUTRITION FACTS: 1 piece equals 357 calories, 12 g fat (5 g saturated fat), 45 mg cholesterol, 864 mg sodium, 37 g carbohydrate, 3 g fiber, 23 g protein. **DIABETIC EXCHANGES:** 3 lean meat, 2 starch, 1 vegetable, 1 fat.

asian vegetable pasta

PREP/TOTAL TIME: 20 minutes

Mitzi Sentiff | ANNAPOLIS, MARYLAND

A little peanut butter and a sprinkling of peanuts give this dish plenty of flavor. While red pepper flakes offer a little kick, brown sugar balances it out with a hint of sweetness.

- 4 quarts water
- 8 ounces uncooked angel hair pasta
- 1 pound fresh asparagus, trimmed and cut into 1-inch pieces
- 3/4 cup julienned carrots
- 1/3 cup reduced-fat creamy peanut butter
- 3 tablespoons rice vinegar
- 3 tablespoons reduced-sodium soy sauce
- 2 tablespoons brown sugar
- 1/2 teaspoon crushed red pepper flakes
- 1/4 cup unsalted peanuts, chopped

- In a Dutch oven, bring the water to a boil. Add pasta and asparagus; cook for 3 minutes. Stir in carrots; cook for 1 minute or until pasta is tender. Drain and keep warm.

- In a saucepan, combine the peanut butter, vinegar, soy sauce, brown sugar and pepper flakes. Bring to a boil over medium heat, stirring constantly. Pour over pasta mixture; toss to coat. Sprinkle with peanuts.

YIELD: 5 servings.

NUTRITION FACTS: 1 cup equals 358 calories, 10 g fat (2 g saturated fat), 0 cholesterol, 472 mg sodium, 54 g carbohydrate, 5 g fiber, 15 g protein.

ASIAN VEGETABLE PASTA

358 CALORIES

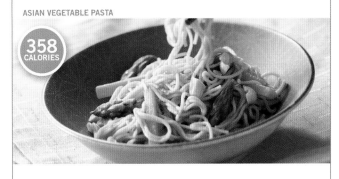

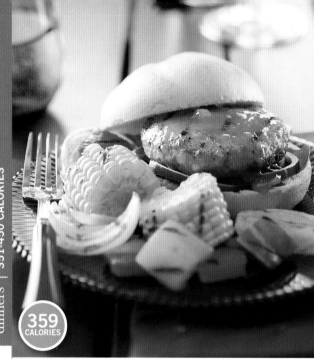

359 CALORIES

CHUTNEY TURKEY BURGERS

chutney turkey burgers

PREP/TOTAL TIME: 20 minutes

Jeanne Lueders | WATERLOO, IOWA
The secret to these burgers is the tangy chutney, but the arugula adds a special "wow" to the sandwich.

- 1/2 cup chutney, *divided*
- 1 tablespoon Dijon mustard
- 2 teaspoons lime juice
- 1/4 cup minced fresh parsley
- 2 green onions, chopped
- 1/2 teaspoon salt
- 1/4 teaspoon pepper
- 1 pound lean ground turkey
- 4 hamburger buns, split
- 16 fresh arugula *or* baby spinach leaves
- 4 slices red onion

- Combine 1/4 cup chutney, mustard and lime juice; set aside. In a large bowl, combine the parsley, onions, salt, pepper and remaining chutney. Crumble turkey over mixture and mix well. Shape into four patties.

- Using long-handled tongs, moisten a paper towel with cooking oil and lightly coat the grill rack. Grill burgers, covered, over medium heat or broil 4 in. from

the heat for 5-7 minutes on each side or until a meat thermometer reads 165° and juices run clear.

- Serve on buns with arugula, onion and reserved chutney mixture.

YIELD: 4 servings.

NUTRITION FACTS: 1 burger equals 359 calories, 12 g fat (3 g saturated fat), 90 mg cholesterol, 749 mg sodium, 38 g carbohydrate, 3 g fiber, 25 g protein. **DIABETIC EXCHANGES:** 3 lean meat, 2-1/2 starch.

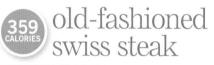

359 CALORIES

old-fashioned swiss steak

PREP: 20 minutes | **BAKE:** 1-1/2 hours

Vera Kleiber | RALEIGH, NORTH CAROLINA
The comforting sauce is wonderful, and this classic dish always brings back great memories.

- 2 tablespoons all-purpose flour
- 1/2 to 1 teaspoon salt
- 1/4 teaspoon pepper
- 1-1/2 pounds beef top round steak
- 2 tablespoons canola oil
- 2 medium onions, chopped
- 2 cans (5-1/2 ounces *each*) tomato juice
- 1 cup diced tomatoes
- 4 teaspoons lemon juice
- 4 teaspoons Worcestershire sauce
- 2 to 3 teaspoons packed brown sugar
- 1 teaspoon prepared mustard

- In a large resealable plastic bag, combine the flour, salt and pepper. Cut steak into four pieces. Add beef, a few pieces at a time, and shake to coat. Remove meat from bag and pound with a mallet to tenderize.

- In a skillet, brown meat in oil on both sides. Transfer to a shallow 2-qt. baking dish coated with cooking spray.

- In the same skillet, saute onions in drippings until tender. Stir in the remaining ingredients. Pour over meat. Cover and bake at 350° for 1-1/2 hours or until tender.

YIELD: 4 servings.

NUTRITION FACTS: 1 serving equals 359 calories, 12 g fat (2 g saturated fat), 96 mg cholesterol, 721 mg sodium, 20 g carbohydrate, 3 g fiber, 41 g protein. **DIABETIC EXCHANGES:** 5 lean meat, 2 vegetable, 1-1/2 fat, 1/2 starch.

I attended the gym on a regular basis, taking Zumba and spinning classes. I kept track of my caloric intake and output, ate more produce and stayed away from fast food. In seven months, I went from 190 pounds to 125. It was liberating to reach my goal without crash dieting but with sheer determination! —**Allison Johnson, Ohio**

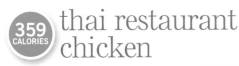

thai restaurant chicken

359 CALORIES

PREP/TOTAL TIME: 30 minutes

Trisha Kruse | EAGLE, IDAHO

You'll love this versatile recipe because you can add any veggies you like, making it your own Thai specialty!

- 2 tablespoons cornstarch
- 1 tablespoon brown sugar
- 1/4 teaspoon pepper
- 1 can (14-1/2 ounces) reduced-sodium chicken broth
- 2 tablespoons rice vinegar
- 2 tablespoons reduced-sodium soy sauce
- 2 tablespoons reduced-fat peanut butter
- 1 pound boneless skinless chicken breasts, cut into 1-inch cubes
- 2 teaspoons sesame oil, *divided*
- 1 large onion, halved and sliced
- 1 medium sweet red pepper, julienned
- 1 cup sliced fresh mushrooms
- 2 garlic cloves, minced
- 2 cups hot cooked rice

- In a large bowl, combine the cornstarch, brown sugar and pepper. Add broth; stir until smooth. Stir in the vinegar, soy sauce and peanut butter; set aside.

- In a nonstick skillet or wok, stir-fry chicken in 1 teaspoon oil until no longer pink. Remove and keep warm.

- Stir-fry the onion and red pepper in remaining oil for 2 minutes. Add mushrooms; stir-fry 2-3 minutes or until crisp-tender. Add garlic; cook 1 minute longer.

- Stir cornstarch mixture and add to the pan. Bring to a boil; cook and stir for 1-2 minutes or until thickened. Add chicken; heat through. Serve with rice.

YIELD: 4 servings.

NUTRITION FACTS: 1 cup stir-fry with 1/2 cup rice equals 359 calories, 8 g fat (2 g saturated fat), 63 mg cholesterol, 704 mg sodium, 40 g carbohydrate, 2 g fiber, 31 g protein. **DIABETIC EXCHANGES:** 3 lean meat, 2 starch, 1 vegetable, 1 fat.

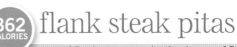

flank steak pitas

362 CALORIES

PREP: 15 minutes + marinating | **GRILL:** 15 minutes

Tammy Kaminski | STANWOOD, WASHINGTON

This sandwich packs so much flavor, you'll be satisfied without eating a huge serving. The marinade makes the most of flavorful ingredients, so you won't even miss the cheese and mayo.

- 1/4 cup balsamic vinegar
- 2 tablespoons water
- 2 tablespoons reduced-sodium soy sauce
- 1 tablespoon hoisin sauce
- 2 garlic cloves, minced
- 1 teaspoon Thai chili sauce
- 3/4 teaspoon pepper
- 1/2 teaspoon sesame oil
- 1 beef flank steak (1 pound)
- 4 whole pita breads
- 4 pieces leaf lettuce, torn
- 1/4 teaspoon sesame seeds

- In a small bowl, combine the first eight ingredients. Pour 1/4 cup marinade into a large resealable plastic bag; add the beef. Seal bag and turn to coat. Refrigerate for at least 8 hours or overnight. Cover and refrigerate remaining marinade.

- Drain and discard marinade. Grill, covered, over medium heat for 6-8 minutes on each side or until meat reaches desired doneness (for medium-rare, a meat thermometer should read 145°; medium, 160°; well-done, 170°). Let stand for 10 minutes.

- Meanwhile, grill pitas, uncovered, over medium heat for 1-2 minutes on each side or until warm. Thinly slice beef across the grain. In a large bowl, toss the beef, lettuce and reserved marinade. Serve in pitas; sprinkle with sesame seeds.

YIELD: 4 servings.

NUTRITION FACTS: 1 filled pita equals 362 calories, 10 g fat (4 g saturated fat), 54 mg cholesterol, 703 mg sodium, 39 g carbohydrate, 2 g fiber, 28 g protein. **DIABETIC EXCHANGES:** 3 lean meat, 2-1/2 starch.

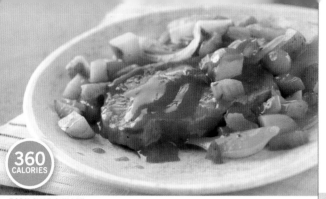

360 CALORIES

PORK CHOP SKILLET

pork chop skillet

PREP: 15 minutes I **COOK:** 30 minutes

Susan Blair I STERLING, MICHIGAN

My husband and I really enjoy this easy supper on busy days when there's little time to spend in the kitchen. It satisfies our meat-and-potato cravings, goes together in a snap, and leftovers taste even better the next day!

    4 medium red potatoes, cubed
  1/2 cup water
1-1/4 cups fresh baby carrots
    2 celery ribs, coarsely chopped
    1 medium onion, cut into wedges
    4 boneless pork loin chops (4 ounces *each*)
    1 tablespoon canola oil

SAUCE:

    1 can (10-3/4 ounces) condensed tomato
       soup, undiluted
  1/2 cup water
    1 teaspoon dried thyme
    1 teaspoon Worcestershire sauce
  1/4 teaspoon pepper
1-1/2 teaspoons all-purpose flour
    2 tablespoons cold water

- Place potatoes and water in a microwave-safe dish; cover and microwave on high for 3 minutes. Add the carrots, celery and onion; cook 4-6 minutes longer or until crisp-tender. Drain.

- In a large skillet over medium heat, brown pork chops in oil on both sides. Top with vegetables.

- Combine the soup, water, thyme, Worcestershire sauce and pepper; pour over the top. Bring to a boil. Reduce heat; cover and simmer for 20-25 minutes or until

meat and vegetables are tender. Remove chops and vegetables; keep warm.

- Combine flour and cold water until smooth; gradually stir into the sauce. Bring to a boil; cook and stir for 2 minutes or until thickened. Serve with chops and vegetables.

YIELD: 4 servings.

EDITOR'S NOTE: This recipe was tested in a 1,100-watt microwave.

NUTRITION FACTS: 1 pork chop with 1-1/2 cups vegetables and 1/4 cup sauce equals 360 calories, 10 g fat (3 g saturated fat), 55 mg cholesterol, 548 mg sodium, 40 g carbohydrate, 5 g fiber, 26 g protein. **DIABETIC EXCHANGES:** 3 lean meat, 2 starch, 1 vegetable, 1/2 fat.

vegetarian tex-mex peppers

PREP: 20 minutes I **BAKE:** 45 minutes

Cele Knight I NACOGDOCHES, TEXAS

Folks who enjoy stuffed peppers will love this delightfully delicious Tex-Mex twist on their old favorite. The veggie filling is hearty enough to satisfy any appetite!

    4 large green peppers
    2 eggs, beaten
    2 cups cooked brown rice
    1 cup frozen vegetarian meat crumbles
    1 cup canned black beans, rinsed and drained
  1/2 teaspoon pepper
  1/4 teaspoon hot pepper sauce
  1/4 teaspoon ground cardamom, optional
    1 can (14-1/2 ounces) diced tomatoes, drained
    1 can (10 ounces) diced tomatoes and
       green chilies
    1 can (8 ounces) no-salt-added tomato sauce
  1/2 cup shredded Colby cheese

- Cut peppers in half lengthwise and remove seeds. Discard stems. In a large kettle, cook peppers in boiling water for 3-5 minutes. Drain and rinse in cold water; set aside.

- In a large bowl, combine the eggs, rice, meat crumbles, beans, pepper, pepper sauce and cardamom if desired. Spoon into peppers. Place in a 13-in. x 9-in. baking dish coated with cooking spray.

- In a small bowl, combine the diced tomatoes, tomatoes and green chilies, and tomato sauce. Spoon over peppers. Cover and bake at 350° for 40-45 minutes or until a thermometer reads 160°. Sprinkle with cheese; bake 5 minutes longer or until cheese is melted.

YIELD: 4 servings.

EDITOR'S NOTE: Vegetarian meat crumbles are a nutritious protein source made from soy. Look for them in the natural foods freezer section.

NUTRITION FACTS: 2 stuffed pepper halves equals 364 calories, 9 g fat (4 g saturated fat), 119 mg cholesterol, 769 mg sodium, 53 g carbohydrate, 11 g fiber, 19 g protein.

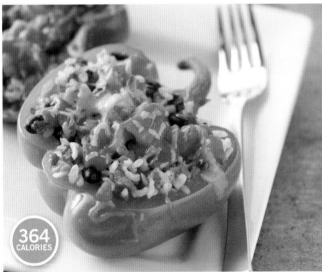

364 CALORIES

VEGETARIAN TEX-MEX PEPPERS

mediterranean shrimp 'n' pasta

PREP: 15 minutes I **COOK:** 20 minutes

Shirley Kunde I RHINELANDER, WISCONSIN
Sun-dried tomatoes and curry take center stage in this dish that's loaded with tender shrimp and pasta.

- 1 cup boiling water
- 1/2 cup dry-pack sun-dried tomatoes, chopped
- 6 ounces uncooked fettuccine
- 1 can (8 ounces) tomato sauce
- 2 tablespoons clam juice
- 2 tablespoons unsweetened apple juice
- 1 teaspoon curry powder
- 1/4 teaspoon pepper
- 1 pound fresh asparagus, trimmed and cut into 1-inch pieces
- 1 tablespoon olive oil
- 1/2 cup thinly sliced green onions
- 2 garlic cloves, minced
- 1 pound uncooked medium shrimp, peeled and deveined

- In a small bowl, pour boiling water over sun-dried tomatoes; let stand for 2 minutes. Drain and set aside. Cook fettuccine according to package directions.

- Meanwhile, in a small bowl, combine the tomato sauce, clam juice, apple juice, curry powder and pepper; set aside. In a large nonstick skillet coated with cooking spray, cook asparagus in oil for 2 minutes. Add green onions and garlic; cook and stir 1 minute longer.

- Stir in shrimp. Cook and stir 3 minutes longer or until shrimp turn pink. Stir in tomato mixture and sun-dried tomatoes; heat through. Drain fettuccine and add to skillet; heat through.

YIELD: 4 servings.

NUTRITION FACTS: 1-1/2 cups equals 368 calories, 6 g fat (1 g saturated fat), 173 mg cholesterol, 702 mg sodium, 46 g carbohydrate, 5 g fiber, 32 g protein. **DIABETIC EXCHANGES:** 3 starch, 3 lean meat, 1/2 fat.

MEDITERRANEAN SHRIMP 'N' PASTA

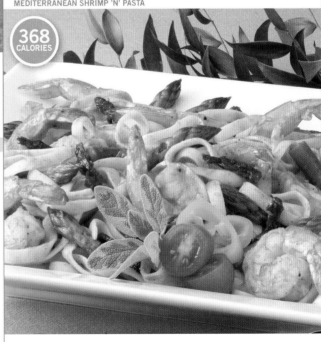

368 CALORIES

> **I've lost weight** by eating smaller portions and baking or broiling my food and cutting out the frying. —Debi N Ga

- In a nonstick skillet coated with cooking spray, saute the onion, red pepper and garlic in oil for 1 minute. Add rice; cook and stir for 4-5 minutes or until lightly browned.
- Stir in the broth, sherry, lemon peel, salt and cayenne. Bring to a boil. Reduce heat; cover and simmer for 15 minutes.
- Stir in the chicken, peas and olives. Cover and simmer 3-6 minutes longer or until rice is tender and chicken is heated through. Sprinkle with cilantro.

YIELD: 4 servings.

NUTRITION FACTS: 1-1/2 cups equals 373 calories, 6 g fat (1 g saturated fat), 54 mg cholesterol, 582 mg sodium, 49 g carbohydrate, 4 g fiber, 28 g protein. **DIABETIC EXCHANGES:** 3 starch, 3 lean meat, 1 vegetable, 1/2 fat.

373 CALORIES

SKILLET ARROZ CON POLLO

skillet arroz con pollo

PREP: 15 minutes I **COOK:** 25 minutes

Cheryl Battaglia I DALTON, PENNSYLVANIA

Serve up a chicken-and-rice dish that's great for both family and special occasion meals. It's a tasty dish made all in one skillet; it smells great while it cooks.

- 1 medium onion, chopped
- 1 medium sweet red pepper, cut into 1/2-inch pieces
- 1 garlic clove, minced
- 2 teaspoons olive oil
- 1 cup uncooked long grain rice
- 1 can (14-1/2 ounces) reduced-sodium chicken broth
- 1/4 cup sherry *or* water
- 1/2 teaspoon grated lemon peel
- 1/4 teaspoon salt
- 1/4 teaspoon cayenne pepper
- 2 cups cubed cooked chicken breast
- 1 cup frozen peas, thawed
- 1/4 cup sliced ripe olives, drained
- 2 tablespoons minced fresh cilantro

370 CALORIES 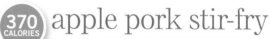 apple pork stir-fry

PREP/TOTAL TIME: 25 minutes

Jo Ann Erpelding I CANTON, MICHIGAN

Try a super stir-fry with a twist. Water chestnuts bring a slight crunch to the tender pork and veggies, while apple pie filling lends a complementary sweetness.

- 1/2 teaspoon cornstarch
- 1/2 cup apple cider *or* unsweetened apple juice
- 2 tablespoons reduced-sodium soy sauce
- 2 boneless pork loin chops (4 ounces *each*), cut into strips
- 2 teaspoons canola oil
- 1/2 cup sliced celery
- 1/3 cup sliced fresh carrots
- 1/3 cup sliced onion
- 1/3 cup julienned sweet red pepper
- 1/3 cup sliced water chestnuts
- 1/4 teaspoon ground ginger
- 1 cup apple pie filling
- 1-1/2 cups hot cooked rice

- In a bowl, combine the cornstarch, cider and soy sauce until smooth; set aside. In a large skillet or wok, stir-fry pork in oil for 5-7 minutes or until no longer pink.

- Add the celery, carrots, onion, red pepper, water chestnuts and ginger; stir-fry until vegetables are tender. Add pie filling.

- Stir cornstarch mixture and stir into pork mixture. Bring to a boil; cook and stir for 1-2 minutes or until thickened. Serve with rice.

YIELD: 3 servings.

NUTRITION FACTS: 1 cup pork mixture with 1/2 cup rice equals 370 calories, 8 g fat (2 g saturated fat), 36 mg cholesterol, 494 mg sodium, 56 g carbohydrate, 3 g fiber, 18 g protein.

turkey burritos with fresh fruit salsa

PREP: 30 minutes | **COOK:** 20 minutes

Lisa Eaton | **KENNEBUNK, MAINE**

Packed with fruit, veggies, nutrition and flavor, this lighter, whole grain twist on traditional burritos is sure to be a big hit with your family. Even our pickiest eater loves these with the sweet-spicy fruit salsa.

> 1 pint grape tomatoes, quartered
> 1 medium mango, peeled and chopped
> 2 medium kiwifruit, peeled and chopped
> 3 green onions, thinly sliced
> 3 tablespoons finely chopped red onion
> 1 jalapeno pepper, seeded and chopped
> 1 tablespoon lime juice

BURRITOS:

> 1 pound lean ground turkey
> 1/2 teaspoon ground turmeric
> 1/4 teaspoon ground cumin
> 1 tablespoon olive oil
> 2 garlic cloves, minced
> 1/2 cup burgundy wine *or* reduced-sodium beef broth
> 1 jar (16 ounces) salsa
> 2 cups frozen corn, thawed
> 1 can (15 ounces) black beans, rinsed and drained
> 10 whole wheat tortillas (8 inches), warmed
> 1 cup (4 ounces) shredded reduced-fat cheddar cheese

- For the salsa, combine the first seven ingredients. Chill until serving.

- In a large nonstick skillet, cook the turkey, turmeric and cumin in oil over medium heat until turkey is no longer pink. Add garlic; cook 1 minute longer. Drain. Stir in wine. Bring to a boil. Reduce heat; simmer, uncovered, for 3-5 minutes or until thickened.

- Stir in the salsa, corn and black beans. Bring to a boil. Reduce heat; simmer, uncovered, for 10-15 minutes or until thickened. Remove from the heat.

- Spoon about 1/2 cup turkey mixture off center on each tortilla. Sprinkle with cheese. Fold sides and ends over filling and roll up. Serve with salsa.

YIELD: 10 servings.

EDITOR'S NOTE: We recommend wearing disposable gloves when cutting hot peppers. Avoid touching your face.

NUTRITION FACTS: 1 burrito equals 371 calories, 11 g fat (3 g saturated fat), 44 mg cholesterol, 553 mg sodium, 47 g carbohydrate, 6 g fiber, 18 g protein. **DIABETIC EXCHANGES:** 3 starch, 2 lean meat.

TURKEY BURRITOS WITH FRESH FRUIT SALSA

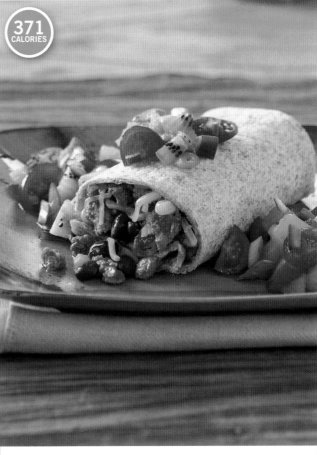

371 CALORIES

390 CALORIES

MEXICAN MANICOTTI

mexican manicotti

PREP: 25 minutes | **BAKE:** 25 minutes

Larry Phillips | SHREVEPORT, LOUISIANA

Enjoy this creative spin on traditional manicotti. The Mexican flavors will leave you dazzled and satisfied!

for 2

- 4 uncooked manicotti shells
- 1 cup cubed cooked chicken breast
- 1 cup salsa, *divided*
- 1/2 cup reduced-fat ricotta cheese
- 2 tablespoons sliced ripe olives
- 4 teaspoons minced fresh parsley
- 1 tablespoon diced pimientos
- 1 green onion, thinly sliced
- 1 small garlic clove, minced
- 1/4 to 1/2 teaspoon hot pepper sauce
- 1/3 cup shredded reduced-fat Monterey Jack cheese *or* reduced-fat Mexican cheese blend

- Cook manicotti according to package directions. In a bowl, combine the chicken, 1/4 cup salsa, ricotta cheese, olives, parsley, pimientos, green onion, garlic and pepper sauce. Drain manicotti; fill with chicken mixture.

- Spread 1/4 cup salsa in an 8-in. square baking dish coated with cooking spray. Top with manicotti shells and remaining salsa.

- Cover and bake at 400° for 20 minutes. Uncover; sprinkle with Monterey Jack cheese and bake 5-10 minutes longer or until cheese is melted and filling is heated through.

YIELD: 2 servings.

NUTRITION FACTS: 2 stuffed manicotti equals 390 calories, 10 g fat (4 g saturated fat), 81 mg cholesterol, 783 mg sodium, 38 g carbohydrate, 2 g fiber, 35 g protein. **DIABETIC EXCHANGES:** 4 lean meat, 2 starch, 1 vegetable.

399 CALORIES

cranberry-orange turkey cutlets

PREP/TOTAL TIME: 20 minutes

Joan Tweed | IRMO, SOUTH CAROLINA

This great company dish is easy to prepare but looks so elegant. People who try it always like it.

- 4 turkey breast tenderloins (4 ounces *each*)
- 1 cup dry bread crumbs
- 1 egg white
- 1 tablespoon fat-free milk
- 1/2 teaspoon salt
- 3/4 cup cranberry-orange *or* whole-berry cranberry sauce
- 1 tablespoon olive oil

- Flatten turkey to 1/4-in. thickness. Place bread crumbs in a shallow bowl. In another shallow bowl, beat the egg white, milk and salt. Dip turkey into egg white mixture, then coat with crumbs. Refrigerate turkey, uncovered, for 10 minutes.

- Meanwhile, in a small saucepan, heat cranberry-orange sauce. In a large nonstick skillet, brown turkey in oil for 3-4 minutes on each side or until no longer pink. Serve sauce with turkey.

YIELD: 4 servings.

NUTRITION FACTS: 1 turkey tenderloin with 3 tablespoons sauce equals 399 calories, 9 g fat (1 g saturated fat), 82 mg cholesterol, 609 mg sodium, 44 g carbohydrate, 1 g fiber, 34 g protein. **DIABETIC EXCHANGES:** 3 starch, 3 lean meat, 1/2 fat.

italian hot dish

PREP: 30 minutes | **BAKE:** 40 minutes

Theresa Smith | SHEBOYGAN, WISCONSIN

My husband had a poor perception of healthy food until he tried this beefy casserole. The combination of pasta, oregano, mushrooms and green peppers makes it a favorite in our house.

- 1-1/2 cups uncooked small pasta shells
- 1 pound lean ground beef (90% lean)
- 1 cup sliced fresh mushrooms, *divided*
- 1/2 cup chopped onion
- 1/2 cup chopped green pepper

1 can (15 ounces) tomato sauce
1 teaspoon dried oregano
1/2 teaspoon garlic powder
1/4 teaspoon onion powder
1/8 teaspoon pepper
1/2 cup shredded part-skim mozzarella cheese, *divided*
4 teaspoons grated Parmesan cheese, *divided*

- Cook pasta according to package directions. Meanwhile, in a large nonstick skillet coated with cooking spray, cook the beef, 1/2 cup mushrooms, onion and green pepper until meat is no longer pink; drain. Stir in the tomato sauce, oregano, garlic powder, onion powder and pepper. Bring to a boil. Reduce heat; cover and simmer for 15 minutes.

- Drain pasta; place in an 8-in. square baking dish coated with cooking spray. Top with meat sauce and remaining mushrooms. Sprinkle with 1/4 cup mozzarella cheese and 2 teaspoons Parmesan cheese.

- Cover and bake at 350° for 35 minutes. Uncover; sprinkle with remaining cheeses. Bake 5-10 minutes longer or until heated through and cheese is melted.

YIELD: 4 servings.

NUTRITION FACTS: 1 serving equals 391 calories, 12 g fat (5 g saturated fat), 65 mg cholesterol, 663 mg sodium, 36 g carbohydrate, 3 g fiber, 33 g protein. **DIABETIC EXCHANGES:** 3 lean meat, 2 starch, 2 vegetable, 1/2 fat.

ITALIAN HOT DISH

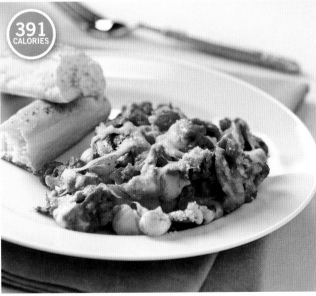

malibu chicken bundles

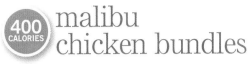

PREP: 25 minutes | **BAKE:** 45 minutes

Beverly Norris | EVANSTON, WYOMING
The first time I made this, it was an instant hit, and we agreed I wouldn't change a thing about the recipe. Mustard might seem like an odd ingredient, but it adds a really nice touch. This rich-tasting dish is surprisingly light.

4 boneless skinless chicken breast halves (4 ounces *each*)
1/2 cup honey Dijon mustard, *divided*
4 thin slices deli ham
4 slices reduced-fat Swiss cheese
1 can (8 ounces) unsweetened crushed pineapple, well drained
1-1/2 cups panko (Japanese) bread crumbs
1/4 teaspoon salt
1/4 teaspoon pepper

SAUCE:
1 can (10-3/4 ounces) reduced-fat reduced-sodium condensed cream of chicken soup, undiluted
1/4 cup reduced-fat sour cream
1/8 teaspoon dried tarragon

- Flatten chicken breasts to 1/4-in. thickness. Spread 1 tablespoon mustard over each; layer with ham, cheese and pineapple. Fold chicken over pineapple; secure with toothpicks. Brush bundles with remaining mustard.

- In a shallow bowl, combine the bread crumbs, salt and pepper. Roll bundles in bread crumb mixture; place in an 11-in. x 7-in. baking dish coated with cooking spray. Bake, uncovered, at 350° for 45-50 minutes or until a meat thermometer reads 170°. Discard toothpicks.

- Meanwhile, in a small saucepan, combine the sauce ingredients. Cook, stirring occasionally, until heated through. Serve with chicken.

YIELD: 4 servings.

NUTRITION FACTS: 1 chicken bundle with 1/3 cup sauce equals 400 calories, 12 g fat (4 g saturated fat), 86 mg cholesterol, 784 mg sodium, 41 g carbohydrate, 2 g fiber, 36 g protein. **DIABETIC EXCHANGES:** 4 lean meat, 2 starch, 1/2 fruit.

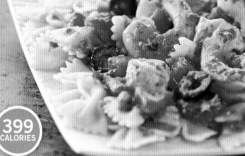

399 CALORIES

BOW TIES WITH CHICKEN & SHRIMP

bow ties with chicken & shrimp

PREP: 20 minutes | **COOK:** 15 minutes

Jan Archer | KANSAS CITY, MISSOURI
What a simple yet savory stovetop supper to keep you warm and satisfied on cold days! It's a delight to serve.

5-1/4 cups uncooked bow tie pasta
3/4 pound boneless skinless chicken breasts, cubed
1 tablespoon *each* butter and olive oil
2 green onions, chopped
2 garlic cloves, minced
2 cans (14-1/2 ounces *each*) Italian diced tomatoes, undrained
2 tablespoons minced fresh parsley, *divided*
1 tablespoon *each* minced fresh basil, thyme and oregano *or* 1 teaspoon *each* dried basil, thyme and oregano
1/4 teaspoon pepper
2 teaspoons cornstarch
1/2 cup reduced-sodium chicken broth
3/4 pound cooked large shrimp, peeled and deveined
3 plum tomatoes, diced
10 large pitted ripe olives, sliced
Minced fresh parsley, optional

- Cook pasta according to package directions. Meanwhile, in a large nonstick skillet, saute chicken in butter and oil until no longer pink. Add onions and garlic; cook 1 minute longer. Stir in the canned tomatoes, parsley, basil, thyme, oregano and pepper.

- Combine cornstarch and broth until smooth; stir into the pan. Bring to a boil; cook and stir for 2 minutes or until thickened. Add the shrimp, plum tomatoes and olives; heat through. Drain pasta; serve with chicken mixture. Sprinkle with parsley if desired.

YIELD: 7 servings.

NUTRITION FACTS: 1 cup pasta with 1 cup sauce equals 399 calories, 8 g fat (2 g saturated fat), 105 mg cholesterol, 661 mg sodium, 54 g carbohydrate, 3 g fiber, 29 g protein.

401 CALORIES

spicy chicken spaghetti

PREP/TOTAL TIME: 25 minutes

LaDonna Reed | PONCA CITY, OKLAHOMA
I look for recipes that serve two. We're also watching our fat grams, so this main course was a great find.

3 ounces uncooked spaghetti
1/2 pound boneless skinless chicken breast, cut into 3/4-inch cubes
1-1/2 teaspoons Cajun seasoning
1 cup sliced fresh mushrooms
1/2 cup chopped green pepper
2 green onions, thinly sliced
1 garlic clove, minced
1 tablespoon cornstarch
1/8 teaspoon *each* salt and pepper
1 cup fat-free half-and-half

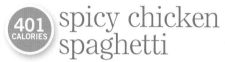

for 2

- Cook spaghetti according to package directions. Meanwhile, sprinkle chicken with Cajun seasoning. In a nonstick skillet coated with cooking spray, cook chicken for 7-9 minutes or until lightly browned and chicken is no longer pink. Remove and keep warm.

- In the same skillet, saute the mushrooms, green pepper and onions until almost tender. Add garlic; cook 1 minute longer. Combine the cornstarch, salt and pepper; sprinkle over vegetables. Cook and stir for 1 minute. Gradually stir in half-and-half. Bring to a boil over medium heat; cook and stir for 1-2 minutes or until thickened.

- Return chicken to the pan; heat through. Drain spaghetti; top with chicken mixture.

YIELD: 2 servings.

NUTRITION FACTS: 1 cup chicken mixture with 3/4 cup spaghetti equals 401 calories, 4 g fat (1 g saturated fat), 63 mg cholesterol, 808 mg sodium, 53 g carbohydrate, 3 g fiber, 34 g protein.

Once a week, I would have a 'splurge' meal where I could eat whatever sounded good to me. Because of my healthier habits, I found that when these meals came around, I was eating less and getting more enjoyment from my food. —**Ashley Latimer, Oregon**

402 CALORIES — asian steak wraps

PREP: 20 minutes + marinating I **COOK:** 10 minutes

Trisha Kruse I EAGLE, IDAHO

A zesty marinade with a splash of fresh lime juice makes these slightly sesame-flavored wraps a treat.

1/4	cup lime juice
3	tablespoons honey
1	tablespoon reduced-sodium soy sauce
2	teaspoons sesame oil
2	teaspoons minced fresh gingerroot
1-1/2	teaspoons minced fresh cilantro
1	pound beef top sirloin steak, cut into thin strips
1/4	teaspoon salt
1/4	teaspoon pepper
1	medium onion, halved and thinly sliced
1	large green pepper, julienned
1	large sweet red pepper, julienned
4	flour tortillas (8 inches), warmed
2	ounces reduced-fat cream cheese
2	teaspoons sesame seeds, toasted

- In a small bowl, combine the first six ingredients. Pour 1/3 cup marinade into a large resealable plastic bag; add the beef. Seal bag and turn to coat; refrigerate for 1 hour. Add salt and pepper to remaining marinade; cover and refrigerate.

- Drain beef and discard marinade. In a nonstick skillet or wok coated with cooking spray, stir-fry beef until no longer pink; remove and keep warm. In the same pan, stir-fry onion and peppers until crisp-tender. Stir in reserved marinade. Return beef to the pan; heat through.

- Spread tortillas with cream cheese; top with beef mixture and sprinkle with sesame seeds. Roll up.

YIELD: 4 servings.

NUTRITION FACTS: 1 wrap equals 402 calories, 14 g fat (5 g saturated fat), 74 mg cholesterol, 575 mg sodium, 41 g carbohydrate, 3 g fiber, 29 g protein. **DIABETIC EXCHANGES:** 3 lean meat, 2 starch, 1 vegetable, 1 fat.

411 CALORIES — citrus fish tacos

PREP: 15 minutes + chilling I **BAKE:** 15 minutes

Maria Baldwin I MESA, ARIZONA

My fun fish tacos bring a deliciously different twist to the Southwestern standby. I combine halibut or cod with a fruity salsa and zesty seasoning, then tuck it all inside wholesome corn tortillas.

1-1/2	cups finely chopped fresh pineapple
1	can (11 ounces) mandarin oranges, drained and cut in half
1	envelope reduced-sodium taco seasoning, *divided*
3	tablespoons thawed orange juice concentrate, *divided*
3	tablespoons lime juice, *divided*
1	jalapeno pepper, seeded and finely chopped
1-1/2	pounds halibut *or* cod, cut into 3/4-inch cubes
8	corn tortillas (6 inches), warmed
3	cups shredded lettuce

- In a large bowl, combine the pineapple, oranges, 1 tablespoon taco seasoning, 1 tablespoon orange juice concentrate, 1 tablespoon lime juice and jalapeno pepper. Cover and refrigerate.

- Place fish in an ungreased shallow 2-qt. baking dish. In a small bowl, combine the remaining orange juice concentrate, lime juice and taco seasoning. Pour over fish; toss gently to coat. Cover and bake at 375° for 12-16 minutes or until fish flakes easily with a fork.

- Place a spoonful of the fish mixture down the center of each tortilla. Top with lettuce and pineapple salsa, roll up.

YIELD: 4 servings.

EDITOR'S NOTE: We recommend wearing disposable gloves when cutting hot peppers. Avoid touching your face.

NUTRITION FACTS: 2 tacos equals 411 calories, 6 g fat (1 g saturated fat), 54 mg cholesterol, 670 mg sodium, 52 g carbohydrate, 5 g fiber, 40 g protein.

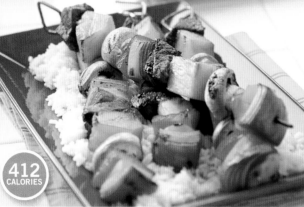

412 CALORIES

PINEAPPLE BEEF KABOBS

pineapple beef kabobs

PREP: 20 minutes + marinating | **GRILL:** 10 minutes

Marguerite Shaeffer | SEWELL, NEW JERSEY

I first tried this recipe after reading a similar one in a medical magazine at my doctor's office. It's easy and colorful, and the basting helps keep the kabobs juicy and tender.

1	can (6 ounces) unsweetened pineapple juice
1/3	cup honey
1/3	cup soy sauce
3	tablespoons cider vinegar
1-1/2	teaspoons minced garlic
1-1/2	teaspoons ground ginger
1-1/2	pounds beef top sirloin steak, cut into 1-inch pieces
1	fresh pineapple, peeled and cut into 1-inch chunks
12	large fresh mushrooms
1	medium sweet red pepper, cut into 1-inch pieces
1	medium sweet yellow pepper, cut into 1-inch pieces
1	medium red onion, cut into 1-inch pieces
2-1/2	cups uncooked instant rice

- In a small bowl, combine the first six ingredients. Pour 3/4 cup into a large resealable plastic bag; add beef. Seal bag and turn to coat; refrigerate for 1-4 hours. Cover and refrigerate remaining marinade for basting.
- Drain and discard marinade. On 12 metal or soaked wooden skewers, alternately thread the beef, pineapple, mushrooms, peppers and onion. Using long-handled tongs, moisten a paper towel with cooking oil and lightly coat the grill rack.
- Grill, covered, over medium-hot heat for 8-10 minutes or until meat reaches desired doneness, turning occasionally and basting frequently with reserved marinade.
- Cook rice according to package directions; serve with the kabobs.

YIELD: 6 servings.

NUTRITION FACTS: 2 kabobs with 3/4 cup rice equals 412 calories, 5 g fat (2 g saturated fat), 46 mg cholesterol, 534 mg sodium, 60 g carbohydrate, 3 g fiber, 31 g protein.

ragu bolognese

PREP: 30 minutes | **COOK:** 1-1/4 hours

Mary Bilyeu | ANN ARBOR, MICHIGAN

I cook this hearty entree slowly, which creates a rich, absolutely delicious sauce. The veggies add fiber, and I use skim milk and turkey sausage to keep it lighter.

1/2	pound Italian turkey sausage links, casings removed
1	large carrot, finely chopped
1	celery rib, finely chopped
1	small onion, finely chopped
1	can (15 ounces) crushed tomatoes
1/2	cup reduced-sodium chicken broth
2	tablespoons balsamic vinegar
1/4	teaspoon crushed red pepper flakes
3/4	cup fat-free milk
4	cups uncooked whole wheat spiral pasta
2	tablespoons prepared pesto
1	tablespoon chopped ripe olives

- Crumble sausage into a nonstick Dutch oven. Add the carrot, celery and onion; cook and stir over medium heat until meat is no longer pink. Drain.
- Stir in the tomatoes, broth, vinegar and pepper flakes. Bring to a boil. Stir in milk. Reduce heat; simmer, uncovered, for 1 to 1-1/4 hours or until thickened, stirring occasionally.
- Cook pasta according to package directions. Stir pesto and olives into meat sauce. Drain pasta; serve with meat sauce.

YIELD: 4 servings.

NUTRITION FACTS: 1 cup pasta with 2/3 cup meat sauce equals 413 calories, 11 g fat (2 g saturated fat), 38 mg cholesterol, 674 mg sodium, 58 g carbohydrate, 6 g fiber, 21 g protein.

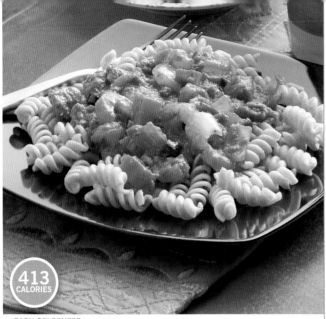

RAGU BOLOGNESE

hearty pasta casserole

PREP: 45 minutes | **BAKE:** 35 minutes

Taste of Home Test Kitchen

Loaded with colorful, flavorful roasted butternut squash, brussels sprouts and onion, this recipe became an instant hit with us. The rustic Italian-inspired casserole is also the perfect main dish "to go" because it transports easily and retains heat well. It's a great make-ahead meal, too!

2	cups cubed peeled butternut squash
1/2	pound fresh brussels sprouts, halved
1	medium onion, cut into wedges
2	teaspoons olive oil
1	package (13-1/4 ounces) whole wheat penne pasta
1	pound Italian turkey sausage links, casings removed
2	garlic cloves, minced
2	cans (14-1/2 ounces *each*) Italian stewed tomatoes
2	tablespoons tomato paste
1-1/2	cups (6 ounces) shredded part-skim mozzarella cheese, *divided*
1/3	cup shredded Asiago cheese, *divided*

- In a large bowl, combine the squash, brussels sprouts and onion; drizzle with oil and toss to coat. Spread vegetables in a single layer in two 15-in. x 10-in. x

1-in. baking pans coated with cooking spray. Bake, uncovered, at 425° for 30-40 minutes or until tender.

- Meanwhile, cook pasta according to package directions. In a large nonstick skillet, cook sausage over medium heat until meat is no longer pink. Add garlic; cook 1 minute longer; drain. Add tomatoes and tomato paste; cook and stir over medium heat until slightly thickened, about 5 minutes.

- Drain pasta and return to the pan. Add sausage mixture, 1 cup mozzarella, 1/4 cup Asiago and the roasted vegetables.

- Transfer to a 13-in. x 9-in. baking dish coated with cooking spray. Cover and bake at 350° for 30-40 minutes or until heated through. Uncover; sprinkle with remaining cheeses. Bake 5 minutes longer or until cheese is melted.

YIELD: 8 servings.

NUTRITION FACTS: 1-1/4 cups equals 416 calories, 13 g fat (5 g saturated fat), 47 mg cholesterol, 816 mg sodium, 53 g carbohydrate, 7 g fiber, 24 g protein.

HEARTY PASTA CASSEROLE

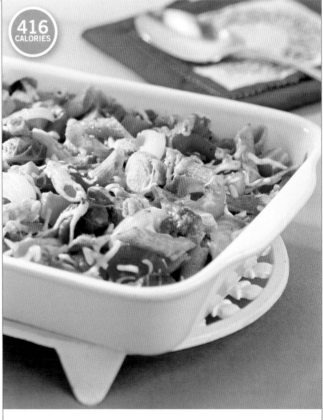

side dishes

Counting calories doesn't mean settling for carrot sticks when it comes to rounding out meals. Dig into classics such as coleslaw, potato salad and even mac 'n' cheese! Make it a 500-calorie dinner by pairing these side dishes with entrees from pages 122 to 171.

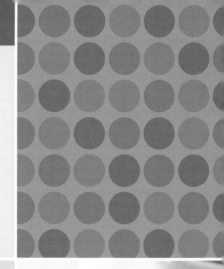

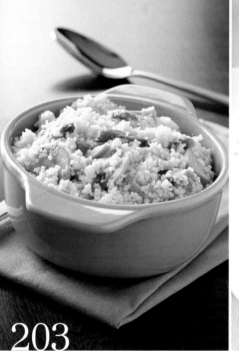

203

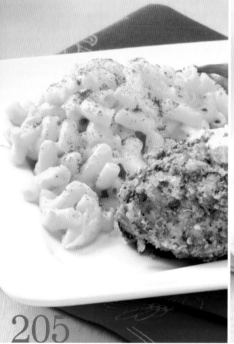

205

192

The first section in this chapter offers items that make it easy to plan calorie-smart meals. Later in the chapter, you'll find more substantial dishes, which can be paired with a lower-in-calorie main dish. Check out readers' comments on how the Comfort Food Diet helped them lose weight.

100 Calories or Less 173
101-200 Calories 187
201-250 Calories 198

100 calories or less

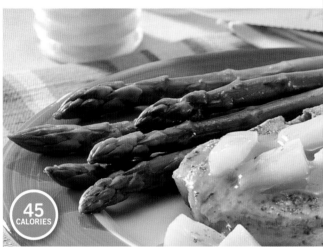

BALSAMIC ASPARAGUS

balsamic asparagus

PREP/TOTAL TIME: 15 minutes

Taste of Home Test Kitchen

Pretty green spears of crisp-tender asparagus are drizzled with a balsamic vinegar mixture for a sensational side dish that's ready in no time.

- 1 cup water
- 1 pound fresh asparagus, trimmed
- 2 tablespoons balsamic vinegar
- 1 tablespoon butter, melted
- 1 teaspoon minced garlic
- 1/4 teaspoon salt
- 1/4 teaspoon pepper

- In a large skillet, bring water to a boil. Add asparagus; cover and cook for 2-4 minutes or until crisp-tender. In a small bowl, combine the vinegar, butter, garlic, salt and pepper. Drain the asparagus; drizzle with the balsamic mixture.

YIELD: 4 servings.

NUTRITION FACTS: 1 serving equals 45 calories, 3 g fat (2 g saturated fat), 8 mg cholesterol, 185 mg sodium, 4 g carbohydrate, 1 g fiber, 2 g protein. **DIABETIC EXCHANGES:** 1 vegetable, 1/2 fat.

citrus spinach salad

PREP/TOTAL TIME: 15 minutes

Edna Lee | GREELEY, COLORADO

A touch of orange in this crisp salad adds a colorful bit of refreshment, and lime lovers will really appreciate its snappy dressing. What a great way to get a healthy vitamin A and C punch for the day.

- 2 tablespoons olive oil
- 1 tablespoon lime juice
- 1 teaspoon sesame seeds, toasted
- 1/2 teaspoon sugar
- 1/2 teaspoon grated lime peel
- 1/4 teaspoon ground ginger
- 4 cups coarsely chopped fresh spinach
- 2 medium navel oranges, peeled and sectioned
- 1 cup sliced fresh mushrooms
- 1/2 small red onion, halved and thinly sliced

- In a small bowl, whisk the first six ingredients.

- In a large salad bowl, combine the spinach, oranges, mushrooms and onion. Just before serving, whisk dressing and pour over salad; toss to coat.

YIELD: 9 servings.

NUTRITION FACTS: 3/4 cup equals 52 calories, 3 g fat (trace saturated fat), 0 cholesterol, 13 mg sodium, 6 g carbohydrate, 1 g fiber, 1 g protein. **DIABETIC EXCHANGES:** 1 vegetable, 1/2 fat.

CITRUS SPINACH SALAD

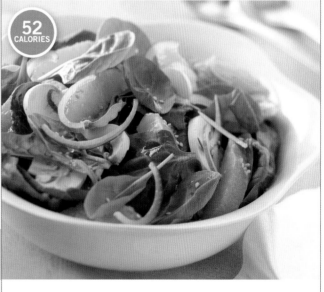

This program is great because the recipes are family-friendly. My husband has loved all the recipes I've tried. It's not hard to make the healthier choice with all the good things we can eat. —**Andrea Johnson, Illinois**

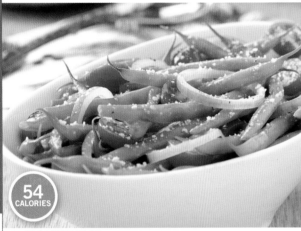

DIJON GREEN BEANS

54 CALORIES

dijon green beans

(also pictured on the cover)

PREP/TOTAL TIME: 20 minutes

Jannine Fisk | MALDEN, MASSACHUSETTS
I love this recipe because it combines the freshness of garden green beans with a warm and tangy dressing.

- 1-1/2 pounds fresh green beans, trimmed
-     2 tablespoons red wine vinegar
-     2 tablespoons olive oil
-     2 teaspoons Dijon mustard
- 1/2 teaspoon salt
- 1/4 teaspoon pepper
-     1 cup grape tomatoes, halved
- 1/2 small red onion, sliced
-     2 tablespoons grated Parmesan cheese

- Place beans in a large saucepan and cover with water. Bring to a boil. Cook, covered, for 10-15 minutes or until crisp-tender.

- Meanwhile, whisk the vinegar, oil, mustard, salt and pepper in a small bowl. Drain beans; place in a large bowl. Add tomatoes and onion. Drizzle with dressing and toss to coat. Sprinkle with cheese.

YIELD: 10 servings.

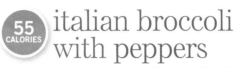

NUTRITION FACTS: 3/4 cup equals 54 calories, 3 g fat (1 g saturated fat), 1 mg cholesterol, 167 mg sodium, 6 g carbohydrate, 2 g fiber, 2 g protein. **DIABETIC EXCHANGES:** 1 vegetable, 1/2 fat.

55 CALORIES

italian broccoli with peppers

PREP/TOTAL TIME: 20 minutes

Maureen McClanahan | ST. LOUIS, MISSOURI
Don't know what side to pair with an entree? Turn to this one that goes with just about anything. And for a satisfying meal, we like it over pasta.

-     6 cups water
-     4 cups fresh broccoli florets
-     1 medium sweet red pepper, julienned
-     1 medium sweet yellow pepper, julienned
-     1 tablespoon olive oil
-     1 garlic clove, minced
-     1 teaspoon dried oregano
- 1/2 teaspoon salt
- 1/4 teaspoon pepper
-     1 medium ripe tomato, cut into wedges and seeded
-     1 tablespoon grated Parmesan cheese

- In a large saucepan, bring water to a boil. Add broccoli; cover and boil for 3 minutes. Drain and immediately place broccoli in ice water. Drain and pat dry.

- In a large nonstick skillet, saute peppers in oil for 3 minutes or until crisp-tender. Add the broccoli, garlic, oregano, salt and pepper; cook 2 minutes longer. Add the tomato; heat through. Sprinkle with cheese.

YIELD: 6 servings.

NUTRITION FACTS: 3/4 cup equals 55 calories, 3 g fat (1 g saturated fat), 1 mg cholesterol, 228 mg sodium, 7 g carbohydrate, 2 g fiber, 2 g protein. **DIABETIC EXCHANGES:** 1 vegetable, 1/2 fat.

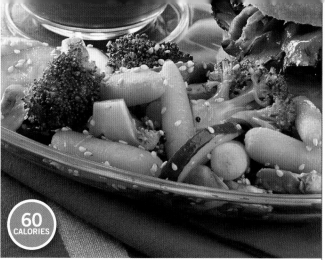

SESAME VEGETABLE MEDLEY

60 CALORIES

sesame vegetable medley

PREP/TOTAL TIME: 10 minutes

Tanya Lamb | TALKING ROCK, GEORGIA

This yummy veggie medley makes a delicious addition to any menu.

1 cup *each* baby carrots, broccoli florets and sliced fresh mushrooms
1 cup sliced zucchini (1/2 inch thick)
1 teaspoon minced garlic
2 tablespoons water
1 tablespoon butter
2 teaspoons sesame seeds, toasted
1/8 teaspoon salt
1/8 teaspoon pepper

- In a large microwave-safe bowl, combine the carrots, broccoli, mushrooms, zucchini, garlic and water. Cover and microwave on high for 3-5 minutes or until vegetables are tender, stirring twice; drain. Stir in the butter, sesame seeds, salt and pepper.

YIELD: 4 servings.

EDITOR'S NOTE: This recipe was tested in a 1,100-watt microwave.

NUTRITION FACTS: 3/4 cup equals 60 calories, 4 g fat (2 g saturated fat), 8 mg cholesterol, 145 mg sodium, 6 g carbohydrate, 2 g fiber, 2 g protein. **DIABETIC EXCHANGES:** 1 vegetable, 1/2 fat.

Here are some typical side dishes and the calories they contain so you can determine how to stay within your goal of a 500-calorie dinner.

- **1/2 cup cooked brown rice,** 108 calories
- **1/2 cup cooked white rice,** 103 calories
- **1 cup cooked egg noodles,** 221 calories
- **1 cup cooked spaghetti,** 200 calories
- **1 cup cooked whole wheat spaghetti,** 176 calories
- **1/2 cup corn,** 83 calories
- **1 small baked russet potato,** 138 calories
- **1 small baked sweet potato,** 128 calories
- **1 medium baked red potato,** 154 calories

- **1/2 cup peas,** 59 calories
- **1/2 cup cooked barley,** 97 calories
- **1/2 cup cooked couscous,** 90 calories
- **1 small buttermilk biscuit,** 154 calories
- **1/2 cup cooked lentils,** 115 calories
- **1/2 cup cooked wild rice,** 83 calories
- **1 cup cooked, mashed acorn squash,** 83 calories
- **1 piece of corn bread prepared from a dry mix,** 188 calories
- **1 small breadstick (4-1/4" long),** 21 calories

- **1 slice whole wheat bread,** 69 calories
- **1 slice reduced-calorie white bread,** 48 calories
- **1 flour tortilla (6" diameter),** 90 calories
- **1 corn tortilla (6" diameter),** 58 calories
- **1 whole wheat dinner roll,** 76 calories
- **1/2 cup 1% cottage cheese,** 81 calories
- **1 saltine cracker,** 13 calories

For the calories of other side items, see the Free Foods Chart on page 53 and the Smart Snacks List on pages 77 and 78. For additional calorie calculations, check the Nutrition Facts labels on food packages.

62 CALORIES

VEGGIE TOSSED SALAD

veggie tossed salad

PREP/TOTAL TIME: 10 minutes

Evelyn Slade | FRUITA, COLORADO

You'll get a dose of veggies and great garden flavor with this simple salad. Feel free to try it with your favorite reduced-fat salad dressing.

- 1-1/2 cups torn romaine
- 1-1/2 cups fresh baby spinach
- 3/4 cup sliced fresh mushrooms
- 3/4 cup grape tomatoes
- 1/2 cup sliced cucumber
- 1/3 cup sliced ripe olives
- 1 tablespoon grated Parmesan cheese
- 1/4 cup reduced-fat Italian salad dressing

- In a large bowl, combine the first seven ingredients. Add salad dressing; toss to coat.

YIELD: 4 servings.

NUTRITION FACTS: 1 cup equals 62 calories, 4 g fat (1 g saturated fat), 1 mg cholesterol, 245 mg sodium, 5 g carbohydrate, 2 g fiber, 2 g protein. **DIABETIC EXCHANGES:** 1 vegetable, 1 fat.

herbed beans and carrots

PREP/TOTAL TIME: 10 minutes

Taste of Home Test Kitchen

A pleasant blend of seasonings accents the fresh taste of this quick, crisp-crunchy side dish.

- 1/2 pound fresh green beans, trimmed
- 3 medium carrots, julienned
- 2 tablespoons water
- 2 tablespoons butter
- 1/2 teaspoon dried rosemary, crushed
- 1/4 teaspoon dried thyme
- 1/4 teaspoon salt
- 1/8 teaspoon lemon-pepper seasoning

- Place the beans and carrots in a microwave-safe 8-in. square dish. Add water. Cover and microwave on high for 3-4 minutes or until crisp-tender; drain. Stir in the butter and seasonings.

YIELD: 4 servings.

EDITOR'S NOTE: This recipe was tested in a 1,100-watt microwave.

NUTRITION FACTS: 3/4 cup (prepared with reduced-fat butter) equals 63 calories, 3 g fat (2 g saturated fat), 10 mg cholesterol, 216 mg sodium, 9 g carbohydrate, 3 g fiber, 2 g protein. **DIABETIC EXCHANGES:** 1-1/2 vegetable, 1/2 fat.

HERBED BEANS AND CARROTS

63 CALORIES

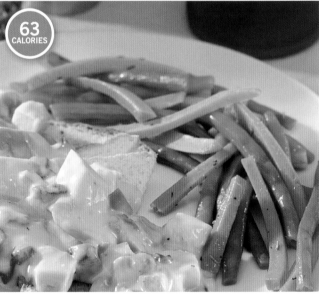

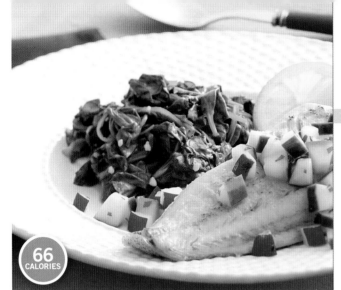

WILTED GARLIC SPINACH

wilted garlic spinach

PREP/TOTAL TIME: 20 minutes

Dotty Egge | PELICAN RAPIDS, MINNESOTA
You don't have to be a spinach fan to happily eat up these greens. Soy sauce gives my energy-packed dish an Asian twist. I serve it over rice or as a side. Try garnishing it with toasted sesame seeds.

1	teaspoon cornstarch
1	teaspoon sugar
2	tablespoons chicken broth
1	tablespoon reduced-sodium soy sauce
1/2	teaspoon sesame oil
6	garlic cloves, minced
1	tablespoon canola oil
3/4	pound fresh spinach, trimmed

- In a small bowl, combine the cornstarch, sugar, broth, soy sauce and sesame oil until smooth; set aside.

- In a small skillet, saute the garlic in canola oil for 1 minute. Stir broth mixture and add to skillet. Cook and stir over medium heat until slightly thickened. Add spinach; cook and stir for 2 minutes or just until spinach is wilted and coated with sauce. Serve with a slotted spoon.

YIELD: 4 servings.

NUTRITION FACTS: 1/2 cup equals 66 calories, 4 g fat (1 g saturated fat), 0 cholesterol, 248 mg sodium, 6 g carbohydrate, 2 g fiber, 3 g protein. **DIABETIC EXCHANGES:** 1 vegetable, 1 fat.

mediterranean summer squash

PREP/TOTAL TIME: 25 minutes

Dawn Bryant | THEDFORD, NEBRASKA
I came up with the recipe when my garden was producing like crazy, and I had a lot of fresh zucchini, yellow squash and tomatoes. I combined the three, added herbs, garlic and feta and created a colorful, flavorful dish that I really love.

1/4	cup chopped onion
1	tablespoon olive oil
1	small yellow summer squash, thinly sliced
1	small zucchini, thinly sliced
1	garlic clove, minced
1	plum tomato, seeded and chopped
1/2	teaspoon dried oregano
1/4	cup crumbled feta cheese
1/4	teaspoon salt
1/4	teaspoon pepper

- In a large skillet, saute onion in oil until tender. Add squash and zucchini; saute 6-8 minutes longer or until tender. Add garlic; cook 1 minute longer. Stir in the remaining ingredients; heat through.

YIELD: 4 servings.

NUTRITION FACTS: 2/3 cup equals 69 calories, 5 g fat (1 g saturated fat), 4 mg cholesterol, 220 mg sodium, 5 g carbohydrate, 2 g fiber, 3 g protein. **DIABETIC EXCHANGES:** 1 vegetable, 1 fat.

MEDITERRANEAN SUMMER SQUASH

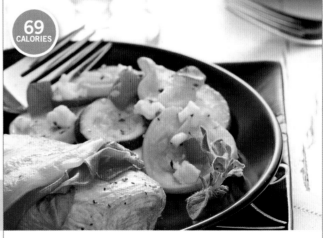

70 CALORIES

MEXICAN VEGGIES

mexican veggies

PREP/TOTAL TIME: 15 minutes

Patricia Mickelson | SAN JOSE, CALIFORNIA
When I needed a side to complement a Mexican dinner I was making, I tossed together this oh-so-easy, colorful combination. Corn, zucchini, salsa and fresh, crunchy flavor make this recipe a keeper!

- 1 medium zucchini, diced
- 1/2 cup fresh *or* frozen corn
- 1/2 cup salsa *or* picante sauce

for 2

- Place 1 in. of water in a small saucepan; add zucchini and corn. Bring to a boil. Reduce heat; cover and simmer for 3-4 minutes or until zucchini is almost tender. Drain. Stir in salsa; heat through.

YIELD: 2 servings.

NUTRITION FACTS: 3/4 cup equals 70 calories, trace fat (trace saturated fat), 0 cholesterol, 284 mg sodium, 13 g carbohydrate, 4 g fiber, 2 g protein. **DIABETIC EXCHANGES:** 1 vegetable, 1/2 starch.

lemon-pepper veggies

PREP/TOTAL TIME: 10 minutes

Linda Bernhagen | PLAINFIELD, ILLINOIS
The microwave makes this no-fuss side a breeze to prepare. I usually pair it with chicken.

- 2 cups fresh broccoli florets
- 2 cups fresh cauliflowerets
- 1 cup sliced carrots
- 2 tablespoons water
- 4-1/2 teaspoons butter, melted
- 1 teaspoon lemon-pepper seasoning
- 1/2 teaspoon garlic powder

- In a microwave-safe bowl, combine the broccoli, cauliflower, carrots and water. Cover and microwave on high for 3-6 minutes or until crisp-tender; drain.

- Combine the remaining ingredients; drizzle over vegetables and toss to coat.

YIELD: 4 servings.

EDITOR'S NOTE: This recipe was tested in a 1,100-watt microwave.

NUTRITION FACTS: 3/4 cup equals 75 calories, 5 g fat (3 g saturated fat), 11 mg cholesterol, 194 mg sodium, 8 g carbohydrate, 3 g fiber, 2 g protein. **DIABETIC EXCHANGES:** 1 vegetable, 1 fat.

LEMON-PEPPER VEGGIES

75 CALORIES

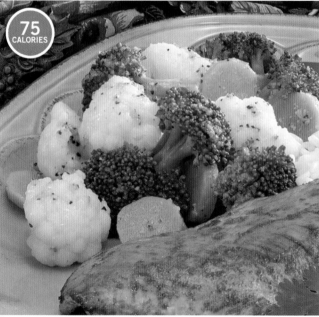

My family and I have tried at least 40 recipes and they are mostly winners! I'm starting to lose pounds and inches by combining the new recipes with daily workouts. We haven't forfeited taste for weight loss, which is the best part of this diet! —**Lisa Miller, Connecticut**

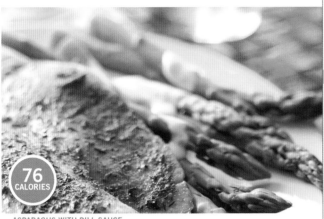

76 CALORIES

ASPARAGUS WITH DILL SAUCE

asparagus with dill sauce

PREP/TOTAL TIME: 15 minutes

Sandy Miller I WIXOM, MICHIGAN
Asparagus with a creamy dill sauce makes a tasty side and is super-easy to make. You'll be delighted with it.

for 2

- 1/2 **pound fresh asparagus, trimmed**
- 1/4 **cup sour cream**
- 1 **teaspoon milk**
- 1/4 **teaspoon dill weed**
- 1/8 **teaspoon salt**
- 1/8 **teaspoon pepper**

- Place asparagus in a steamer basket; place in a large saucepan over 1 in. of water. Bring to a boil; cover and steam for 3-5 minutes or until crisp-tender.

- Meanwhile, in a small microwave-safe bowl, combine the remaining ingredients. Microwave on high for 30-60 seconds or until heated through. Serve with asparagus.

YIELD: 2 servings.

NUTRITION FACTS: 1/4 pound asparagus with 2 tablespoons sauce equals 76 calories, 5 g fat (4 g saturated fat), 20 mg cholesterol, 165 mg sodium, 4 g carbohydrate, 1 g fiber, 3 g protein. **DIABETIC EXCHANGES:** 1 vegetable, 1 fat.

pretty almond green beans

PREP/TOTAL TIME: 25 minutes

Vikki Peck I POLAND, OHIO
Enjoy the traditional flavors of green beans, mushrooms and onions without the calories of a classic green bean casserole! This dish is light, festive and easy to put together. It has become a holiday tradition at our house.

- 1 **pound fresh green beans, trimmed**
- 1 **medium sweet red pepper, julienned**
- 1 **cup sliced fresh mushrooms**
- 1 **small onion, chopped**
- 1 **tablespoon olive oil**
- 1/4 **cup sliced almonds, toasted**

- Place beans in a large saucepan and cover with water. Bring to a boil. Cover and cook for 4-7 minutes or until crisp-tender.

- Meanwhile, in a large nonstick skillet, saute the pepper, mushrooms and onion in oil until tender. Drain beans; stir into vegetable mixture. Sprinkle with almonds.

YIELD: 6 servings.

NUTRITION FACTS: 3/4 cup equals 78 calories, 4 g fat (1 g saturated fat), 0 cholesterol, 6 mg sodium, 9 g carbohydrate, 4 g fiber, 3 g protein. **DIABETIC EXCHANGES:** 1 vegetable, 1 fat.

PRETTY ALMOND GREEN BEANS

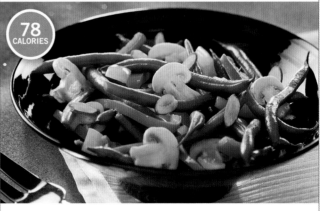

78 CALORIES

78 CALORIES

BRAVO BROCCOLI

bravo broccoli

PREP/TOTAL TIME: 20 minutes

Taste of Home Test Kitchen
Here's a fast, delicious way to dress up crisp-tender broccoli. Just toss with a simple sweet-sour mixture that gets a slight kick from crushed red pepper flakes.

1 bunch broccoli, cut into florets
1 tablespoon butter, melted
1 tablespoon rice vinegar
1-1/2 teaspoons brown sugar
1/4 teaspoon salt
1/4 teaspoon crushed red pepper flakes
1/8 teaspoon garlic powder

- Arrange broccoli in a steamer basket; place in a large saucepan over 1 in. of water. Bring to a boil; cover and steam for 3-4 minutes or until tender. Transfer to a large bowl.

- Combine the remaining ingredients; drizzle over broccoli and gently toss to coat.

YIELD: 4 servings.

NUTRITION FACTS: 3/4 cup equals 78 calories, 3 g fat (2 g saturated fat), 8 mg cholesterol, 210 mg sodium, 10 g carbohydrate, 5 g fiber, 5 g protein. **DIABETIC EXCHANGES:** 2 vegetable, 1/2 fat

italian vegetable medley

PREP/TOTAL TIME: 15 minutes

Margaret Wilson | SUN CITY, CALIFORNIA
Round out a variety of menus with this side dish that lends a wonderful pop of color. The recipe is also a tasty way to use up leftover veggies. People are always surprised at how easy this dish is!

1 package (16 ounces) broccoli stir-fry vegetables
1 tablespoon butter
2 tablespoons grated Parmesan cheese
1 tablespoon seasoned bread crumbs
1/8 teaspoon garlic powder
1/8 teaspoon seasoned salt
1/8 teaspoon pepper

- Microwave vegetables according to package directions; drain. Stir in butter. Meanwhile, in a small bowl, combine the cheese, bread crumbs, garlic powder, salt and pepper; sprinkle over vegetables.

YIELD: 4 servings.

NUTRITION FACTS: 3/4 cup equals 79 calories, 4 g fat (2 g saturated fat), 10 mg cholesterol, 174 mg sodium, 7 g carbohydrate, 2 g fiber, 2 g protein. **DIABETIC EXCHANGES:** 1 vegetable, 1/2 fat.

ITALIAN VEGETABLE MEDLEY

79 CALORIES

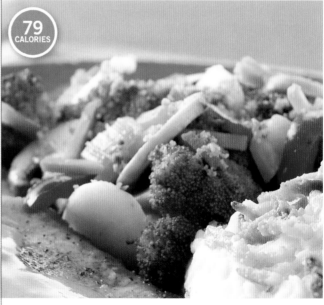

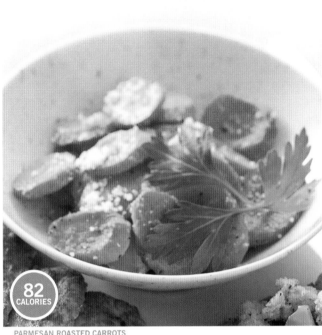

82 CALORIES

PARMESAN ROASTED CARROTS

snow pea medley

PREP/TOTAL TIME: 20 minutes

Lucille Mead | ILION, NEW YORK
Even in frosty weather, I serve up garden-fresh flavor with this pretty side. The crisp-tender veggie combo is so easy to create.

- 1/3 cup chopped red onion
- 2 teaspoons canola oil **for 2**
- 1/3 cup julienned sweet red pepper
- 1/3 cup julienned sweet yellow pepper
- 1/2 cup fresh snow peas
- 1/2 cup sliced fresh mushrooms
- 1/4 teaspoon salt

- In a nonstick skillet coated with cooking spray, saute onion in oil for 1-2 minutes. Add peppers; cook for 2 minutes. Stir in the peas and mushrooms; saute 3-4 minutes longer or until vegetables are crisp-tender. Sprinkle with salt.

YIELD: 2 servings.

NUTRITION FACTS: 3/4 cup equals 83 calories, 5 g fat (trace saturated fat), 0 cholesterol, 299 mg sodium, 8 g carbohydrate, 2 g fiber, 3 g protein. **DIABETIC EXCHANGES:** 1 vegetable, 1 fat.

SNOW PEA MEDLEY

83 CALORIES

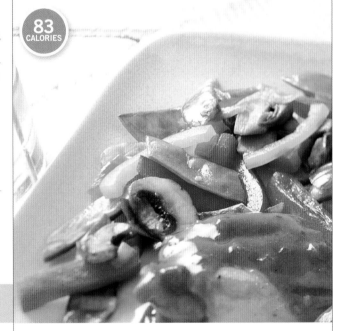

parmesan roasted carrots

PREP/TOTAL TIME: 20 minutes

Pam Ion | GAITHERSBURG, MARYLAND
This oven-baked side dish helped turn my children on to eating carrots. The downsized version of the recipe is just right for two.

- 4 large carrots, cut diagonally into 1/4-inch slices
- 2 tablespoons unsweetened applesauce
- 1 tablespoon finely chopped onion
- 1/4 teaspoon salt

Dash paprika **for 2**

Pepper to taste

- 1 tablespoon grated Parmesan cheese

- In a small bowl, combine the first six ingredients. Transfer to a baking sheet coated with cooking spray.
- Bake at 425° for 10-15 minutes or until golden brown. Sprinkle with Parmesan cheese. Serve immediately.

YIELD: 2 servings.

NUTRITION FACTS: 1/2 cup equals 82 calories, 1 g fat (1 g saturated fat), 2 mg cholesterol, 392 mg sodium, 17 g carbohydrate, 5 g fiber, 3 g protein. **DIABETIC EXCHANGE:** 1 starch.

Using Comfort Food Diet recipes, I can still make good food that my picky husband will eat while lowering my calorie intake. Using those recipes along with exercise, I've lost a good amount of weight in six months. I don't feel deprived and I can still eat the foods I love! —Jennifer Watson Spence

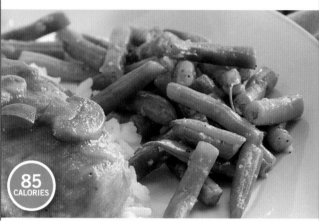

85 CALORIES

ITALIAN GREEN BEANS

italian green beans

PREP/TOTAL TIME: 15 minutes

Rudy Martino | LOMBARD, ILLINOIS

The sharpness of the Parmesan cheese is a nice accent to these beans. This has been a family favorite for many years.

- 1/2 pound fresh *or* frozen cut green beans
- 2 tablespoons water
- 2-1/4 teaspoons grated Parmesan cheese
- 2-1/4 teaspoons seasoned bread crumbs
- 1/4 teaspoon garlic salt
- 1/8 teaspoon pepper
- 1-1/2 teaspoons olive oil

for 2

- Place beans and water in a microwave-safe dish. Cover and microwave on high for 4-5 minutes or until crisp-tender. Meanwhile, in a small bowl, combine the cheese, bread crumbs, garlic salt and pepper. Drain beans; drizzle with olive oil. Sprinkle with cheese mixture and toss to coat.

YIELD: 2 servings.

EDITOR'S NOTE: This recipe was tested in a 1,100-watt microwave.

NUTRITION FACTS: 3/4 cup equals 85 calories, 4 g fat (1 g saturated fat), 1 mg cholesterol, 309 mg sodium, 10 g carbohydrate, 4 g fiber, 3 g protein. **DIABETIC EXCHANGES:** 1 vegetable, 1/2 fat.

sauteed corn with tomatoes & basil

PREP/TOTAL TIME: 15 minutes

Patricia Nieh | PORTOLA VALLY, CALIFORNIA

In the summer, we harvest the veggies and basil from our backyard garden just minutes before fixing this recipe! It's so fresh and simple.

- 1 cup fresh *or* frozen corn
- 1 tablespoon olive oil
- 2 cups cherry tomatoes, halved
- 1/4 teaspoon salt
- 1/4 teaspoon pepper
- 3 fresh basil leaves, thinly sliced

- In a large skillet, saute corn in oil until crisp-tender. Stir in the tomatoes, salt and pepper; cook 1 minute longer. Remove from the heat; sprinkle with basil.

YIELD: 4 servings.

NUTRITION FACTS: 3/4 cup equals 85 calories, 4 g fat (1 g saturated fat), 0 cholesterol, 161 mg sodium, 12 g carbohydrate, 2 g fiber, 2 g protein.

SAUTEED CORN WITH TOMATOES & BASIL

85 CALORIES

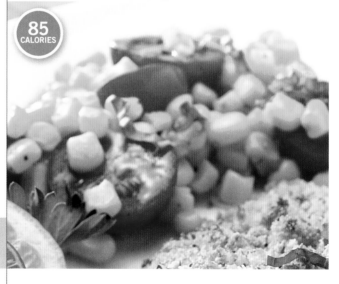

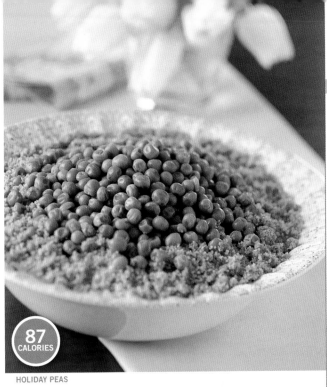

HOLIDAY PEAS

holiday peas

PREP/TOTAL TIME: 20 minutes

Sue Gronholz | BEAVER DAM, WISCONSIN

My mom used to dress up peas with buttered cracker crumbs when I was little, and it still remains one of my favorite dishes. Just about any type of savory crackers can be substituted, including herb-flavored varieties.

 2 **packages (16 ounces *each*) frozen peas**
 2 **teaspoons salt**
 1 **cup finely crushed wheat crackers**
 2 **tablespoons grated Parmesan cheese**
 2 **tablespoons butter, melted**

- Place peas in a large saucepan; add salt. Cover with water. Bring to a boil. Reduce heat; cover and simmer for 5-6 minutes or until tender.

- Meanwhile, toss the cracker crumbs, cheese and butter. Drain the peas and place in a serving bowl; top with the crumb mixture.

YIELD: 12 servings.

NUTRITION FACTS: 3/4 cup equals 87 calories, 3 g fat (1 g saturated fat), 6 mg cholesterol, 523 mg sodium, 12 g carbohydrate, 4 g fiber, 4 g protein. **DIABETIC EXCHANGES:** 1 starch, 1/2 fat.

home-style coleslaw

PREP: 20 minutes + chilling

Joy Cochran | ROY, WASHINGTON

This recipe is a staple at our house. The flecks of color get the kids' attention, especially when I use red and green cabbage.

 8 **cups finely shredded cabbage**
 1/2 **cup shredded carrot**
DRESSING:
 1/3 **cup reduced-fat mayonnaise**
 1/3 **cup fat-free sour cream**
 1 **tablespoon sugar**
 2 **teaspoons cider vinegar**
 1/2 **teaspoon salt**
 1/4 **teaspoon pepper**

- In a large bowl, combine cabbage and carrot. In a small bowl, combine the dressing ingredients. Pour over cabbage mixture; toss to coat. Cover and refrigerate for 6-8 hours or overnight.

YIELD: 7 servings.

NUTRITION FACTS: 2/3 cup equals 88 calories, 4 g fat (1 g saturated fat), 5 mg cholesterol, 292 mg sodium, 12 g carbohydrate, 3 g fiber, 2 g protein. **DIABETIC EXCHANGES:** 1 vegetable, 1 fat, 1/2 starch.

HOME-STYLE COLESLAW

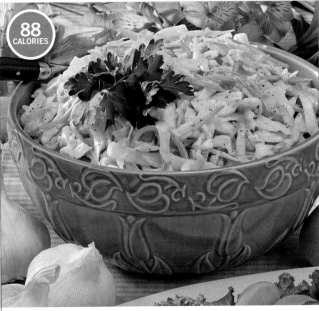

88 CALORIES

pineapple peach soup

PREP: 25 minutes + chilling

Teresa Lynn | KERRVILLE, TEXAS

I like to take this one-of-a-kind, chilled soup to potlucks and other events where I need to bring a dish to pass. It's usually different than the dishes other people bring, and everyone raves about the flavors.

- 6 medium peaches, peeled and sliced
- 1 can (8 ounces) crushed unsweetened pineapple, undrained
- 1/4 cup white grape juice
- 1/4 cup lemon juice
- 2 tablespoons honey
- 3/4 teaspoon ground cinnamon
- 1/4 teaspoon ground nutmeg
- 1 medium cantaloupe, peeled, seeded and cubed
- 1 cup orange juice

Fresh strawberries and whipped cream, optional

- In 3-qt. saucepan, combine peaches, pineapple, grape juice, lemon juice, honey, cinnamon and nutmeg; bring to a boil over medium heat. Reduce heat and simmer, uncovered, for 10 minutes. Remove from the heat; cool to room temperature. Stir in three-fourths of the cantaloupe and the orange juice.

- In a blender or food processor, puree the mixture in batches until smooth.

- Pour into a large bowl. Add remaining cantaloupe. Cover and refrigerate for at least 3 hours. Garnish with strawberries and whipped cream if desired.

YIELD: 9 servings (2-1/4 quarts).

NUTRITION FACTS: 1 cup equals 88 calories, trace fat (trace saturated fat), 0 cholesterol, 6 mg sodium, 22 g carbohydrate, 2 g fiber, 1 g protein. **DIABETIC EXCHANGE:** 1-1/2 fruit.

dilly vegetable medley

PREP: 25 minutes | **GRILL:** 20 minutes

Rebecca Barjonah | CORALVILLE, IOWA

I love to eat what I grow, and I have tried many combinations of the fresh vegetables from my garden. This one is really delectable! I never have leftovers when I make this tasty side.

- 1/4 cup olive oil
- 2 tablespoons minced fresh basil
- 2 teaspoons dill weed
- 1/2 teaspoon salt
- 1/2 teaspoon pepper
- 7 small yellow summer squash, cut into 1/2-inch slices
- 1 pound Yukon Gold potatoes, cut into 1/2-inch cubes
- 5 small carrots, cut into 1/2-inch slices

- In a very large bowl, combine the first five ingredients. Add vegetables and toss to coat.

- Place half of the vegetables on a double thickness of heavy-duty foil (about 18 in. square). Fold the foil around the vegetables and seal tightly. Repeat with the remaining vegetables.

- Grill, covered, over medium heat for 20-25 minutes or until potatoes are tender, turning once. Open foil carefully to allow steam to escape.

YIELD: 13 servings.

NUTRITION FACTS: 3/4 cup equals 91 calories, 4 g fat (1 g saturated fat), 0 cholesterol, 109 mg sodium, 12 g carbohydrate, 2 g fiber, 2 g protein. **DIABETIC EXCHANGES:** 1 vegetable, 1 fat, 1/2 starch.

DILLY VEGETABLE MEDLEY

91 CALORIES

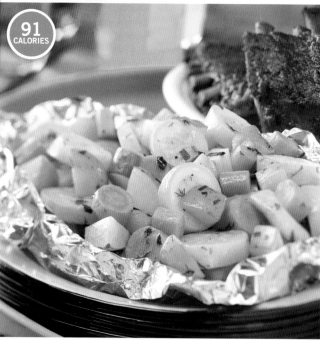

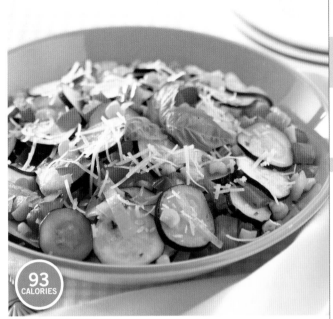

93 CALORIES

ITALIAN VEGGIE SKILLET

italian veggie skillet

PREP/TOTAL TIME: 20 minutes

Sue Spencer | COARSEGOLD, CALIFORNIA
This vibrant blend of sauteed vegetables is as pretty as it is delicious. The recipe was given to me by a dear friend, and it's become a family favorite.

- 1 medium onion, halved and sliced
- 1 medium sweet red pepper, chopped
- 1 tablespoon olive oil
- 3 medium zucchini, thinly sliced
- 1 garlic clove, minced
- 1-1/2 cups frozen corn, thawed
- 1 large tomato, chopped
- 2 teaspoons minced fresh basil
- 1/2 teaspoon salt
- 1/2 teaspoon Italian seasoning
- 1/4 cup shredded Parmesan cheese

- In a large nonstick skillet, saute onion and red pepper in oil for 2 minutes. Add zucchini; saute 4-5 minutes or until vegetables are crisp-tender. Add the garlic; cook 1 minute longer.

- Stir in corn, tomato, basil, salt and Italian seasoning; cook and stir until heated through. Sprinkle with the cheese. Serve immediately.

YIELD: 6 servings.

NUTRITION FACTS: 1 cup equals 93 calories, 4 g fat (1 g saturated fat), 3 mg cholesterol, 266 mg sodium, 14 g carbohydrate, 3 g fiber, 4 g protein. **DIABETIC EXCHANGES:** 2 vegetable, 1/2 starch.

lemon garlic mushrooms

PREP/TOTAL TIME: 25 minutes

Diane Hixon | NICEVILLE, FLORIDA
I baste whole mushrooms with a lemony sauce for a superb side dish. Using skewers or a grill basket makes it easy to turn the mushrooms.

- 1/4 cup lemon juice
- 3 tablespoons minced fresh parsley
- 2 tablespoons olive oil
- 3 garlic cloves, minced

Pepper to taste

- 1 pound large fresh mushrooms

- In a small bowl, combine the first five ingredients; set aside. Grill the mushrooms, covered, over medium-hot heat for 5 minutes. Brush generously with the lemon mixture. Turn the mushrooms; grill 5-8 minutes longer or until tender. Brush with the remaining lemon mixture before serving.

YIELD: 4 servings.

NUTRITION FACTS: 1 serving equals 96 calories, 7 g fat, 0 cholesterol, 7 mg sodium, 8 g carbohydrate, 2 g fiber, 3 g protein. **DIABETIC EXCHANGES:** 1-1/2 fat, 1 vegetable. 1/2 fat.

LEMON GARLIC MUSHROOMS

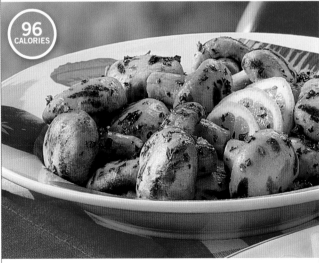

96 CALORIES

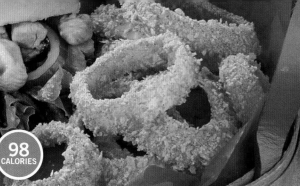

98 CALORIES

BAKED ONION RINGS

baked onion rings

PREP: 15 minutes | **BAKE:** 20 minutes

Marilyn Lee | RICHMOND, MISSOURI
If you love onion rings but not the fat from deep-frying them, try baking them instead. These crisp rings round out a meal or make a scrumptious snack.

> 2 large sweet onions
> 2 eggs
> 1-1/2 cups crushed cornflakes
> 2 teaspoons sugar
> 1 teaspoon paprika
> 1/4 teaspoon garlic salt
> 1/4 teaspoon seasoned salt

- Cut onions into 1/2-in. slices; separate into rings. In a shallow dish, whisk eggs. In another shallow dish, combine the cornflake crumbs, sugar, paprika, garlic salt and seasoned salt. Dip onion rings into eggs, then coat with cornflake mixture.

- Arrange the rings in a single layer on greased baking sheets. Bake at 375° for 20-25 minutes or until tender.

YIELD: 8 servings.

NUTRITION FACTS: 5 onion rings equals 98 calories, 1 g fat (trace saturated fat), 53 mg cholesterol, 241 mg sodium, 18 g carbohydrate, 1 g fiber, 4 g protein. **DIABETIC EXCHANGES:** 1 starch, 1 vegetable.

italian squash casserole

PREP: 45 minutes | **BAKE:** 30 minutes

Paul VanSavage | BINGHAMTON, NEW YORK
You can assemble these garlic-kissed veggies in advance, but wait to bake them until just before serving. The aroma from the oven will lure everyone to the kitchen.

> 1 whole garlic bulb
> 2 tablespoons olive oil, *divided*
> 1 medium butternut squash (about 3-1/2 pounds), cut into 1-inch cubes
> 2 large sweet red peppers, cut into 1-inch pieces
> 1 large red onion, cut into wedges
> 2 medium tomatoes, cut into wedges
> 1/4 cup dry bread crumbs
> 3 tablespoons minced fresh parsley
> 1-1/2 teaspoons minced fresh rosemary *or* 1/2 teaspoon dried rosemary, crushed
> 1 teaspoon salt
> 1/2 teaspoon pepper
> 1/2 cup grated Parmesan cheese

- Remove papery outer skin from garlic (do not peel or separate cloves). Cut top off of garlic bulb. Brush with 1/2 teaspoon oil. Wrap bulb in heavy-duty foil. Bake at 425° for 30-35 minutes or until softened. Reduce heat to 400°. Cool garlic for 10 minutes. Squeeze softened garlic into a bowl and mash.

- Meanwhile, in a large skillet, saute the squash in 1 tablespoon oil until golden brown; transfer to a large bowl. In the same skillet, saute peppers and onion in remaining oil until crisp-tender. Add to squash.

- Stir in the tomatoes, garlic, bread crumbs, parsley, rosemary, salt and pepper. Transfer to a greased 13-in. x 9-in. baking dish; sprinkle with cheese. Bake, uncovered, for 30-40 minutes or until squash is tender.

YIELD: 14 servings.

NUTRITION FACTS: 3/4 cup equals 99 calories, 3 g fat (1 g saturated fat), 3 mg cholesterol, 234 mg sodium, 17 g carbohydrate, 4 g fiber, 3 g protein. **DIABETIC EXCHANGES:** 1 starch, 1 vegetable.

ITALIAN SQUASH CASSEROLE

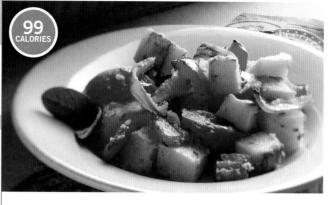

99 CALORIES

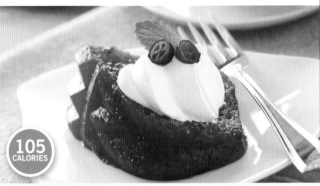

HOLIDAY GELATIN MOLD

105 CALORIES

holiday gelatin mold

PREP: 25 minutes + chilling

Mareen Robinson I SPANISH FORK, UTAH
Because I care for a teenager with diabetes, I decided to change my annual Thanksgiving salad so she could enjoy a serving of it.

- 1 package (.3 ounce) sugar-free lemon gelatin
- 1 package (.3 ounce) sugar-free strawberry gelatin
- 1 package (.3 ounce) sugar-free cherry gelatin
- 1-3/4 cups boiling water
- 1 can (20 ounces) unsweetened crushed pineapple
- 1 can (14 ounces) whole-berry cranberry sauce
- 1 medium navel orange, peeled and sectioned
- 3/4 cup reduced-fat whipped topping
- 1/4 cup fat-free sour cream

- In a large bowl, dissolve the gelatins in boiling water. Drain pineapple, reserving juice in a 2-cup measuring cup; add enough cold water to measure 2 cups. Stir into gelatin mixture.

- Place the pineapple, cranberry sauce and orange in a food processor; cover and pulse until blended. Stir into gelatin mixture. Transfer to an 8-cup ring mold coated with cooking spray. Refrigerate until firm.

- In a small bowl, combine whipped topping and sour cream. Unmold gelatin; serve with topping.

YIELD: 12 servings (3/4 cup topping).

NUTRITION FACTS: 2/3 cup gelatin with 1 tablespoon topping equals 105 calories, 1 g fat (1 g saturated fat), 1 mg cholesterol, 62 mg sodium, 24 g carbohydrate, 1 g fiber, 1 g protein. **DIABETIC EXCHANGES:** 1 fruit, 1/2 starch.

baked veggie chips

PREP: 15 minutes I **BAKE:** 20 minutes

Christine Schenher I SAN CLEMENTE, CALIFORNIA
Roasted root vegetable chips are a fun, festive snack or side. These perfectly seasoned chips are so good they don't even need dip!

- 1/2 pound fresh beets (about 2 medium)
- 1 medium potato
- 1 medium sweet potato
- 1 medium parsnip
- 2 tablespoons canola oil
- 2 tablespoons grated Parmesan cheese
- 1/2 teaspoon salt
- 1/2 teaspoon garlic powder
- 1/2 teaspoon dried oregano

Dash pepper

- Peel vegetables and cut into 1/8-in. slices. Place in a large bowl. Drizzle with oil. Combine the remaining ingredients; sprinkle over vegetables and toss to coat.

- Arrange in a single layer in two ungreased 15-in. x 10-in. x 1-in. baking pans. Bake at 375° for 15-20 minutes or until golden brown, turning once.

YIELD: 3-1/2 cups.

NUTRITION FACTS: 1/2 cup equals 108 calories, 5 g fat (1 g saturated fat), 1 mg cholesterol, 220 mg sodium, 15 g carbohydrate, 2 g fiber, 2 g protein. **DIABETIC EXCHANGES:** 1 starch, 1 fat.

BAKED VEGGIE CHIPS

108 CALORIES

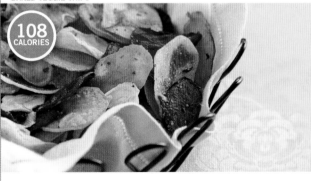

I have the Comfort Food Diet Cookbook and use a lot of the recipes. I've started to lose weight even in the first few weeks. I'm doing it the healthy way so it will stay off. No rebounding for me! —Ruth Woodman York

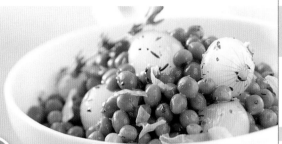

112 CALORIES

PEAS A LA FRANCAISE

peas a la francaise

PREP/TOTAL TIME: 30 minutes

Christine Frazier | AUBURNDALE, FLORIDA
I love peas, and this is one of my favorite ways to prepare them. It features tiny pearl onions touched with thyme and chervil, and its presentation is delightful.

- 1-1/2 cups pearl onions, trimmed
- 1/4 cup butter, cubed
- 1/4 cup water
- 1 tablespoon sugar
- 1 teaspoon salt
- 1/4 teaspoon dried thyme
- 1/4 teaspoon dried chervil
- 1/4 teaspoon pepper
- 2 packages (16 ounces *each*) frozen peas, thawed
- 2 cups shredded lettuce

- In a large saucepan, bring 6 cups water to a boil. Add onions; boil for 5 minutes. Drain and rinse in cold water; peel.

- In the same saucepan, melt butter over medium heat. Stir in the onions, water, sugar and seasonings. Add peas and lettuce; stir until blended. Cover and cook for 6-8 minutes or until tender.

- Serve with a slotted spoon.

YIELD: 12 servings.

NUTRITION FACTS: 1/2 cup equals 112 calories, 4 g fat (2 g saturated fat), 10 mg cholesterol, 315 mg sodium, 15 g carbohydrate, 4 g fiber, 4 g protein. **DIABETIC EXCHANGES:** 1 starch, 1 fat.

flavorful corn

PREP/TOTAL TIME: 15 minutes

Taste of Home Test Kitchen
A pinch of sage and thyme season this quick and easy treatment for frozen corn. It is versatile enough to serve with most any entree.

- 2-1/2 cups frozen corn
- 1/4 cup water
- 1 tablespoon butter
- 1/4 teaspoon rubbed sage
- 1/8 teaspoon dried thyme
- 1/8 teaspoon pepper

- In a large saucepan, bring the corn and water to a boil. Reduce heat; cover and simmer for 4-6 minutes or until corn is tender. Drain; add butter and seasonings. Stir until butter is melted.

YIELD: 4 servings.

NUTRITION FACTS: 1/2 cup equals 116 calories, 4 g fat (2 g saturated fat), 8 mg cholesterol, 32 mg sodium, 21 g carbohydrate, 3 g fiber, 3 g protein. **DIABETIC EXCHANGES:** 1-1/2 starch, 1/2 fat.

FLAVORFUL CORN

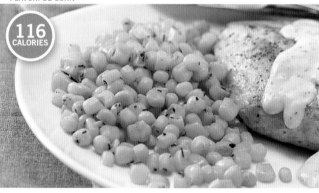
116 CALORIES

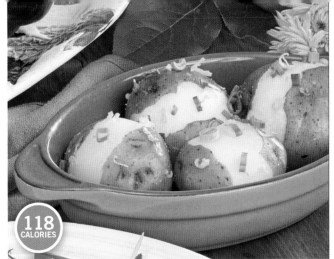

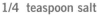

LEMONY NEW POTATOES

lemony new potatoes

PREP/TOTAL TIME: 25 minutes

Cheryl Tichenor | ELGIN, ILLINOIS
I can't recall where this recipe came from, but I know my family has enjoyed it for years.

```
      6  to 8 small red potatoes
      1  teaspoon butter
  1-1/2  teaspoons lemon juice       for 2
    1/4  teaspoon salt
    1/4  teaspoon grated lemon peel
      1  tablespoon sliced green onion (green part only)
```

- Peel a strip from around each potato. Place potatoes in a small saucepan; cover with water. Bring to a boil. Reduce heat; cover and simmer for 15-20 minutes or until tender. Drain. Add the butter, lemon juice, salt and lemon peel; toss to coat. Sprinkle with green onion.

YIELD: 2 servings.

NUTRITION FACTS: 1 serving equals 118 calories, 2 g fat (1 g saturated fat), 5 mg cholesterol, 317 mg sodium, 23 g carbohydrate, 2 g fiber, 3 g protein. **DIABETIC EXCHANGES:** 1-1/2 starch, 1/2 fat.

parmesan cauliflower

PREP/TOTAL TIME: 15 minutes

Brenda Biron | SYDNEY, NOVA SCOTIA
Need a last-minute side dish to round out your meal? This cheesy recipe can be table-ready in minutes! It's also yummy with broccoli instead of cauliflower.

```
  1-1/2  cups fresh caulifllowerets
      5  teaspoons reduced-fat butter      for 2
      2  teaspoons all-purpose flour
      3  tablespoons reduced-fat sour cream
      2  tablespoons shredded Parmesan cheese
    1/4  teaspoon salt
    1/8  teaspoon white pepper
```
Minced fresh parsley, optional

- Place cauliflower in a steamer basket; place in a small saucepan over 1 in. of water. Bring to a boil; cover and steam for 4-5 minutes or until crisp-tender.

- Meanwhile, in another small saucepan, melt butter. Stir in flour until smooth. Remove from the heat; stir in the sour cream, Parmesan cheese, salt and pepper.

- Add cauliflower to the cream sauce. Cook and stir over low heat for 1-2 minutes or until heated through. Sprinkle with parsley if desired.

YIELD: 2 servings.

EDITOR'S NOTE: This recipe was tested with Land O'Lakes light stick butter.

NUTRITION FACTS: 3/4 cup equals 121 calories, 8 g fat (6 g saturated fat), 28 mg cholesterol, 476 mg sodium, 8 g carbohydrate, 2 g fiber, 6 g protein. **DIABETIC EXCHANGES:** 1-1/2 fat, 1 vegetable.

PARMESAN CAULIFLOWER

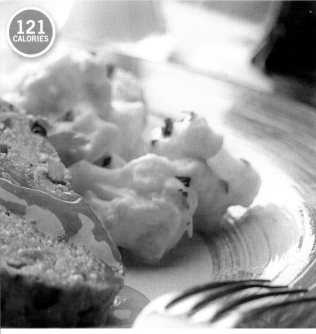

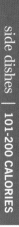

side dishes | 101-200 CALORIES

seasoned yukon gold wedges

PREP: 10 minutes | **BAKE:** 40 minutes

Jane Lynch | SCARBOROUGH, ONTARIO

These zesty potatoes are a snap to make. My two boys and husband just love them. They're good with roast or chops but can also be served as an appetizer with dip.

- 1-1/2 **pounds Yukon Gold potatoes (about 3 medium), cut into wedges**
- 1 **tablespoon olive oil**
- 1/4 **cup dry bread crumbs**
- 1-1/2 **teaspoons paprika**
- 3/4 **teaspoon salt**
- 1/4 **teaspoon dried oregano**
- 1/4 **teaspoon dried thyme**
- 1/4 **teaspoon ground cumin**
- 1/8 **teaspoon pepper**
- 1/8 **teaspoon cayenne pepper**

- In a large bowl, toss potatoes with oil. Combine the remaining ingredients; sprinkle over the potatoes and toss to coat.

- Arrange potatoes in a single layer in a 15-in. x 10-in. x 1-in. baking pan coated with cooking spray.

- Bake, uncovered, at 425° for 40-45 minutes or until tender, stirring once.

YIELD: 6 servings.

NUTRITION FACTS: 3/4 cup equals 121 calories, 3 g fat (trace saturated fat), 0 cholesterol, 339 mg sodium, 21 g carbohydrate, 2 g fiber, 3 g protein. **DIABETIC EXCHANGES:** 1-1/2 starch, 1/2 fat.

SEASONED YUKON GOLD WEDGES

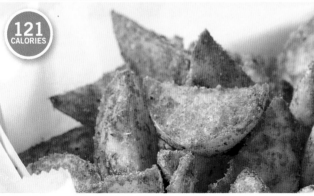

121 CALORIES

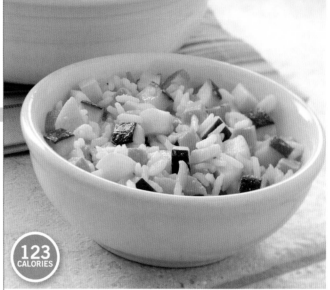

123 CALORIES

RICE WITH SUMMER SQUASH

rice with summer squash

PREP: 15 minutes | **COOK:** 25 minutes

Heather Ratigan | KAUFMAN, TEXAS

I don't usually create my own recipes, but this one passed my palate test. It offers a buttery flavor that those of us who are watching our weight miss at times.

- 1 **cup chopped carrots**
- 1/2 **cup chopped onion**
- 1 **tablespoon butter**
- 1 **cup reduced-sodium chicken broth** *or* **vegetable broth**
- 1/3 **cup uncooked long grain rice**
- 1/4 **teaspoon salt**
- 1/4 **teaspoon pepper**
- 1 **medium yellow summer squash, chopped**
- 1 **medium zucchini, chopped**

- In a large saucepan coated with cooking spray, cook carrots and onion in butter until tender. Stir in the broth, rice, salt and pepper. Bring to a boil. Reduce heat; cover and simmer for 13 minutes.

- Stir in yellow squash and zucchini. Cover and simmer 6-10 minutes longer or until the rice and vegetables are tender.

YIELD: 4 servings.

NUTRITION FACTS: 3/4 cup equals 123 calories, 3 g fat (2 g saturated fat), 8 mg cholesterol, 346 mg sodium, 21 g carbohydrate, 3 g fiber, 4 g protein. **DIABETIC EXCHANGES:** 1 starch, 1 vegetable, 1/2 fat.

glazed orange carrots

PREP/TOTAL TIME: 25 minutes

Marilyn Hash | ENUMCLAW, WASHINGTON

Want your kids to eat more carrots? These have a pleasant citrus flavor and a pretty orange glaze. It's a must at our family gatherings.

2	pounds fresh carrots, sliced
2	tablespoons butter
1/4	cup thawed orange juice concentrate
2	tablespoons brown sugar
2	tablespoons minced fresh parsley

- Place 1 in. of water in a saucepan; add carrots. Bring to a boil. Reduce heat; cover and simmer for 7-9 minutes or until crisp-tender. Drain.

- Melt butter in a large skillet; stir in orange juice concentrate and brown sugar. Add carrots and parsley; stir to coat. Cook and stir for 1-2 minutes or until glaze is thickened.

YIELD: 6 servings.

NUTRITION FACTS: 2/3 cup equals 132 calories, 4 g fat (2 g saturated fat), 10 mg cholesterol, 134 mg sodium, 24 g carbohydrate, 4 g fiber, 2 g protein. **DIABETIC EXCHANGES:** 1 vegetable, 1 fat, 1/2 starch.

GLAZED ORANGE CARROTS

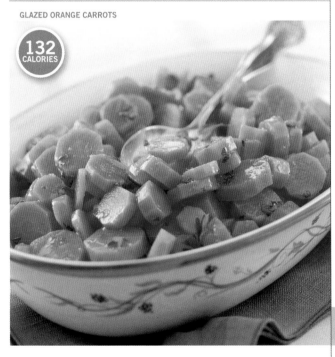

132 CALORIES

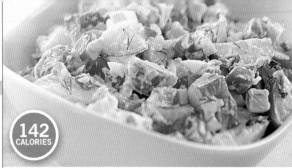

142 CALORIES

HERBED POTATO SALAD

herbed potato salad

PREP: 40 minutes + chilling

Judy Grebetz | RACINE, WISCONSIN

Calcium-rich cheese and potatoes and peppers packed with vitamin C make this potluck favorite something to smile about!

3	pounds small red potatoes, cubed
1/2	cup cubed reduced-fat cheddar cheese
1/4	cup chopped dill pickle
1/4	cup chopped red onion
1/4	cup chopped green pepper
1/4	cup chopped sweet red pepper
1	jalapeno pepper, seeded and minced
3/4	cup fat-free mayonnaise
1	tablespoon minced fresh basil
1	tablespoon snipped fresh dill
1	tablespoon minced fresh tarragon
1/2	teaspoon salt
1/2	teaspoon pepper
1	hard-cooked egg, chopped

- Place potatoes in a large saucepan and cover with water. Bring to a boil. Reduce heat; cover and simmer for 10-15 minutes or until tender. Drain and cool to room temperature.

- In a large bowl, combine the potatoes, cheese, pickle, onion and peppers. In a small bowl, combine the mayonnaise, basil, dill, tarragon, salt and pepper. Pour over salad and toss to coat. Cover and refrigerate until chilled. Garnish with chopped egg.

YIELD: 10 servings.

EDITOR'S NOTE: We recommend wearing disposable gloves when cutting hot peppers. Avoid touching your face.

NUTRITION FACTS: 3/4 cup equals 142 calories, 3 g fat (1 g saturated fat), 27 mg cholesterol, 371 mg sodium, 25 g carbohydrate, 3 g fiber, 5 g protein. **DIABETIC EXCHANGE:** 1-1/2 starch.

flavorful mashed potatoes

PREP: 20 minutes | **COOK:** 25 minutes

Mary Relyea | CANASTOTA, NEW YORK

Earthy herbs bring a full chorus of flavor to creamy red potatoes, making this side dish anything but ordinary. Save it for special occasions or serve as a dressy accompaniment to a weeknight meal.

      4   pounds red potatoes (about 12 medium)
      6   garlic cloves, peeled and thinly sliced
    1/2   cup fat-free milk
    1/2   cup reduced-fat sour cream
      2   tablespoons butter, melted
      2   tablespoons minced fresh parsley
          or 2 teaspoons dried parsley flakes
      2   tablespoons minced fresh thyme
          or 2 teaspoons dried thyme
      1   tablespoon minced fresh rosemary
          or 1 teaspoon dried rosemary, crushed
  1-1/4   teaspoons salt

- Scrub and quarter potatoes; place in a large saucepan and cover with water. Add the garlic. Bring to a boil. Reduce heat; cover and cook for 15-20 minutes or until potatoes are tender; drain.

- In a large bowl, mash the potato mixture. Stir in the remaining ingredients.

YIELD: 12 servings.

NUTRITION FACTS: 3/4 cup equals 146 calories, 3 g fat (2 g saturated fat), 9 mg cholesterol, 280 mg sodium, 26 g carbohydrate, 3 g fiber, 4 g protein. **DIABETIC EXCHANGES:** 2 starch, 1/2 fat.

FLAVORFUL MASHED POTATOES

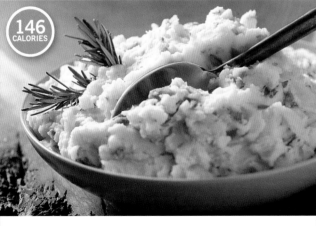

146 CALORIES

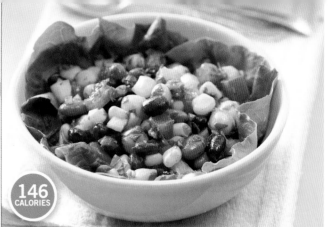

146 CALORIES

ALFRESCO BEAN SALAD

alfresco bean salad

PREP/TOTAL TIME: 25 minutes

Cristina Vives | PALM BEACH GARDENS, FLORIDA

If you're bored with the usual greens, whip up this super healthy version of classic three bean salad. It's so terrific that I sometimes fill my plate and eat it as a meal.

    1/4   cup lime juice
  4-1/2   teaspoons olive oil
    1/2   teaspoon chili powder
Dash salt and pepper
      1   can (16 ounces) red beans, rinsed and drained
      1   can (15-1/4 ounces) whole kernel corn, drained
      1   can (15 ounces) garbanzo beans *or* chickpeas, rinsed and drained
      1   can (15 ounces) black beans, rinsed and drained
      2   medium tomatoes, seeded and chopped
      1   cup coarsely chopped fresh cilantro
      1   small yellow onion, chopped
      1   small red onion, chopped
      1   jalapeno pepper, seeded and chopped

- In a large bowl, whisk the lime juice, oil, chili powder, salt and pepper. Add the remaining ingredients and toss to coat. Chill until serving.

YIELD: 12 servings.

EDITOR'S NOTE: We recommend wearing disposable gloves when cutting hot peppers. Avoid touching your face.

NUTRITION FACTS: 2/3 cup equals 146 calories, 3 g fat (trace saturated fat), 0 cholesterol, 360 mg sodium, 23 g carbohydrate, 6 g fiber, 6 g protein. **DIABETIC EXCHANGES:** 1-1/2 starch, 1 lean meat.

I have lost significant weight over the last year by counting calories and changing my portion sizes. For dinner, I fix what I normally would for my family, but I just limit my intake. If I get hungry between meals, I'll snack on fruit or a 100-calorie snack, and I only drink water. If I can lose weight by doing this, anyone can. —**Michelle Nichols, West Virginia**

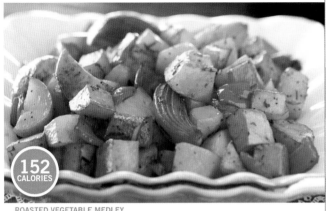

152 CALORIES

ROASTED VEGETABLE MEDLEY

roasted vegetable medley

PREP: 25 minutes | **BAKE:** 30 minutes

Shirley Beauregard | GRAND JUNCTION, COLORADO
Pork pairs well with this veggie combo. And because the vegetables can be prepared in advance, I have more time to enjoy the company of my dinner guests.

- 3 Yukon Gold potatoes, cut into small wedges
- 2 medium sweet red peppers, cut into 1-inch pieces
- 1 small butternut squash, peeled and cubed
- 1 medium sweet potato, peeled and cubed
- 1 medium red onion, quartered
- 3 tablespoons olive oil
- 2 tablespoons balsamic vinegar
- 2 tablespoons minced fresh rosemary *or* 2 teaspoons dried rosemary, crushed
- 1 tablespoon minced fresh thyme *or* 1 teaspoon dried thyme
- 1 teaspoon salt
- 1/2 teaspoon pepper

- In a large bowl, combine the potatoes, red peppers, squash, sweet potato and onion. In a small bowl, whisk the oil, vinegar and seasonings. Pour over vegetables and toss to coat.

- Transfer to two greased 15-in. x 10-in. x 1-in. baking pans. Bake, uncovered, at 425° for 30-40 minutes or until tender, stirring occasionally.

YIELD: 7 servings.

NUTRITION FACTS: 1 cup equals 152 calories, 6 g fat (1 g saturated fat), 0 cholesterol, 347 mg sodium, 24 g carbohydrate, 4 g fiber, 2 g protein. **DIABETIC EXCHANGES:** 1 starch, 1 vegetable, 1 fat.

147 CALORIES

mashed potato cakes

PREP/TOTAL TIME: 25 minutes

Taste of Home Test Kitchen
This is a great way to use up any remaining mashed potatoes. These light cakes cook up golden brown and have a wonderful butter-and-onion flavor. Kids and adults alike will love our spin on a classic!

- 1 egg white, lightly beaten
- 1 cup mashed potatoes (with added milk and butter)
- 1 tablespoon all-purpose flour
- 2-1/2 teaspoons finely chopped green onion
- 1/2 teaspoon minced fresh parsley
- 1/8 teaspoon salt
- 1/8 teaspoon pepper
- Butter-flavored cooking spray
- 1 teaspoon reduced-fat butter

for 2

- In a small bowl, combine the first seven ingredients. In a large nonstick skillet coated with butter-flavored cooking spray, melt butter over medium heat.

- Drop potato mixture by 1/4 cupfuls into skillet; press lightly to flatten. Cook over medium heat for 4-5 minutes on each side or until golden brown. Serve warm.

YIELD: 2 servings.

EDITOR'S NOTE: This recipe was tested with Land O'Lakes light stick butter.

NUTRITION FACTS: 2 potato cakes equals 147 calories, 6 g fat (4 g saturated fat), 16 mg cholesterol, 497 mg sodium, 21 g carbohydrate, 2 g fiber, 4 g protein. **DIABETIC EXCHANGES:** 1-1/2 starch, 1 fat.

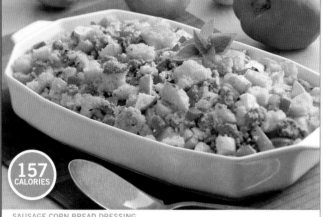

157 CALORIES

SAUSAGE CORN BREAD DRESSING

sausage corn bread dressing

PREP: 30 minutes | **BAKE:** 50 minutes

Rebecca Baird | SALT LAKE CITY, UTAH

You can enjoy this stuffing without any guilt since it is made with turkey sausage, herbs, fruit and veggies.

- 1 cup all-purpose flour
- 1 cup cornmeal
- 1/4 cup sugar
- 3 teaspoons baking powder
- 1 teaspoon salt
- 1 cup buttermilk
- 1/4 cup unsweetened applesauce
- 2 egg whites

DRESSING:

- 1 pound turkey Italian sausage links, casings removed
- 4 celery ribs, chopped
- 1 medium onion, chopped
- 1 medium sweet red pepper, chopped
- 2 medium tart apples, chopped
- 1 cup chopped roasted chestnuts
- 3 tablespoons minced fresh parsley
- 2 garlic cloves, minced
- 1/2 teaspoon dried thyme
- 1/2 teaspoon pepper
- 1 cup reduced-sodium chicken broth
- 1 egg white

- For corn bread, combine first five ingredients in a large bowl. Combine buttermilk, applesauce and egg whites; stir into dry ingredients just until moistened. Pour into an

8-in. square baking dish coated with cooking spray. Bake at 400° 20-25 minutes or until a toothpick inserted near the center comes out clean. Cool on a wire rack.

- In a large nonstick skillet, cook the sausage, celery, onion and red pepper over medium heat until meat is no longer pink; drain. Transfer to a large bowl. Crumble corn bread over mixture. Add the apples, chestnuts, parsley, garlic, thyme and pepper. Stir in broth and egg white.

- Transfer to a 13-in. x 9-in. baking dish coated with cooking spray. Cover and bake at 325° for 40 minutes. Uncover; bake 10 minutes longer or until lightly browned.

YIELD: 16 servings.

NUTRITION FACTS: 3/4 cup equals 157 calories, 3 g fat (1 g saturated fat), 18 mg cholesterol, 464 mg sodium, 24 g carbohydrate, 2 g fiber, 8 g protein. **DIABETIC EXCHANGES:** 1-1/2 starch, 1 lean meat.

154 CALORIES

great grain pilaf

PREP: 5 minutes | **COOK:** 30 minutes

Joyce Graves | STERLING HEIGHTS, MICHIGAN

Bored with boiled rice? This pilaf is mild tasting and a great way to include fiber in your diet.

- 1/2 cup chopped green onions
- 2 garlic cloves, minced
- 2 teaspoons butter
- 1 cup uncooked long grain rice
- 1/2 cup bulgur
- 1/4 cup quick-cooking barley
- 3 cups reduced-sodium chicken broth *or* vegetable broth
- 1/2 teaspoon salt

Dash pepper

- 1/3 cup minced fresh parsley

- In a large saucepan, saute onions and garlic in butter until tender. Add the rice, bulgur and barley; cook and stir for 5 minutes. Gradually stir in the broth, salt and pepper. Bring to a boil. Reduce heat; cover and simmer for 25 minutes or until grains are tender and broth is absorbed. Stir in parsley.

YIELD: 8 servings.

NUTRITION FACTS: 2/3 cup equals 154 calories, 2 g fat (1 g saturated fat), 4 mg cholesterol, 202 mg sodium, 30 g carbohydrate, 3 g fiber, 5 g protein. **DIABETIC EXCHANGE:** 2 starch.

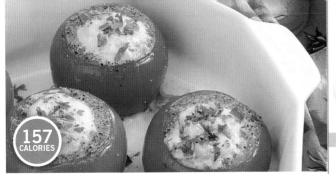

CORN PUDDING STUFFED TOMATOES

corn pudding stuffed tomatoes

PREP: 15 minutes | **BAKE:** 40 minutes

Jean Smalls | COOPER CITY, FLORIDA

I use tomatoes and sweet corn I grow to make this delightful side. Everyone at your table will agree: Nothing beats garden-fresh produce!

- 8 medium tomatoes
- 1 teaspoon salt, *divided*
- 1/2 teaspoon pepper, *divided*
- 2 tablespoons all-purpose flour
- 2 tablespoons sugar
- 1/2 teaspoon baking powder
- 2 eggs, lightly beaten
- 1 cup half-and-half cream
- 1 cup whole kernel corn
- 2 tablespoons butter, melted

Minced fresh parsley

- Cut a thin slice off the top of each tomato; scoop out and discard pulp. Sprinkle inside of tomatoes with half of the salt and pepper. Invert on paper towels to drain.

- In a large bowl, combine the flour, sugar, baking powder and remaining salt and pepper. Combine the eggs, cream, corn and butter; stir into dry ingredients. Spoon into tomatoes.

- Place in a shallow baking dish. Bake, uncovered, at 350° for 38-40 minutes or until a knife inserted near the center of corn pudding comes out clean. Sprinkle with parsley.

YIELD: 8 servings.

NUTRITION FACTS: 1 stuffed tomato equals 157 calories, 8 g fat (4 g saturated fat), 76 mg cholesterol, 397 mg sodium, 18 g carbohydrate, 2 g fiber, 5 g protein. **DIABETIC EXCHANGES:** 1-1/2 fat, 1 vegetable, 1/2 starch.

wholesome apple-hazelnut stuffing

PREP: 20 minutes | **BAKE:** 30 minutes

Donna Noel | GRAY, MAINE

Try this whole grain, fruit and nut stuffing for a delicious new slant. Herbs balance the sweetness of the apples and give this dish a wonderful flavor.

- 2 celery ribs, chopped
- 1 large onion, chopped
- 1 tablespoon olive oil
- 1 small carrot, shredded
- 3 tablespoons minced fresh parsley *or* 1 tablespoon dried parsley flakes
- 1 tablespoon minced fresh rosemary *or* 1 teaspoon dried rosemary, crushed
- 2 garlic cloves, minced
- 4 cups cubed day-old whole wheat bread
- 1-1/2 cups shredded peeled tart apples (about 2 medium)
- 1/2 cup chopped hazelnuts, toasted
- 1 egg, lightly beaten
- 3/4 cup apple cider *or* unsweetened apple juice
- 1/2 teaspoon coarsely ground pepper
- 1/4 teaspoon salt

- In a large nonstick skillet, saute celery and onion in oil for 4 minutes. Add the carrot, parsley and rosemary; saute 2-4 minutes longer or until vegetables are tender. Add garlic; cook 1 minute longer.

- In a large bowl, combine the vegetable mixture, bread cubes, apples and hazelnuts. In a small bowl, combine the egg, cider, pepper and salt. Add to stuffing mixture and mix well.

- Transfer to an 8-in. square baking dish coated with cooking spray. Cover and bake at 350° for 20 minutes. Uncover; bake 10-15 minutes longer or until a thermometer reads 160°.

YIELD: 6 cups.

NUTRITION FACTS: 3/4 cup equals 159 calories, 8 g fat (1 g saturated fat), 27 mg cholesterol, 195 mg sodium, 20 g carbohydrate, 4 g fiber, 4 g protein. **DIABETIC EXCHANGES:** 1-1/2 fat, 1 starch.

> **I use many of the recipes** from the Comfort Food Diet Cookbook, eat lots of fruits and veggies and watch portion sizes. In recent years, I've had weight loss success!
> —Crystol McGrath Burnett

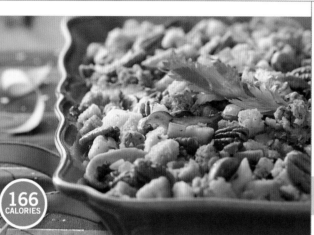

166 CALORIES

SAUSAGE BREAD DRESSING

sausage bread dressing

PREP: 30 minutes I **BAKE:** 40 minutes

Bette Votral I BETHLEHEM, PENNSYLVANIA

My husband and father go crazy for this dressing. Although leftovers are rare, it freezes quite well. To save time, chop the veggies and prepare the stuffing mix ahead of time.

- 4 cups seasoned stuffing cubes
- 1 cup corn bread stuffing mix
- 1/2 pound bulk Italian sausage
- 1 large onion, chopped
- 1 large tart apple, peeled and chopped
- 1-1/3 cups sliced fresh shiitake mushrooms
- 1-1/4 cups sliced fresh mushrooms
- 1 celery rib, chopped
- 1/8 teaspoon salt
- 1/8 teaspoon pepper
- 3 tablespoons butter
- 1 can (14-1/2 ounces) chicken broth
- 1 cup pecan halves
- 1/2 cup minced fresh parsley
- 1 tablespoon fresh sage *or* 1 teaspoon dried sage leaves

- In a large bowl, combine stuffing cubes and stuffing mix; set aside. In a large skillet, cook the sausage, onion, apple, mushrooms, celery, salt and pepper in butter over medium heat until sausage is no longer pink. Add to stuffing mixture. Stir in the broth, pecans, parsley and sage; toss to coat.

- Transfer to a greased 3-qt. baking dish. Cover and bake at 325° for 30 minutes. Uncover; bake 10 minutes longer or until lightly browned.

YIELD: about 12 cups.

NUTRITION FACTS: 3/4 cup equals 166 calories, 10 g fat (2 g saturated fat), 12 mg cholesterol, 455 mg sodium, 17 g carbohydrate, 2 g fiber, 4 g protein.

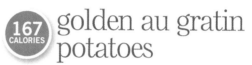

167 CALORIES

golden au gratin potatoes

PREP: 35 minutes I **BAKE:** 1-1/2 hours

Janice Elder I CHARLOTTE, NORTH CAROLINA

With its golden, crunchy topping and gooey, cheesy interior, this comforting spin on a classic side dish is brimming with robust flavors. Horseradish and nutmeg add that extra-special touch.

- 2 large onions, thinly sliced
- 2 tablespoons butter
- 1 cup half-and-half cream
- 1 cup canned pumpkin
- 1 tablespoon prepared horseradish
- 1/2 teaspoon ground nutmeg
- 1 teaspoon salt
- 1/2 teaspoon pepper
- 2-1/4 pounds potatoes, peeled and cut into 1/4-inch slices
- 2 cups soft bread crumbs
- 8 ounces Gruyere *or* Swiss cheese, shredded
- 2 tablespoons chopped fresh sage

- In a large skillet, cook onions in butter over medium heat for 15-20 minutes or until onions are golden brown, stirring frequently.

- In a large bowl, combine the cream, pumpkin, horseradish, nutmeg, salt and pepper. In a greased 13-in. x 9-in. baking pan, layer with potato slices and onions. Spread with pumpkin mixture. Cover and bake at 350° for 1-1/4 hours.

- Increase temperature to 400°. In a large bowl, combine the bread crumbs, cheese and sage. Sprinkle over the top. Bake, uncovered, 15-20 minutes longer or until golden brown.

YIELD: 15 servings.

NUTRITION FACTS: 1 serving equals 167 calories, 8 g fat (5 g saturated fat), 29 mg cholesterol, 274 mg sodium, 16 g carbohydrate, 2 g fiber, 7 g protein. **DIABETIC EXCHANGES:** 1 starch, 1 lean meat, 1 fat.

sweet potato casserole

PREP: 30 minutes | **BAKE:** 35 minutes

Kathy Rairigh | MILFORD, INDIANA
I am always looking for ways to use sweet potatoes. This recipe is my own creation that I have made many times. I take it to family potlucks and it never fails to bring compliments!

2-1/4 pounds sweet potatoes (about 3 large), peeled and cubed
   3 egg whites, lightly beaten
   3 tablespoons maple syrup
   1 teaspoon vanilla extract

TOPPING:
1/4 cup chopped pecans
   1 tablespoon brown sugar
   1 tablespoon butter, melted
1/8 teaspoon ground cinnamon
1/3 cup dried apricots, chopped
1/3 cup dried cherries, chopped

- Place sweet potatoes in a Dutch oven and cover with water. Bring to a boil. Reduce heat; cover and simmer for 15-20 minutes or until tender. Drain and place in a large bowl; mash. Cool slightly. Stir in the egg whites, syrup and vanilla.

- Transfer to an 8-in. square baking dish coated with cooking spray. Combine the pecans, brown sugar, butter and cinnamon; sprinkle over the top.

- Bake, uncovered, at 350° for 30 minutes. Sprinkle with apricots and cherries. Bake 5-7 minutes longer or until a thermometer reads 160° and the fruits are heated through.

YIELD: 8 servings.

NUTRITION FACTS: 1/2 cup equals 186 calories, 4 g fat (1 g saturated fat), 4 mg cholesterol, 40 mg sodium, 34 g carbohydrate, 3 g fiber, 3 g protein. **DIABETIC EXCHANGES:** 1-1/2 starch, 1 fat, 1/2 fruit.

gruyere mashed potatoes

PREP/TOTAL TIME: 25 minutes

Preci D'Silva | DUBAI, UNITED ARAB EMIRATES
Gruyere cheese and chives take mashed potatoes to a whole new level this holiday season. Don't have chives? Just use extra green onion instead.

   2 pounds potatoes, peeled and cubed
1/2 cup sour cream
1/3 cup whole milk
1/4 cup butter, cubed
1/4 cup shredded Gruyere *or* Swiss cheese
1/4 cup chopped green onions
1/4 cup minced chives
   1 teaspoon minced garlic
1/2 teaspoon garlic salt
1/4 teaspoon pepper

- Place potatoes in a Dutch oven and cover with water. Bring to a boil. Reduce heat; cover and cook for 10-15 minutes or until tender. Drain.

- In a large bowl, mash potatoes with remaining ingredients.

YIELD: 8 servings.

NUTRITION FACTS: 3/4 cup equals 193 calories, 9 g fat (6 g saturated fat), 29 mg cholesterol, 175 mg sodium, 23 g carbohydrate, 2 g fiber, 4 g protein.

GRUYERE MASHED POTATOES

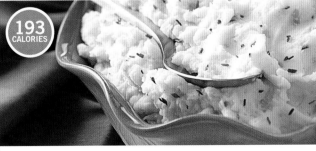

201-250 calories

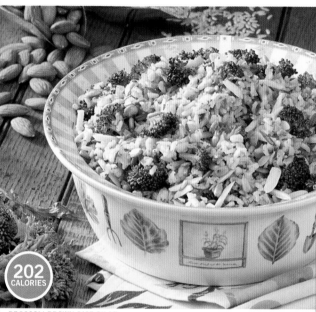

202 CALORIES

BROCCOLI BROWN RICE PILAF

broccoli brown rice pilaf

PREP: 5 minutes | **COOK:** 50 minutes

Marie Condit | BROOKLYN CENTER, MINNESOTA
This is one of my favorite low-fat dishes!

- 1 cup uncooked brown rice
- 2-1/4 cups reduced-sodium chicken broth
  or vegetable broth
- 2 tablespoons minced fresh rosemary
  or 2 teaspoons dried rosemary, crushed
- 2 garlic cloves, minced
- 2 cups chopped fresh broccoli
- 1/4 cup slivered almonds
- 1/4 cup unsalted sunflower kernels
- 1/2 teaspoon salt
- 1/8 teaspoon pepper

- In a large nonstick skillet coated with cooking spray, saute rice until lightly browned. Add the broth, rosemary and garlic; bring to a boil. Reduce heat; cover and simmer for 40 minutes or until rice is almost tender.

- Stir in the broccoli, almonds, sunflower kernels, salt and pepper. Cover and cook 3-5 minutes longer or until rice is tender and broccoli is crisp-tender. Fluff with a fork.

YIELD: 6 servings.

NUTRITION FACTS: 2/3 cup equals 202 calories, 6 g fat (1 g saturated fat), 0 cholesterol, 414 mg sodium, 31 g carbohydrate, 2 g fiber, 7 g protein. **DIABETIC EXCHANGES:** 2 starch, 1 fat.

cranberry couscous

PREP/TOTAL TIME: 15 minutes

Taste of Home Test Kitchen
Although it looks like a grain, couscous is a form of pasta made by steaming and drying cracked wheat.

- 1 can (14-1/2 ounces) chicken broth
- 1 tablespoon butter
- 1-1/2 cups uncooked couscous
- 1/4 cup dried cranberries, chopped
- 3 tablespoons chopped green onions

- In a large saucepan, bring broth and butter to a boil. Stir in the couscous, cranberries and onions. Remove from the heat. Cover and let stand for 5 minutes or until broth is absorbed. Fluff with a fork.

YIELD: 6 servings.

NUTRITION FACTS: 3/4 cup equals 202 calories, 3 g fat (1 g saturated fat), 5 mg cholesterol, 295 mg sodium, 39 g carbohydrate, 2 g fiber, 7 g protein.

CRANBERRY COUSCOUS

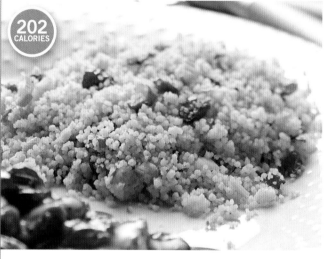

202 CALORIES

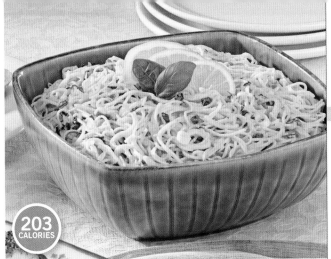

203 CALORIES

BASIL-PARMESAN ANGEL HAIR

basil-parmesan angel hair

PREP/TOTAL TIME: 30 minutes

Barbara Dorsett | SAN DIEGO, CALIFORNIA
I've given this crowd-pleasing recipe to many people, and they all love how quick and simple it is.

- 1 package (16 ounces) angel hair pasta
- 2 tablespoons olive oil
- 1 can (12 ounces) fat-free evaporated milk
- 2/3 cup shredded Parmesan cheese
- 1/2 cup thinly sliced green onions
- 1/4 cup minced fresh basil
- 1 teaspoon grated lemon peel
- 1/2 teaspoon salt
- 1/2 teaspoon garlic powder
- 1/4 teaspoon pepper
Additional fresh basil
- 12 lemon slices

- Cook pasta according to package directions. Drain and return to the pan. Add oil; toss to coat. Add the milk, cheese, onions, basil, lemon peel, salt, garlic powder and pepper. Cook and stir over medium heat until heated through. Sprinkle with additional basil. Serve with lemon.

YIELD: 12 servings.

NUTRITION FACTS: 2/3 cup equals 203 calories, 5 g fat (1 g saturated fat), 5 mg cholesterol, 219 mg sodium, 32 g carbohydrate, 2 g fiber, 9 g protein. **DIABETIC EXCHANGES:** 2 starch, 1/2 fat.

makeover patrician potatoes

PREP: 45 minutes | **BAKE:** 20 minutes

Kathy Fleming | LISLE, ILLINOIS
The Thanksgiving table just isn't complete without a steaming side of mashed potatoes. This makeover transformed high-fat Patrician Potatoes into a light side that still tastes decadent.

- 5 pounds medium potatoes, peeled and quartered
- 2 tablespoons butter, melted
- 1 package (8 ounces) fat-free cream cheese
- 1 cup (8 ounces) reduced-fat sour cream
- 2 teaspoons salt
- 2 teaspoons minced chives
- 1/4 cup shredded Parmesan cheese
- 1 teaspoon paprika

- Place potatoes in a Dutch oven and cover with water. Bring to a boil. Reduce heat; cover and simmer for 15-20 minutes or until tender.

- Drain potatoes and place in a large bowl; mash with butter. In a small bowl, beat the cream cheese, sour cream and salt until light and fluffy; add to potatoes. Stir in chives.

- Transfer to a 13-in. x 9-in. baking dish coated with cooking spray. Sprinkle with cheese and paprika. Bake, uncovered, at 350° for 20-25 minutes or until heated through.

YIELD: 12 servings.

NUTRITION FACTS: 1 cup equals 207 calories, 4 g fat (3 g saturated fat), 14 mg cholesterol, 563 mg sodium, 35 g carbohydrate, 3 g fiber, 8 g protein. **DIABETIC EXCHANGES:** 2 starch, 1 fat.

MAKEOVER PATRICIAN POTATOES

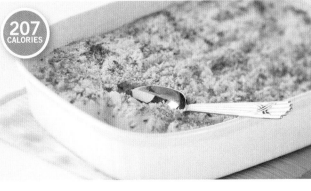

207 CALORIES

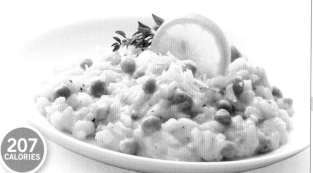

207 CALORIES

LEMON RISOTTO WITH PEAS

lemon risotto with peas

PREP: 10 minutes | **COOK:** 30 minutes

Suzanne Dannahower | FORT PIERCE, FLORIDA

Lemon adds a refreshing taste to this lovely risotto dish that's ideal for spring. This easy side is festively sprinkled with baby peas.

- 4 to 4-1/2 cups reduced-sodium chicken broth
- 2 shallots, finely chopped
- 1 tablespoon butter
- 1-1/2 cups uncooked arborio rice
- 1/2 teaspoon dried thyme
- 1/4 teaspoon pepper
- 1/3 cup white wine *or* additional reduced-sodium chicken broth
- 3 tablespoons lemon juice
- 1 cup frozen peas, thawed
- 1/2 cup grated Parmesan cheese
- 1-1/2 teaspoons grated lemon peel

- In a small saucepan, heat broth and keep warm. In a large nonstick skillet, saute shallots in butter for 2-3 minutes or until tender. Add the rice, thyme and pepper; cook and stir for 2-3 minutes. Stir in wine and lemon juice. Cook and stir until all of the liquid is absorbed.

- Stir in heated broth, 1/2 cup at a time, stirring constantly. Allow liquid to absorb between additions. Cook just until risotto is creamy and rice is almost tender. Total cooking time is about 20 minutes. Add the peas, cheese and lemon peel; cook and stir until heated through. Serve immediately.

YIELD: 8 servings.

NUTRITION FACTS: 1/2 cup equals 207 calories, 3 g fat (2 g saturated fat), 8 mg cholesterol, 440 mg sodium, 35 g carbohydrate, 1 g fiber, 7 g protein. **DIABETIC EXCHANGES:** 2 starch, 1/2 fat.

makeover fancy bean casserole

PREP: 15 minutes | **BAKE:** 35 minutes

Venola Sharpe | CAMPBELLSVILLE, KENTUCKY

I've shared this recipe with many friends. This lighter version retains all its crunchy, creamy goodness.

- 3 cups frozen French-style green beans, thawed
- 1 can (10-3/4 ounces) reduced-fat reduced-sodium condensed cream of chicken soup, undiluted
- 1-1/2 cups frozen corn, thawed
- 1 can (8 ounces) sliced water chestnuts, drained
- 1 medium onion, chopped
- 1/2 cup reduced-fat sour cream
- 1/4 cup cubed reduced-fat process cheese (Velveeta)
- 5 teaspoons reduced-fat butter
- 1/3 cup crushed butter-flavored crackers
- 2 tablespoons slivered almonds

- In a large bowl, combine the first seven ingredients. Transfer to an 11-in. x 7-in. baking dish coated with cooking spray.

- In a small skillet, melt butter. Add cracker crumbs and almonds; cook and stir until lightly browned. Sprinkle over the top.

- Bake, uncovered, at 350° for 35-40 minutes or until heated through and topping is golden brown.

YIELD: 6 servings.

EDITOR'S NOTE: This recipe was tested with Land O'Lakes light stick butter.

NUTRITION FACTS: 2/3 cup equals 213 calories, 8 g fat (3 g saturated fat), 17 mg cholesterol, 355 mg sodium, 32 g carbohydrate, 5 g fiber, 7 g protein. **DIABETIC EXCHANGES:** 1-1/2 starch, 1 vegetable, 1 fat.

MAKEOVER FANCY BEAN CASSEROLE

213 CALORIES

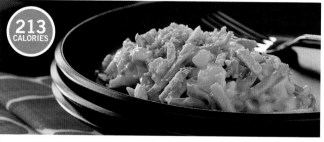

My weight soared when a medical condition left me unable to exercise. When I got my strength back, I started to cook and bake and lose weight. I only enjoy a small piece for myself (I need to make sure it is good enough to share!) and give the rest to my husband to take to work. I count calories and choose low-calorie options at restaurants. Now I can do all the things I love. —**Regina Lindsey, Texas**

224 CALORIES potato smashers

PREP/TOTAL TIME: 20 minutes

Janet Steiger | BUCYRUS, OHIO

Try this dressed-up version of stuffed potato skins for a great side dish that no one will ever guess is light!

- 6 small red potatoes (about 3/4 pound)
- 1/2 cup water
- 2 center-cut bacon strips
- 2 tablespoons reduced-fat Italian salad dressing
- 1/4 cup shredded sharp cheddar cheese

Reduced-fat sour cream, optional

- Place potatoes in a small microwave-safe dish; add water. Microwave, uncovered, on high for 8-9 minutes or until tender, stirring once.

- Meanwhile, in a large nonstick skillet, cook bacon over medium heat until crisp. Remove to paper towels to drain. Crumble bacon and set aside.

- With the bottom of a glass, flatten potatoes to 1/2-in. thickness. In the same skillet coated with cooking spray, cook potatoes in dressing over medium heat for 2-3 minutes or until bottoms are golden brown.

- Turn potatoes; sprinkle with cheese and reserved bacon. Cover and cook 2-3 minutes longer or until cheese is melted. Serve with sour cream if desired.

YIELD: 2 servings.

EDITOR'S NOTE: This recipe was tested in a 1,100-watt microwave.

NUTRITION FACTS: 3 potatoes (calculated without sour cream) equals 224 calories, 8 g fat (4 g saturated fat), 23 mg cholesterol, 314 mg sodium, 29 g carbohydrate, 3 g fiber, 9 g protein. **DIABETIC EXCHANGES:** 2 starch, 1 medium-fat meat, 1/2 fat.

springtime barley

PREP/TOTAL TIME: 30 minutes

Sharon Helmick | COLFAX, WASHINGTON

As a sorority house mother, I found the girls really liked low-fat dishes like this attractive medley.

- 1 small onion, chopped
- 1 medium carrot, chopped
- 1 tablespoon butter
- 1 cup quick-cooking barley
- 2 cups reduced-sodium chicken broth, *divided*
- 1/2 pound fresh asparagus, trimmed and cut into 1-inch pieces
- 1/4 teaspoon dried marjoram
- 1/8 teaspoon pepper
- 2 tablespoons shredded Parmesan cheese

- In a large skillet, saute onion and carrot in butter until crisp-tender. Stir in barley; cook and stir for 1 minute. Stir in 1 cup broth. Bring to a boil. Reduce heat; cook and stir until liquid is absorbed.

- Add asparagus. Cook for 15-20 minutes or until barley is tender and liquid is absorbed, stirring occasionally and adding more broth as needed. Stir in marjoram and pepper; sprinkle with cheese.

YIELD: 4 servings.

NUTRITION FACTS: 3/4 cup equals 226 calories, 5 g fat (2 g saturated fat), 9 mg cholesterol, 396 mg sodium, 39 g carbohydrate, 9 g fiber, 9 g protein. **DIABETIC EXCHANGES:** 2 starch, 1 vegetable, 1/2 fat.

SPRINGTIME BARLEY

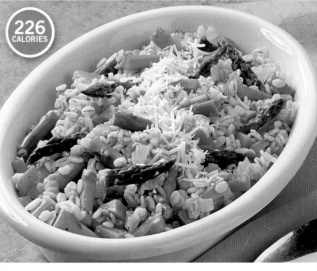

226 CALORIES

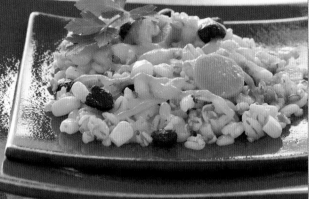

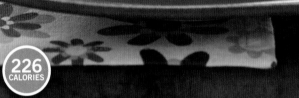

226 CALORIES

GO FOR THE GRAINS CASSEROLE

go for the grains casserole

PREP: 25 minutes | **BAKE:** 55 minutes

Melanie Blair | WARSAW, INDIANA

This casserole is hearty and delicious. A friend of mine gave me the recipe when I was compiling a file for healthier dishes. This colorful medley has "good-for-you" written all over it.

- 5 medium carrots, thinly sliced
- 2 cups frozen corn, thawed
- 1 medium onion, diced
- 1 cup quick-cooking barley
- 1/2 cup bulgur
- 1/3 cup minced fresh parsley
- 1 teaspoon salt
- 1/2 teaspoon pepper
- 3 cups vegetable broth
- 1 can (15 ounces) black beans, rinsed and drained
- 1-1/2 cups (6 ounces) shredded reduced-fat cheddar cheese

- In a large bowl, combine the carrots, corn, onion, barley, bulgur, parsley, salt and pepper. Stir in broth and beans. Transfer to a 13-in. x 9-in. baking dish coated with cooking spray.

- Cover and bake at 350° for 50-55 minutes or until grains are tender, stirring once. Sprinkle with cheese. Bake, uncovered, 3-5 minutes longer or until cheese is melted.

YIELD: 10 servings.

NUTRITION FACTS: 3/4 cup equals 226 calories, 5 g fat (3 g saturated fat), 12 mg cholesterol, 741 mg sodium, 38 g carbohydrate, 8 g fiber, 12 g protein.

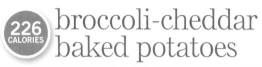

226 CALORIES

broccoli-cheddar baked potatoes

PREP: 20 minutes | **BAKE:** 70 minutes

Mary Bauer | WICHITA, KANSAS

Bring a dash of holiday color to the table with this green and red side. Adding a cup of leftover diced chicken to the vegetables makes this a quick lunch or meal in itself.

- 1 large baking potato
- 1/4 cup chopped fresh broccoli
- 1/4 cup sliced fresh mushrooms
- 1 tablespoon diced pimientos
- 1 teaspoon canola oil
- 1/4 cup shredded reduced-fat cheddar cheese, *divided*
- 1/4 cup fat-free plain yogurt
- 1/4 teaspoon salt
- 1/8 teaspoon garlic powder
- 1/8 teaspoon paprika

Pepper to taste

for 2

- Scrub and pierce potato. Bake at 375° for 1 hour or until tender. Meanwhile, in a small skillet, saute the broccoli, mushrooms and pimientos in oil until vegetables are tender; set aside.

- When potato is cool enough to handle, cut in half lengthwise. Scoop out pulp, leaving a thin shell.

- In a small bowl, mash the pulp. Stir in 2 tablespoons cheese, yogurt, salt, garlic powder, paprika and pepper. Stir in broccoli mixture. Spoon into potato shells. Sprinkle with remaining cheese. Place on a baking sheet.

- Bake at 375° for 10 minutes or until cheese is melted.

YIELD: 2 servings.

NUTRITION FACTS: 1 stuffed potato half equals 226 calories, 6 g fat (2 g saturated fat), 11 mg cholesterol, 417 mg sodium, 37 g carbohydrate, 3 g fiber, 9 g protein.

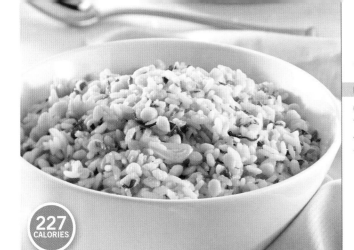

227 CALORIES

GARLIC-HERB ORZO PILAF

garlic-herb orzo pilaf

PREP: 10 minutes | **COOK:** 30 minutes

Mary Relyea | CANASTOTA, NEW YORK

Mildly flavored and flecked with garlic and fresh herbs, this creamy, versatile pilaf can accompany a wide variety of entrees. Plus, it's a cinch to put together.

   8 garlic cloves, peeled and thinly sliced
   1 tablespoon olive oil
 1/2 cup uncooked orzo pasta
 1/2 cup uncooked long grain rice
   1 can (14-1/2 ounces) reduced-sodium chicken broth *or* vegetable broth
 1/3 cup water
   3 green onions, thinly sliced
 1/3 cup thinly sliced fresh basil leaves
 1/4 cup minced fresh parsley
 1/4 teaspoon salt

- In a large nonstick skillet coated with cooking spray, cook garlic in oil over medium-high heat for 1 minute. Add orzo and rice; cook 4-6 minutes longer or until lightly browned.

- Stir in broth and water. Bring to a boil. Reduce heat; cover and simmer for 15-20 minutes or until rice is tender and liquid is absorbed. Stir in the onions, basil, parsley and salt.

YIELD: 4 servings.

NUTRITION FACTS: 3/4 cup equals 227 calories, 4 g fat (1 g saturated fat), 0 cholesterol, 426 mg sodium, 40 g carbohydrate, 1 g fiber, 7 g protein. **DIABETIC EXCHANGES:** 2-1/2 starch, 1/2 fat.

couscous with mushrooms

PREP/TOTAL TIME: 15 minutes

Claudia Ruiss | MASSAPEQUA, NEW YORK

This fluffy and tasty couscous lends itself to whatever vegetables you have on hand.

1-1/4 cups water
   2 tablespoons butter
   2 teaspoons chicken bouillon granules
 1/4 teaspoon salt
 1/4 teaspoon pepper
   1 cup uncooked couscous
   1 can (7 ounces) mushroom stems and pieces, drained

- In a large saucepan, bring the water, butter, bouillon, salt and pepper to a boil. Stir in the couscous and mushrooms. Cover and remove from the heat; let stand for 5 minutes. Fluff with a fork.

YIELD: 4 servings.

NUTRITION FACTS: 3/4 cup equals 230 calories, 6 g fat (4 g saturated fat), 15 mg cholesterol, 794 mg sodium, 37 g carbohydrate, 3 g fiber, 8 g protein.

COUSCOUS WITH MUSHROOMS

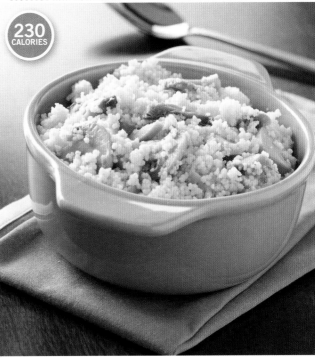

230 CALORIES

> **I have learned to love eating lighter** because I love how my weight loss has made me feel: fit, strong, proud and healthy! —Jessica Santistevan Martinez

southwestern pasta & cheese

PREP: 30 minutes | **BAKE:** 20 minutes

Naomi Reed | MCMINNVILLE, OREGON

I decided to give my old mac 'n' cheese recipe a new twist by including some of my favorite Southwestern ingredients. I especially like the smoky flavors of the chipotle and bacon—my family loves it all!

- 3-1/3 cups uncooked bow tie pasta
- 1 medium sweet red pepper, chopped
- 8 green onions, chopped
- 1 tablespoon olive oil
- 1/4 cup all-purpose flour
- 1 teaspoon chili powder
- 1 teaspoon minced chipotle pepper in adobo sauce
- 1/2 teaspoon salt
- 1/2 teaspoon ground cumin
- 2-1/4 cups fat-free milk
- 1 cup (4 ounces) shredded sharp cheddar cheese, *divided*
- 4 center-cut bacon strips, cooked and crumbled
- 2 tablespoons minced fresh cilantro

SOUTHWESTERN PASTA & CHEESE

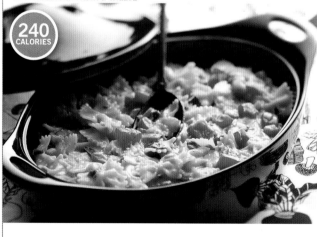

240 CALORIES

- Cook pasta according to package directions.
- Meanwhile, in a large skillet, saute pepper and onions in oil until tender. Stir in the flour, chili powder, chipotle pepper, salt and cumin until blended. Gradually stir in milk. Bring to a boil; cook and stir for 2 minutes or until thickened. Stir in 1/4 cup cheese until melted.
- Drain pasta; toss with sauce. Stir in the bacon and cilantro. Transfer to a 2-qt. baking dish coated with cooking spray. Sprinkle with remaining cheese. Bake, uncovered, at 400° for 20-25 minutes or until bubbly.

YIELD: 8 servings.

NUTRITION FACTS: 3/4 cup equals 240 calories, 8 g fat (4 g saturated fat), 20 mg cholesterol, 327 mg sodium, 32 g carbohydrate, 2 g fiber, 12 g protein. **DIABETIC EXCHANGES:** 2 starch, 1 medium-fat meat, 1/2 fat.

makeover corn 'n' green bean bake

PREP: 20 minutes | **BAKE:** 40 minutes

Donna Brockett | KINGFISHER, OKLAHOMA

The result of this makeover is a delicious, creamy and cheesy casserole perfect for any night of the year. While the original is so decadent that you might make it only for those really special occasions, this lightened-up version is great year round, yet tasty enough for those festive times, too.

- 3-1/2 cups frozen corn, thawed
- 2 cans (14-1/2 ounces *each*) French-style green beans, drained
- 2 cans (10-3/4 ounces *each*) reduced-fat reduced-sodium condensed cream of mushroom soup, undiluted
- 1 cup (8 ounces) reduced-fat sour cream
- 1 cup (8 ounces) plain yogurt
- 1 cup (4 ounces) shredded sharp cheddar cheese
- 1 large onion, chopped
- 1 celery rib, chopped
- 1 small green pepper, chopped

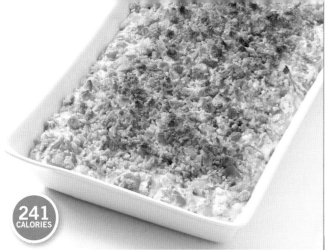

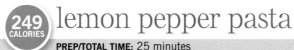

241 CALORIES

MAKEOVER CORN 'N' GREEN BEAN BAKE

> 2 cups crushed reduced-fat butter-flavored crackers (about 50 crackers)
> 1/3 cup reduced-fat butter, melted

- In a large bowl, combine the first nine ingredients. Transfer to a 13-in. x 9-in. baking dish coated with cooking spray.
- Toss the cracker crumbs and butter; sprinkle over vegetable mixture. Bake, uncovered, at 350° for 40-45 minutes or until bubbly.

YIELD: 12 servings.

EDITOR'S NOTE: This recipe was tested with Land O'Lakes light stick butter.

NUTRITION FACTS: 3/4 cup equals 241 calories, 11 g fat (6 g saturated fat), 32 mg cholesterol, 679 mg sodium, 30 g carbohydrate, 3 g fiber, 8 g protein.

249 CALORIES

lemon pepper pasta

PREP/TOTAL TIME: 25 minutes

Jolinda Whittle | BEAVER, PENNSYLVANIA
A full-size version of this pretty pasta was cut down to make it ideal for two to enjoy.

> 2 ounces uncooked vermicelli
> 1/4 cup fat-free milk
> 2 ounces reduced-fat process cheese (Velveeta), cubed
> 1/8 teaspoon salt
> 1 medium sweet red pepper, cut into 1/8-inch strips
> 1 medium sweet yellow pepper, cut into 1/8-inch strips

 for 2

> 2 teaspoons olive oil
> 1-1/2 teaspoons grated lemon peel
> 1/8 teaspoon pepper

- Cook pasta according to package directions. Meanwhile, in a saucepan, combine milk, cheese and salt; cook and stir over medium-low heat until cheese is melted. Drain pasta. Add cheese sauce; toss to coat. Keep warm.
- In a nonstick skillet, saute peppers in oil for 5 minutes or until crisp-tender. Sprinkle with lemon peel and pepper; mix well. Toss with pasta mixture.

YIELD: 2 servings.

NUTRITION FACTS: 1 cup equals 249 calories, 8 g fat (3 g saturated fat), 13 mg cholesterol, 617 mg sodium, 34 g carbohydrate, 3 g fiber, 12 g protein. **Diabetic Exchanges:** 2 starch, 1-1/2 fat, 1 vegetable

250 CALORIES

low-fat macaroni and cheese

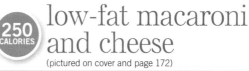

(pictured on cover and page 172)

PREP: 15 minutes | **BAKE:** 1 hour

Joanie Elbourn | GARDNER, MASSACHUSETTS
When I want a dish that's real, old-fashioned comfort food, I make a batch of this macaroni and cheese.

> 1 cup fat-free milk
> 1-1/4 cups shredded reduced-fat cheddar cheese
> 2/3 cup fat-free cottage cheese
> 3 tablespoons all-purpose flour
> Pepper to taste
> 2-1/2 cups cooked elbow macaroni
> 1 tablespoon grated onion
> Paprika

- In a blender or food processor, combine the milk, cheeses, flour and pepper. Cover and process until creamy. Pour into a bowl; stir in macaroni and onion.
- Transfer to a 1-1/2-qt. baking dish coated with cooking spray. Sprinkle with paprika. Bake, uncovered, at 350° for 1 hour or until heated through.

YIELD: 4 servings.

NUTRITION FACTS: 3/4 cup equals 250 calories, 8 g fat (5 g saturated fat), 28 mg cholesterol, 395 mg sodium, 27 g carbohydrate, 1 g fiber, 19 g protein. **DIABETIC EXCHANGES:** 2 medium-fat meat, 1-1/2 starch.

desserts

There's always room for dessert...particularly classics such as cupcakes, cookies, bars, pudding and more! When planning your meals for the day, remember to set a few calories aside so you can treat yourself to a sweet bite and still land within the 1,400-calorie daily guideline.

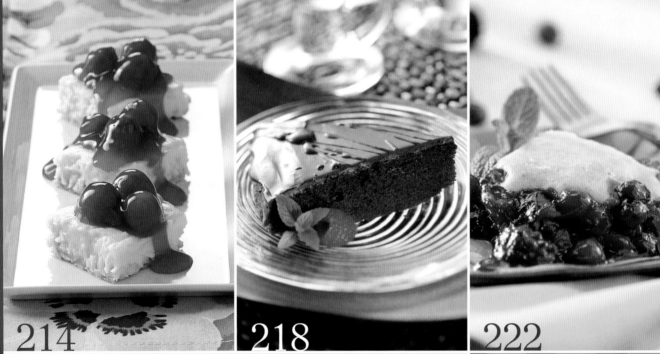

214 218 222

Looking for a snack between meals? Consider the lower-calorie options at the start of this chapter. When you'd like to cap off a meal with something a bit more impressive, see the desserts toward the end of the section. Regardless, you're sure to find a bite to tickle your sweet tooth!

100 Calories or Less 207
101-150 Calories 210
151-250 Calories 218

100 calories or less

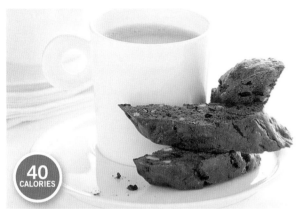

40 CALORIES

CHOCOLATE DUNK-SHOT BISCOTTI

chocolate dunk-shot biscotti

PREP: 30 minutes | **BAKE:** 30 minutes + cooling

Nancy Whitford | EDWARDS, NEW YORK
These crunchy cookies are great with a hot drink! They're perfect with after-dinner coffee or as a morning treat. They're just as yummy dunked in milk.

- 2 cups all-purpose flour
- 1/2 cup sugar blend
- 1/3 cup baking cocoa
- 1/2 teaspoon salt
- 1/2 teaspoon baking soda
- 2 eggs
- 3 egg whites, *divided*
- 1 teaspoon vanilla extract
- 1 teaspoon instant coffee granules
- 1 tablespoon grated orange peel
- 1/2 cup chopped almonds, toasted
- 1/4 cup miniature semisweet chocolate chips
- 1 teaspoon water

- In a large bowl, combine the flour, sugar blend, cocoa, salt and baking soda. In a small bowl, whisk the eggs, 2 egg whites, vanilla and coffee granules; let stand for 3-4 minutes or until granules are dissolved. Stir in

orange peel. Stir into flour mixture and mix well. Stir in almonds and chocolate chips.

- Divide dough in half. On a baking sheet coated with cooking spray, shape each half into a 14-in. x 1-3/4-in. rectangle. Combine water and remaining egg white; brush over rectangles. Bake at 350° for 20-25 minutes or until cracked and firm to the touch. Carefully remove to wire racks; cool for 5 minutes.

- Transfer to a cutting board; cut diagonally with a serrated knife into 1/2-in. slices. Place cut side down on ungreased baking sheets. Bake for 5-7 minutes on each side or until firm. Remove to wire racks to cool. Store in an airtight container.

YIELD: 4-1/2 dozen.

EDITOR'S NOTE: This recipe was tested with Splenda sugar blend.

NUTRITION FACTS: 1 cookie equals 40 calories, 1 g fat (trace saturated fat), 8 mg cholesterol, 39 mg sodium, 6 g carbohydrate, trace fiber, 1 g protein. **DIABETIC EXCHANGE:** 1/2 starch.

cinnamon blueberry sauce

50 CALORIES

PREP/TOTAL TIME: 20 minutes

Linda Johnson | MONTESANO, WASHINGTON
Having frozen yogurt for dessert? Top it with this nutrient-packed sauce. It's fruity and delicious over pancakes, too.

Sugar substitute equivalent to 1/4 cup sugar
- 2 teaspoons cornstarch
- 2 cups frozen unsweetened blueberries
- 1/4 cup water
- 2 tablespoons lemon juice
- 1/2 teaspoon ground cinnamon

- In a small saucepan, combine sugar substitute and cornstarch. Add the blueberries, water, lemon juice and cinnamon. Cook and stir until mixture comes to a boil. Reduce heat; simmer, uncovered, for 5 minutes, stirring frequently. Serve warm. Refrigerate leftovers.

YIELD: 1 cup.

EDITOR'S NOTE: This recipe was tested with Splenda no-calorie sweetener.

NUTRITION FACTS: 1/4 cup equals 50 calories, 1 g fat (trace saturated fat), 0 cholesterol, 1 mg sodium, 12 g carbohydrate, 2 g fiber, trace protein. **DIABETIC EXCHANGE:** 1 fruit.

66 CALORIES

LEMON ANISE BISCOTTI

lemon anise biscotti

PREP: 25 minutes | **BAKE:** 40 minutes + cooling

Carrie Sherrill | FORESTVILLE, WISCONSIN

With the growing popularity of gourmet coffees, cappuccino and espresso, I'm finding lots of people who enjoy these classic Italian dipping cookies.

- 2 eggs
- 1 cup sugar
- 1/4 cup canola oil
- 1/2 teaspoon lemon extract
- 1/4 teaspoon vanilla extract
- 2 cups all-purpose flour
- 1 teaspoon baking powder
- 1/2 teaspoon salt
- 4 teaspoons grated lemon peel
- 2 teaspoons aniseed, crushed

- In a small bowl, beat eggs and sugar for 2 minutes or until thickened. Add oil and extracts; mix well. Combine the flour, baking powder and salt; beat into egg mixture. Stir in lemon peel and aniseed.

- Divide dough in half. On a lightly floured surface, shape each portion into a 12-in. x 2-in. rectangle. Transfer to a baking sheet lined with parchment paper. Flatten to 1/2-in. thickness.

- Bake at 350° for 30-35 minutes or until golden and tops begin to crack. Carefully remove to wire racks; cool for 5 minutes.

- Transfer to a cutting board; cut with a serrated knife into scant 3/4-in. slices. Place cut side down on ungreased

baking sheets. Bake for 5 minutes. Turn and bake 5-7 minutes longer or until firm and golden brown. Remove to wire racks to cool. Store in an airtight container.

YIELD: 3 dozen.

NUTRITION FACTS: 1 cookie equals 66 calories, 2 g fat (trace saturated fat), 12 mg cholesterol, 48 mg sodium, 11 g carbohydrate, trace fiber, 1 g protein. **DIABETIC EXCHANGES:** 1/2 starch, 1/2 fat.

75 CALORIES

peanut butter-chocolate chip cookies

PREP: 15 minutes + chilling | **BAKE:** 10 minutes/batch

Muriel Mableson | WINNIPEG, MANITOBA

I stir in a few chocolate chips to give these peanut butter cookies some chocolaty goodness.

- 1/2 cup butter, cubed
- 1/3 cup reduced-fat creamy peanut butter
- 1/4 cup unsweetened applesauce
- 3/4 cup sugar
- 3/4 cup packed brown sugar
- 2 eggs
- 1-1/2 teaspoons vanilla extract
- 2-1/4 cups all-purpose flour
- 1/2 teaspoon baking soda
- 1/2 teaspoon ground cinnamon
- 1/4 teaspoon salt
- 1/2 cup semisweet chocolate chips

- In a small microwave-safe bowl, microwave butter and peanut butter until butter is melted; stir until smooth. Stir in applesauce.

- Transfer to a large bowl. Beat in the sugars until blended. Beat in eggs and vanilla. Combine the flour, baking soda, cinnamon and salt; gradually add to peanut butter mixture and mix well. Stir in chocolate chips. Cover and refrigerate for at least 2 hours.

- Drop by tablespoonfuls 2 in. apart onto baking sheets coated with cooking spray. Bake at 350° for 7-9 minutes or until lightly browned. Remove to wire racks. Store in an airtight container.

YIELD: 4-1/2 dozen.

NUTRITION FACTS: 1 cookie equals 75 calories, 3 g fat (2 g saturated fat), 12 mg cholesterol, 47 mg sodium, 11 g carbohydrate, trace fiber, 1 g protein. **DIABETIC EXCHANGES:** 1 starch, 1/2 fat.

broiled fruit dessert

PREP/TOTAL TIME: 15 minutes

Jim Gales | GLENDALE, WISCONSIN

I'm happy to share the recipe for this super dessert. It's a quick, guilt-free treat.

- 1 medium peach
- 1 medium fresh nectarine **for 2**
- 1 tablespoon brown sugar

Whipped cream *or* vanilla ice cream, optional

- Halve and pit the peach and nectarine. Line a shallow baking dish with foil; coat foil with cooking spray. Place fruit cut side down in prepared dish.

- Broil 6 in. from the heat for 3 minutes; turn fruit over and sprinkle with brown sugar. Broil 2-3 minutes longer or until sugar is melted and bubbly. Serve warm with whipped cream or ice cream if desired.

YIELD: 2 servings.

NUTRITION FACTS: 1 serving (calculated without whipped cream or ice cream) equals 80 calories, trace fat (trace saturated fat), 0 cholesterol, 3 mg sodium, 20 g carbohydrate, 2 g fiber, 1 g protein. **DIABETIC EXCHANGE:** 1 fruit.

BROILED FRUIT DESSERT

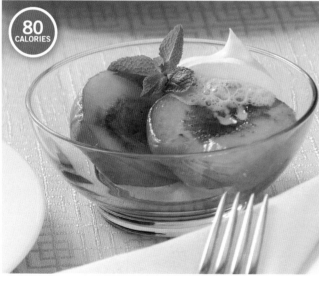

80 CALORIES

CHOCOLATE CHIP COOKIES

chocolate chip cookies

PREP: 15 minutes | **BAKE:** 10 minutes/batch + cooling

Bethany Thayer | TROUTVILLE, VIRGINIA

Chocolate chip cookies are almost everyone's favorites, and these are sure to please!

- 1/2 cup reduced-fat margarine
- 3/4 cup sugar
- 3/4 cup packed brown sugar
- 2 eggs
- 1/4 cup (2 ounces) reduced-fat plain yogurt
- 2 teaspoons vanilla extract
- 2-1/2 cups all-purpose flour
- 1 teaspoon baking soda
- 1 teaspoon salt
- 1-1/2 cups miniature semisweet chocolate chips
- 1/2 cup chopped walnuts, toasted

- In a large bowl, lightly cream the margarine and sugars. Add eggs, one at a time, beating well after each addition. Beat in yogurt and vanilla. Combine the flour, baking soda and salt; gradually add to creamed mixture. Stir in chocolate chips and walnuts.

- Drop by heaping tablespoonfuls 2 in. apart onto baking sheets coated with cooking spray. Bake at 375° for 8-10 minutes or until golden brown. Remove to wire racks.

YIELD: 4 dozen.

NUTRITION FACTS: 1 cookie equals 94 calories, 4 g fat (1 g saturated fat), 9 mg cholesterol, 93 mg sodium, 15 g carbohydrate, 1 g fiber, 1 g protein. **DIABETIC EXCHANGES:** 1 starch, 1/2 fat.

94 CALORIES

101-150 calories

cappuccino pudding

PREP/TOTAL TIME: 20 minutes

Cindy Bertrand | FLOYDADA, TEXAS

With its fun combination of chocolate, coffee and cinnamon, this smooth dessert is one of my favorites. A garnish of whipped topping and chocolate wafer crumbs provides additional appeal.

      4 teaspoons instant coffee granules
      1 tablespoon boiling water
  1-1/2 cups cold fat-free milk
      1 package (1.4 ounces) sugar-free instant chocolate (fudge) pudding mix
    1/2 teaspoon ground cinnamon
      1 cup reduced-fat whipped topping
         Additional whipped topping and chocolate wafer crumbs, optional

- Dissolve coffee in water; set aside. In a bowl, combine milk, pudding mix and cinnamon. Beat on low speed for 2 minutes. Stir in coffee. Fold in whipped topping. Spoon into serving dishes. Garnish with whipped topping and wafer crumbs if desired.

YIELD: 4 servings.

NUTRITION FACTS: 1/2 cup (calculated without optional ingredients) equals 105 calories, 2 g fat (0 saturated fat), 2 mg cholesterol, 48 mg sodium, 17 g carbohydrate, 0 fiber, 3 g protein. **DIABETIC EXCHANGES:** 1/2 starch, 1/2 fat-free milk.

CAPPUCCINO PUDDING

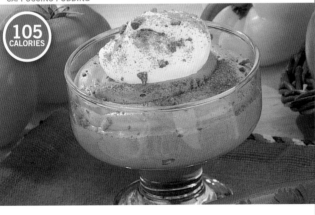

105 CALORIES

peach-topped cake

121 CALORIES

PREP: 20 minutes + chilling | **BAKE:** 10 minutes

Chris Lafser | RICHMOND, VIRGINIA

It's easy to love the tender yellow cake on the bottom and the delightful peach-filled gelatin on top of this treat. This bright orange dessert is perfect for year-round menus.

      2 tablespoons butter, softened
    1/2 cup sugar
      1 egg
    1/2 teaspoon vanilla extract
    3/4 cup cake flour
    3/4 teaspoon baking powder
    1/4 teaspoon salt
    1/4 cup fat-free milk

TOPPING:

      1 envelope unflavored gelatin
  1-3/4 cups cold water, *divided*
    1/4 cup sugar
      1 envelope sugar-free orange soft drink mix
      2 medium ripe peaches, thinly sliced *or* 1 can (15 ounces) sliced peaches
    1/2 cup reduced-fat whipped topping

- In a small bowl, beat butter and sugar until crumbly. Beat in the egg and vanilla. Combine the flour, baking powder and salt; add to sugar mixture alternately with milk.

- Spread into a 9-in. springform pan coated with cooking spray. Bake at 350° for 10-15 minutes or until a toothpick inserted near the center comes out clean. Cool on a wire rack.

- In a small saucepan, sprinkle gelatin over 1/2 cup cold water. Let stand for 1 minute. Stir in sugar and soft drink mix; cook and stir over low heat until gelatin is dissolved. Transfer to a large bowl; stir in remaining cold water. Refrigerate until partially set, about 1-1/2 hours.

- Line outside of springform pan with foil. Arrange peaches over top of cake. Pour gelatin over peaches. Chill overnight. Just before serving, remove foil and sides of pan. Garnish with whipped topping. Refrigerate leftovers.

YIELD: 12 servings.

NUTRITION FACTS: 1 slice equals 121 calories, 3 g fat (2 g saturated fat), 23 mg cholesterol, 103 mg sodium, 22 g carbohydrate, trace fiber, 2 g protein. **DIABETIC EXCHANGES:** 1-1/2 starch, 1/2 fat.

desserts | 101-150 CALORIES

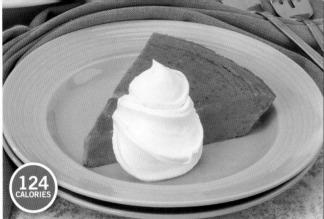

124 CALORIES

LOW-CALORIE PUMPKIN PIE

low-calorie pumpkin pie

PREP: 10 minutes | **BAKE:** 35 minutes + cooling

Diane Jessen | BAYFIELD, COLORADO

I've brought this crustless pie to the office, and no one guessed it's sugar-free. Even the guy who says he doesn't eat anything healthy likes its traditional pumpkin flavor.

    1   egg
    2   egg whites
    1   can (15 ounces) solid-pack pumpkin
Sugar substitute equivalent to 3/4 cup sugar
  1/2   cup reduced-fat biscuit/baking mix
    1   teaspoon vanilla extract
    1   teaspoon ground cinnamon
  1/2   teaspoon ground ginger
  1/4   teaspoon ground cloves
    1   can (12 ounces) fat-free evaporated milk
    1   cup reduced-fat whipped topping

- In a large bowl, combine the egg, egg whites, pumpkin, sugar substitute, biscuit mix, vanilla and spices until smooth. Gradually stir in evaporated milk.

- Pour into a 9-in. pie plate coated with cooking spray. Bake at 350° for 35-40 minutes or until knife inserted near the center comes out clean. Cool on a wire rack. Dollop with whipped topping before serving. Refrigerate leftovers.

YIELD: 8 servings.

EDITOR'S NOTE: This recipe was tested with Splenda no-calorie sweetener.

NUTRITION FACTS: 1 piece equals 124 calories, 2 g fat (1 g saturated fat), 28 mg cholesterol, 160 mg sodium, 19 g carbohydrate, 3 g fiber, 6 g protein. **DIABETIC EXCHANGE:** 1-1/2 starch.

makeover oatmeal bars

PREP: 10 minutes | **BAKE:** 15 minutes + cooling

Clyde Williams | CHAMBERSBURG, PENNSYLVANIA

These delicious bars are even more moist and chewy than the original recipe, but with all the old-fashioned oatmeal flavor and only half the fat!

  2/3   cup sugar
  1/2   cup unsweetened applesauce
  1/3   cup canola oil
    1   tablespoon maple syrup
    2   cups quick-cooking oats
    1   cup all-purpose flour
    1   teaspoon baking soda
  1/2   teaspoon salt
  1/2   teaspoon ground allspice
  1/2   cup raisins

- In a large bowl, beat the sugar, applesauce, oil and syrup until well blended.

- In a small bowl, combine the oats, flour, baking soda, salt and allspice; gradually beat into applesauce mixture until blended. Stir in raisins.

- Spread batter into a 13-in. x 9-in. baking pan coated with cooking spray. Bake at 350° for 15-20 minutes or until edges begin to brown. Cool completely on a wire rack. Cut into bars.

YIELD: 20 servings.

NUTRITION FACTS: 1 bar equals 127 calories, 4 g fat (trace saturated fat), 0 cholesterol, 123 mg sodium, 21 g carbohydrate, 1 g fiber, 2 g protein. **DIABETIC EXCHANGES:** 1 starch, 1 fat.

MAKEOVER OATMEAL BARS

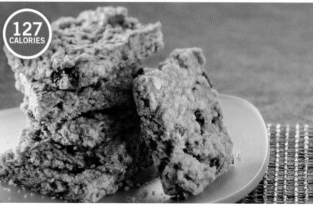

127 CALORIES

Moderation is the key to keeping our desserts light and low-calorie.
I prepare mini cupcakes instead of full-size ones or cut full-size ones into smaller pieces.
—Lisa Painter Starkey

129 CALORIES
ladyfinger cream sandwiches

PREP: 25 minutes + chilling

Taste of Home Test Kitchen
Dainty and delicious, these elegant finger-sandwich treats make the perfect finish to any luncheon. Enjoy!

- 1/4 cup all-purpose flour
- 1/4 cup sugar
- Sugar substitute equivalent to 1/4 cup sugar
- 1/4 teaspoon salt
- 2-3/4 cups 2% milk, *divided*
- 3 eggs
- 3/4 teaspoon vanilla extract
- 2 packages (3 ounces *each*) ladyfingers, split
- 2 teaspoons coarse sugar

- In a saucepan, combine flour, sugar, sugar substitute, salt and 2-1/2 cups milk until smooth. Cook and stir over medium-high heat until thickened and bubbly. Reduce heat; stir 2 minutes longer. Remove from the heat.

- In a small bowl, whisk 2 eggs. Stir a small amount of hot filling into eggs; return all to the pan, stirring constantly. Bring to a gentle boil; cook and stir 2 minutes longer. Remove from the heat. Gently stir in vanilla. Transfer to a bowl; press plastic wrap onto surface of custard. Refrigerate until chilled.

- Place tops of ladyfingers on an ungreased baking sheet. In a small bowl, whisk remaining egg and milk; lightly brush over ladyfingers. Sprinkle with coarse sugar. Broil 4 in. from the heat for 1-2 minutes or until golden brown.

- Spread custard over the bottoms of ladyfingers. Replace tops. Serve immediately. Refrigerate leftovers.

YIELD: 2 dozen.

EDITOR'S NOTE: This recipe was tested with Splenda no-calorie sweetener.

NUTRITION FACTS: 2 filled ladyfingers equals 129 calories, 4 g fat (2 g saturated fat), 109 mg cholesterol, 114 mg sodium, 19 g carbohydrate, trace fiber, 5 g protein.
DIABETIC EXCHANGES: 1 starch, 1/2 fat.

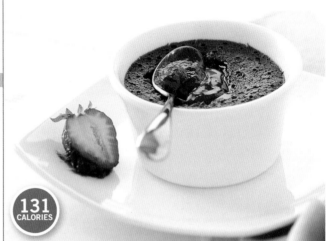

131 CALORIES

WARM CHOCOLATE MELTING CUPS

warm chocolate melting cups

PREP: 20 minutes | **BAKE:** 20 minutes

Kissa Vaughn | TROY, TEXAS
Our guests rave about these chocolate desserts. It's surprising to everyone that they're so light and healthy.

- 1-1/4 cups sugar, *divided*
- 1/2 cup baking cocoa
- 2 tablespoons all-purpose flour
- 1/8 teaspoon salt
- 3/4 cup water
- 3/4 cup plus 1 tablespoon semisweet chocolate chips
- 1 tablespoon brewed coffee
- 1 teaspoon vanilla extract
- 2 eggs
- 1 egg white
- 10 fresh strawberry halves, optional

- In a small saucepan, combine 3/4 cup sugar, cocoa, flour and salt. Gradually stir in water. Bring to a boil; cook and stir for 2 minutes or until thickened. Remove from the heat; stir in the chocolate chips, coffee and vanilla until smooth. Transfer to a large bowl.

- In another bowl, beat eggs and egg white until slightly thickened. Gradually add remaining sugar, beating until thick and lemon-colored. Fold into chocolate mixture.

- Transfer to ten 4-oz. ramekins coated with cooking spray. Place ramekins in a baking pan; add 1 in. of boiling water to pan. Bake, uncovered, at 350° for 20-25 minutes or just until centers are set. Garnish with strawberry halves if desired. Serve immediately.

YIELD: 10 servings.

NUTRITION FACTS: 1 serving equals 131 calories, 1 g fat (trace saturated fat), 42 mg cholesterol, 49 mg sodium, 29 g carbohydrate, 1 g fiber, 3 g protein. **DIABETIC EXCHANGE:** 2 starch.

blondies with chips

133 CALORIES

PREP: 5 minutes | **BAKE:** 20 minutes + cooling

Kai Skupinski | CANTON, MICHIGAN
My friends and family request these scrumptious bars. They love this pared-down version of the classic snack and never suspect that I use whole wheat flour.

- 1/3 cup all-purpose flour
- 1/3 cup whole wheat flour
- 1/4 cup packed brown sugar
- 1/2 teaspoon baking powder
- 1/4 teaspoon salt
- 1 egg
- 1/4 cup canola oil
- 2 tablespoons honey
- 1 teaspoon vanilla extract
- 1/2 cup semisweet chocolate chips

- In a small bowl, combine the flours, brown sugar, baking powder and salt.

- In another bowl, whisk the egg, oil, honey and vanilla; stir into dry ingredients just until combined. Stir in chocolate chips (batter will be thick).

- Spread into an 8-in. square baking dish coated with cooking spray. Bake at 350° for 20-22 minutes or until a toothpick inserted near the center comes out clean. Cool on a wire rack. Cut into bars.

YIELD: 1 dozen.

NUTRITION FACTS: 1 bar equals 133 calories, 7 g fat (2 g saturated fat), 18 mg cholesterol, 67 mg sodium, 17 g carbohydrate, 1 g fiber, 2 g protein. **DIABETIC EXCHANGES:** 1 starch, 1 fat.

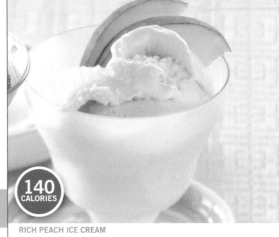

140 CALORIES

RICH PEACH ICE CREAM

rich peach ice cream

PREP: 15 minutes | **PROCESS:** 20 minutes/batch + freezing

Catherine MacRae Lyerly | WINSTON-SALEM, NORTH CAROLINA
Our family enjoys ice cream, and this homemade one is a favorite. I came up with the recipe when I needed to use up the fruit from our peach trees.

- 2 cups cold fat-free milk
- 1 package (3.4 ounces) instant vanilla pudding mix
- 4 medium peaches, peeled and chopped
- 2 cans (12 ounces *each*) fat-free evaporated milk
- 1 can (14 ounces) sweetened condensed milk
- 1/2 cup sugar
- 1/4 cup lemon juice
- 1 teaspoon vanilla extract
- 1/2 teaspoon almond extract
- 1/8 teaspoon salt
- 1 carton (8 ounces) fat-free frozen whipped topping, thawed

- In a large bowl, beat milk and pudding mix on low speed for 2 minutes. Beat in the peaches, evaporated milk, condensed milk, sugar, lemon juice, extracts and salt. Beat in whipped topping just until combined.

- Fill cylinder of ice cream freezer two-thirds full; freeze according to manufacturer's directions. Refrigerate remaining mixture until ready to freeze. Transfer to freezer containers; freeze for 2-4 hours before serving.

YIELD: 4 quarts.

NUTRITION FACTS: 2/3 cup equals 140 calories, 2 g fat (1 g saturated fat), 7 mg cholesterol, 139 mg sodium, 27 g carbohydrate, trace fiber, 4 g protein. **DIABETIC EXCHANGE:** 2 starch.

no-bake cheesecake pie

141 CALORIES

PREP: 20 minutes + chilling

Norma Jo Reynolds | GOLDWAITE, TEXAS
You won't miss the traditional graham cracker crust with this fluffy lemon dessert. The texture is wonderful, and the citrus taste is great, plus it's easy to prepare.

- 2 tablespoons graham cracker crumbs, *divided*
- 1 package (.3 ounce) sugar-free lemon gelatin
- 2/3 cup boiling water
- 1 package (8 ounces) reduced-fat cream cheese, cubed
- 1 cup (8 ounces) 1% cottage cheese
- 2 cups reduced-fat whipped topping

- Coat the bottom and sides of a 9-in. pie plate with cooking spray. Sprinkle with 1 tablespoon cracker crumbs; set aside.

- In a small bowl, dissolve gelatin in boiling water; cool slightly. Pour into a blender; add cream cheese and cottage cheese. Cover and process until smooth. Transfer to a large bowl. Fold in whipped topping. Pour into prepared pie plate. Sprinkle with remaining cracker crumbs. Cover and refrigerate until set.

YIELD: 8 servings.

NUTRITION FACTS: 1 slice equals 141 calories, 8 g fat (6 g saturated fat), 21 mg cholesterol, 272 mg sodium, 9 g carbohydrate, trace fiber, 7 g protein. **DIABETIC EXCHANGES:** 1-1/2 fat, 1/2 starch.

coconut-cherry cream squares

PREP: 30 minutes + chilling

Taste of Home Test Kitchen
You'll be wowed by these cherry-topped delights. With a delectable coconut-custard filling, one square will satisfy your sweet tooth for less than 150 calories.

- 3/4 cup all-purpose flour
- 1/3 cup flaked coconut
- 3 tablespoons brown sugar
- 3 tablespoons cold reduced-fat butter

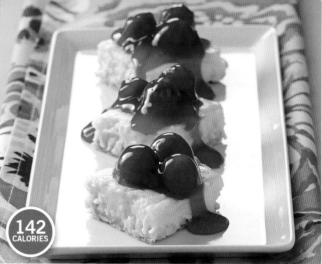

142 CALORIES

COCONUT-CHERRY CREAM SQUARES

FILLING:
- 1/3 cup all-purpose flour
- 1/4 cup sugar
- Sugar substitute equivalent to 1/4 cup sugar
- 1/4 teaspoon salt
- 2-1/2 cups fat-free milk
- 2 eggs, lightly beaten
- 1/2 cup flaked coconut
- 2 teaspoons coconut extract
- 1 can (20 ounces) reduced-sugar cherry pie filling

- In a small bowl, combine the flour, coconut and brown sugar; cut in butter until crumbly. Press into a 9-in. square baking pan coated with cooking spray. Bake at 400° for 7-10 minutes or until lightly browned. Cool on a wire rack.

- In a small saucepan, combine the flour, sugar, sugar substitute and salt. Stir in milk until smooth. Cook and stir over medium-high heat until thickened and bubbly. Reduce heat; cook and stir 2 minutes longer. Remove from the heat.

- Stir a small amount of hot filling into eggs; return all to the pan, stirring constantly. Bring to a gentle boil; cook and stir 2 minutes longer. Remove from the heat.

- Gently stir in coconut and extract. Pour over crust. Refrigerate until set. Top with pie filling. Refrigerate for at least 2 hours before cutting.

YIELD: 16 servings.

NUTRITION FACTS: 1 square equals 142 calories, 4 g fat (3 g saturated fat), 31 mg cholesterol, 95 mg sodium 24 g carbohydrate, 1 g fiber, 3 g protein. **DIABETIC EXCHANGES:** 1-1/2 starch, 1/2 fat.

colorful frozen yogurt

PREP: 20 minutes + freezing

Tiffany Blepp | OLATHE, KANSAS

Here's a beautiful, low-fat recipe for sunny days. Not only is it a pretty dessert, but blending the berries into the vanilla yogurt is simple. I serve the honey-topped yogurt in martini glasses with mint leaves for garnishes.

> 3 pints low-fat vanilla frozen yogurt, softened, *divided*
>
> 1-1/2 cups frozen unsweetened sliced peaches, thawed
>
> 1-1/4 cups frozen unsweetened blueberries, thawed
>
> 1-1/4 cups frozen unsweetened strawberries, thawed
>
> 12 teaspoons honey

- Place one pint of frozen yogurt in a blender; add peaches. Cover and process until smooth. Transfer to a freezer-safe container; cover and freeze. Repeat twice, making a batch of blueberry frozen yogurt and a batch of strawberry frozen yogurt.

- Using a small scoop or melon baller, scoop each flavor of yogurt onto a waxed paper-lined baking sheet. Freeze until firm.

- For each serving, place two scoops of each flavor in individual dessert dishes. Drizzle each with 1 teaspoon honey.

YIELD: 12 servings.

NUTRITION FACTS: 1/2 cup equals 143 calories, 1 g fat (1 g saturated fat), 5 mg cholesterol, 60 mg sodium, 29 g carbohydrate, 1 g fiber, 5 g protein. **DIABETIC EXCHANGE:** 2 starch.

COLORFUL FROZEN YOGURT

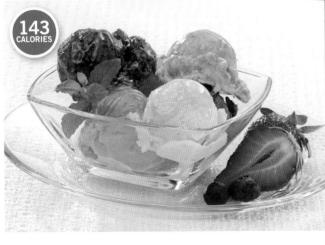

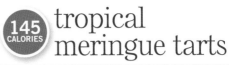

145 CALORIES tropical meringue tarts

PREP: 30 minutes + standing | **BAKE:** 50 minutes + cooling

Taste of Home Test Kitchen

What a special treat! These tender meringue shells are filled with creamy pudding, then topped with fresh fruit and coconut. This dessert is a showstopper.

> 4 egg whites
>
> 1 teaspoon white vinegar
>
> 1 teaspoon vanilla extract
>
> 1 teaspoon cornstarch
>
> 1 cup sugar
>
> 1-1/4 cups cold fat-free milk
>
> 1 package (1 ounce) sugar-free instant vanilla pudding mix
>
> 1 cup reduced-fat whipped topping
>
> 1 cup cubed fresh pineapple
>
> 2 medium kiwifruit, peeled and sliced
>
> 2 tablespoons flaked coconut, toasted

- Place egg whites in a large bowl; let stand at room temperature for 30 minutes. Meanwhile, line a baking sheet with parchment paper or foil. Draw ten 3-in. circles on paper; set aside.

- Add vinegar and vanilla to egg whites; beat on medium speed until soft peaks form. Beat in cornstarch. Gradually beat in sugar, 2 tablespoons at a time, on high until stiff glossy peaks form and sugar is dissolved.

- Cut a small hole in the corner of pastry or plastic bag; insert a large star pastry tip (#6B). Fill the bag with meringue. Pipe meringue in a spiral fashion to fill in circles on prepared pan. Pipe twice around the base of each shell in a spiral fashion to make the sides.

- Bake at 275° for 50-60 minutes or until set and dry. Turn oven off and leave door closed; leave meringues in oven for 1 hour.

- For filling, in a large bowl, whisk milk and pudding mix for 2 minutes. Let stand for 2 minutes or until soft-set. Fold in whipped topping. Spoon into meringue shells. Top with the pineapple, kiwi and coconut.

YIELD: 10 servings.

NUTRITION FACTS: 1 tart equals 145 calories, 2 g fat (1 g saturated fat), 1 mg cholesterol, 157 mg sodium, 30 g carbohydrate, 1 g fiber, 3 g protein. **DIABETIC EXCHANGE:** 2 starch.

147 CALORIES

BERRIES WITH SOUR CREAM SAUCE

berries with sour cream sauce

PREP/TOTAL TIME: 10 minutes

Linda Franceschi | ELDRED, NEW YORK
Delightfully dressed-up sour cream makes a delicious topping for fruit in this simple dish.

- 1 quart fresh strawberries, halved
- 1 pint fresh raspberries
- 1 pint fresh blueberries
- 1 pint fresh blackberries
- 2 cups (16 ounces) reduced-fat sour cream
- 1/4 cup honey

- In a large bowl, combine the first four ingredients. In another bowl, combine the sour cream and honey. Serve with berries.

YIELD: 10 servings.

NUTRITION FACTS: 3/4 cup fruit with 3 tablespoons sauce equals 147 calories, 4 g fat (3 g saturated fat), 15 mg cholesterol, 32 mg sodium, 25 g carbohydrate, 6 g fiber, 4 g protein. **DIABETIC EXCHANGES:** 1 fruit, 1/2 starch, 1/2 fat.

149 CALORIES fresh fruit parfaits

PREP/TOTAL TIME: 30 minutes

Karin Christian | PLANO, TEXAS
I fix this great recipe when I want to prepare something impressive for company. It makes a low-calorie dessert or breakfast that feels indulgent.

- 1/2 cup mixed berry yogurt
- 3/4 cup reduced-fat whipped topping
- 1 cup sliced ripe banana
- 1 cup sliced fresh strawberries
- 1 cup cubed fresh pineapple
- 1 cup fresh blueberries
- 4 whole strawberries

- In a small bowl, combine yogurt and whipped topping; set aside 4 teaspoons for topping. Spoon half of the remaining yogurt mixture into four parfait glasses; layer with half of the banana, sliced strawberries, pineapple and blueberries. Repeat layers.

- Top each parfait with reserved yogurt mixture and a whole strawberry. Chill until serving.

YIELD: 4 servings.

NUTRITION FACTS: 1 parfait equals 149 calories, 2 g fat (2 g saturated fat), 2 mg cholesterol, 22 mg sodium, 31 g carbohydrate, 4 g fiber, 2 g protein. **DIABETIC EXCHANGES:** 1-1/2 fruit, 1/2 starch.

makeover frosted banana bars

PREP: 15 minutes | **BAKE:** 20 minutes + cooling

Susan Stuff | MERCERSBURG, PENNSYLVANIA
I've made these banana bars many times, always with favorable comments and requests for the recipe. With this light makeover, you don't have to be shy about having a treat!

- 3 tablespoons butter, softened
- 1-1/2 cups sugar
- 2 eggs
- 1-1/2 cups mashed ripe bananas (about 3 medium)
- 1/4 cup unsweetened applesauce
- 1 teaspoon vanilla extract
- 2 cups all-purpose flour
- 1 teaspoon baking soda

Dash salt
FROSTING:
- 1 package (8 ounces) reduced-fat cream cheese
- 1/3 cup butter, softened
- 3 cups confectioners' sugar
- 2 teaspoons vanilla extract

I ate a cookie the other day and then thought 'I better log that cookie.' When I found the nutrition information, I almost cried. So many calories in one cookie! Before, I would have eaten five or six of them, but now I'm much more careful.

—Michelle Wyland, Pennsylvania

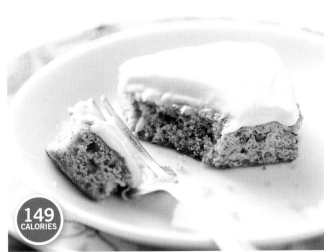

149 CALORIES

MAKEOVER FROSTED BANANA BARS

- In a large bowl, beat butter and sugar until crumbly, about 2 minutes. Add eggs, one at a time, beating well after each addition. Beat in the bananas, applesauce and vanilla. Combine the flour, baking soda and salt; stir into butter mixture just until blended.

- Transfer to a 15-in. x 10-in. x 1-in. baking pan coated with cooking spray. Bake at 350° for 20-25 minutes or until a toothpick inserted near the center comes out clean. Cool in pan on a wire rack.

- For frosting, in a small bowl, beat cream cheese and butter until fluffy. Add confectioners' sugar and vanilla; beat until smooth. Frost bars. Refrigerate leftovers.

YIELD: 3 dozen.

NUTRITION FACTS: 1 bar equals 149 calories, 4 g fat (3 g saturated fat), 23 mg cholesterol, 89 mg sodium, 26 g carbohydrate, trace fiber, 2 g protein. **DIABETIC EXCHANGES:** 2 starch, 1 fat.

fruit juice pops

PREP: 25 minutes + freezing

Barbara Stewart | GARLAND, TEXAS

I've used this recipe for years. My children enjoyed these refreshing pops more than any store-bought ones. They taste great with pineapple or orange juice.

2 cups water
1-1/2 cups sugar
4 cups unsweetened apple juice
1 cup unsweetened pineapple *or* orange juice
1/2 cup lemon juice
12 Popsicle molds *or* paper cups (3 ounces *each*) and Popsicle sticks

- In a large saucepan, combine water and sugar; bring to a boil. Reduce heat; simmer, uncovered, for 3-4 minutes or until sugar is dissolved, stirring occasionally. Remove from the heat; stir in juices.

- Fill molds or cups with 1/4 cup juice mixture; top with holders or insert sticks into cups. Freeze.

YIELD: 1 dozen.

NUTRITION FACTS: 1 juice pop equals 149 calories, trace fat (trace saturated fat), 0 cholesterol, 3 mg sodium, 38 g carbohydrate, trace fiber, trace protein.

FRUIT JUICE POPS

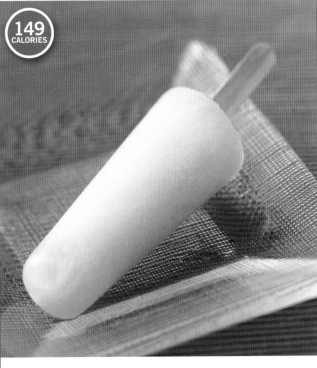

149 CALORIES

151-250 calories

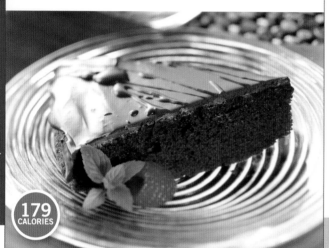

179 CALORIES

CHOCOLATE GANACHE CAKE

chocolate ganache cake

PREP: 20 minutes I **BAKE:** 20 minutes + cooling

Taste of Home Test Kitchen
Although this cake looks very elegant and like something you'd serve only for special occasions, it's really not tricky to prepare. Everyone loves the rich chocolate ganache poured over the top.

- 2 ounces 53% cacao dark baking chocolate, coarsely chopped
- 2 tablespoons butter
- 3/4 cup boiling water
- 3/4 cup sugar
- 1/4 cup buttermilk
- 1 egg
- 1 teaspoon vanilla extract
- 1/2 teaspoon orange extract
- 1 cup all-purpose flour
- 1 teaspoon baking soda
- 1/2 teaspoon salt

GANACHE:
- 3 ounces 53% cacao dark baking chocolate, coarsely chopped
- 1/4 cup half-and-half cream

- Place chocolate and butter in a large bowl; add boiling water and stir until smooth. Stir in the sugar, buttermilk, egg and extracts. Combine the flour, baking soda and salt; beat into chocolate mixture just until blended.

- Transfer to a 9-in. round baking pan coated with cooking spray. Bake at 350° for 18-22 minutes or until a toothpick inserted near the center comes out clean. Cool for 10 minutes before removing from pan to a wire rack to cool completely. Place rack on a waxed paper-lined baking sheet.

- For ganache, place chocolate in a small bowl. In a small saucepan, bring cream just to a boil. Pour over chocolate; whisk until smooth. Cool for 10 minutes or until slightly thickened.

- Slowly pour ganache over cake, allowing some ganache to drape over the sides. Refrigerate until serving. Cut into wedges.

YIELD: 12 servings.

NUTRITION FACTS: 1 slice equals 179 calories, 7 g fat (4 g saturated fat), 26 mg cholesterol, 236 mg sodium, 28 g carbohydrate, 1 g fiber, 3 g protein. **DIABETIC EXCHANGES:** 2 starch, 1 fat.

cranberry apple tart

PREP: 30 minutes + rising I **BAKE:** 15 minutes + chilling

Taste of Home Test Kitchen
No one will ever guess this impressive and luscious fruit tart is sweetened with sugar substitute.

- 1/2 teaspoon active dry yeast
- 1 tablespoon warm water (110° to 115°)
- 2 tablespoons beaten egg
- 2 tablespoons butter, softened
- 4-1/2 teaspoons sugar
- 1 teaspoon grated orange peel
- 3/4 cup plus 2 tablespoons all-purpose flour
- 1/4 teaspoon salt

FILLING:
- 1 package (12 ounces) fresh *or* frozen cranberries
- 1-1/2 cups chopped dried apples
- 1-1/2 cups unsweetened apple juice
- 1-1/4 cups sugar
- Sugar substitute equivalent to 1 cup sugar
- 1/2 cup water

1/4 teaspoon salt
1/4 cup cornstarch
1/3 cup cold water

- In a small bowl, dissolve yeast in warm water. Beat in the egg, butter, sugar and orange peel. Combine flour and salt; beat into yeast mixture on low speed just until mixture holds together.

- Shape into a ball. Place in a small bowl coated with cooking spray, turning once to coat top. Cover and let rise in a warm place for 1-1/4 hours (dough will not double, but will leave a slight indentation when pressed).

- Coat an 11-in. fluted tart pan with removable bottom with cooking spray; set aside. Place dough on a piece of waxed paper. Lightly flour dough and roll into a 13-in. circle. Invert into prepared pan; gently peel off waxed paper.

- Line unpricked tart shell with a double thickness of heavy-duty foil. Bake at 375° for 8 minutes. Remove foil; bake 6 minutes longer or until golden brown. Cool on a wire rack.

- In a large saucepan, combine the first seven filling ingredients. Cook and stir until mixture comes to a boil and cranberries pop. Combine cornstarch and cold water until smooth; gradually stir into cranberry mixture. Cook 2 minutes longer or until thickened. Cool for 20 minutes. Pour into crust. Refrigerate for at least 3 hours before cutting.

YIELD: 14 servings.

EDITOR'S NOTE: This recipe was tested with Splenda no-calorie sweetener.

NUTRITION FACTS: 1 piece equals 183 calories, 2 g fat (1 g saturated fat), 14 mg cholesterol, 113 mg sodium, 41 g carbohydrate, 2 g fiber, 1 g protein.

CRANBERRY APPLE TART

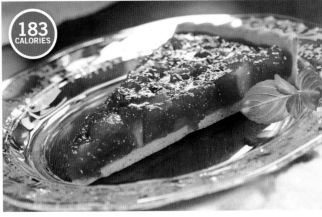

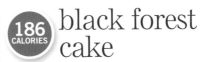

black forest cake

186 CALORIES

PREP: 40 minutes | BAKE: 35 minutes + cooling

Nancy Zimmerman | CAPE MAY COURT HOUSE, NEW JERSEY

Applesauce is used to keep this light version of Black Forest Cake healthy. Now, even people who are on a diet can enjoy a slice of rich chocolate cake!

2 cups cherry juice blend
1-3/4 cups sugar
1/2 cup unsweetened applesauce
1/4 cup canola oil
2 eggs
2 tablespoons cider vinegar
3 teaspoons vanilla extract
3 cups all-purpose flour
1/3 cup baking cocoa
2 teaspoons baking soda
1 teaspoon salt
1-1/2 cups cold fat-free milk
1 package (1.4 ounces) sugar-free instant chocolate pudding mix
1 can (20 ounces) reduced-sugar cherry pie filling
1-1/2 cups frozen fat-free whipped topping, thawed

- In a large bowl, beat the cherry juice, sugar, applesauce, oil, eggs, vinegar and vanilla until well blended. In a large bowl, combine the flour, cocoa, baking soda and salt; gradually beat into cherry juice mixture until blended.

- Pour into a 13-in. x 9-in. baking pan coated with cooking spray. Bake at 350° for 35-40 minutes or until a toothpick inserted near the center comes out clean. Cool completely on a wire rack.

- In a small bowl, whisk milk and pudding mix for 2 minutes. Let stand for 2 minutes or until soft-set. Frost top of cake with pudding. Cover and refrigerate for 15 minutes. Top with pie filling. Chill until serving. Serve with whipped topping.

YIELD: 24 servings.

NUTRITION FACTS: 1 piece with 1 tablespoon whipped topping equals 186 calories, 3 g fat (trace saturated fat), 18 mg cholesterol, 272 mg sodium, 36 g carbohydrate, 1 g fiber, 3 g protein.

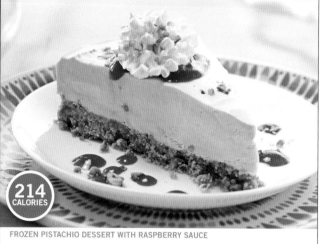

214 CALORIES

FROZEN PISTACHIO DESSERT WITH RASPBERRY SAUCE

frozen pistachio dessert with raspberry sauce

PREP: 35 minutes + freezing

Suzette Jury | KEENE, CALIFORNIA

Raspberry sauce brings bright flavor and a touch of festive color to this cool and creamy treat, while pistachios add a lick of saltiness. It will make you happy you chose to spend calories on dessert!

1-1/2	cups crushed vanilla wafers (about 45 wafers)
1/4	cup finely chopped pistachios
1/4	cup reduced-fat butter, melted
1-1/4	cups fat-free milk
1	package (1 ounce) sugar-free instant pistachio pudding mix
6	ounces reduced-fat cream cheese
1	carton (8 ounces) frozen fat-free whipped topping, thawed, *divided*
1	package (12 ounces) frozen unsweetened raspberries, thawed
2	tablespoons sugar
2	tablespoons orange liqueur *or* orange juice
2	tablespoons chopped pistachios

- In a small bowl, combine the wafers, finely chopped pistachios and butter. Press onto the bottom of a 9-in. springform pan coated with cooking spray. Place pan on a baking sheet. Bake at 350° for 10 minutes or until lightly browned. Cool on a wire rack.

- Meanwhile, in a small bowl, whisk milk and pudding mix for 2 minutes. Let stand for 2 minutes or until soft-set. In a large bowl, beat cream cheese until smooth. Beat in the pudding.

- Set aside 3/4 cup whipped topping for garnish; fold remaining whipped topping into cream cheese mixture. Pour filling over crust. Freeze for 5 hours or overnight. Cover and refrigerate remaining whipped topping.

- For sauce, place the raspberries, sugar and liqueur in a food processor. Cover and process for 1-2 minutes or until smooth. Strain and discard seeds and pulp. Refrigerate until serving.

- Remove dessert from the freezer 15 minutes before serving. Remove sides of pan. Garnish with chopped pistachios and remaining whipped topping. Serve with sauce.

YIELD: 12 servings.

EDITOR'S NOTE: This recipe was tested with Land O'Lakes light stick butter.

NUTRITION FACTS: 1 slice with 4 teaspoons sauce equals 214 calories, 9 g fat (4 g saturated fat), 18 mg cholesterol, 268 mg sodium, 28 g carbohydrate, 2 g fiber, 4 g protein. **DIABETIC EXCHANGES:** 2 starch, 2 fat.

chocolate bliss marble cake

PREP: 40 minutes | **BAKE:** 30 minutes + cooling

Josephine Piro | EASTON, PENNSYLVANIA

This cake is served at all of our family parties. It's low in fat, yet still delicious.

5	egg whites
1/4	cup baking cocoa
1/4	cup hot water
1	cup sugar, *divided*
1	cup fat-free milk
3	tablespoons canola oil
1	teaspoon vanilla extract
3/4	teaspoon almond extract
2-1/2	cups all-purpose flour
3	teaspoons baking powder
1/2	teaspoon salt
1-1/2	cups reduced-fat whipped topping
4	ounces semisweet chocolate
1-1/2	cups fresh raspberries

- Let egg whites stand at room temperature for 30 minutes. Dissolve cocoa in water; let stand until cool.

> **I decided that** I had to start preparing lean substitutes for foods that I crave and keep them on hand so I'm not stuck grabbing the high-fat and high-calorie versions.
> —Cathy Hodge Smith

- In a large bowl, beat 3/4 cup sugar, milk, oil and extracts until well blended. Combine the flour, baking powder and salt; gradually beat into sugar mixture until blended.

- In another bowl with clean beaters, beat egg whites on medium speed until soft peaks form. Beat in remaining sugar, 1 tablespoon at a time, on high until stiff peaks form. Gradually fold into batter. Remove 2 cups batter; stir in reserved cocoa mixture.

- Coat a 10-in. fluted tube pan with cooking spray. Alternately spoon the plain and chocolate batters into pan. Cut through batter with a knife to swirl.

- Bake at 350° for 30-35 minutes or until a toothpick inserted near the center comes out clean. Cool for 10 minutes before removing from pan to a wire rack to cool completely.

- For topping, in a microwave, melt whipped topping and chocolate; stir until smooth.

- Place cake on a serving plate. Drizzle with topping. Arrange raspberries in center of cake.

YIELD: 16 servings.

NUTRITION FACTS: 1 slice equals 215 calories, 6 g fat (2 g saturated fat), trace cholesterol, 172 mg sodium, 37 g carbohydrate, 2 g fiber, 4 g protein.

CHOCOLATE BLISS MARBLE CAKE

215 CALORIES

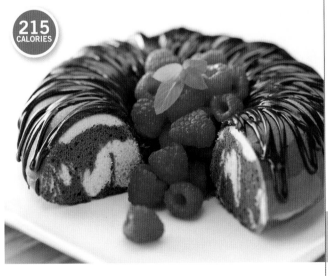

216 CALORIES fruit pizza

PREP: 35 minutes + chilling

Julie Meyer | MADISON, WISCONSIN

I enjoy desserts ... but not the calories that come with them. My roommates and I don't feel guilty about savoring a slice of dessert pizza with good-for-you fruit toppings.

- 1 **sheet refrigerated pie pastry**
- 1 **cup water**
- 1 **package (.8 ounce) cook-and-serve vanilla pudding mix**
- 1 **package (.3 ounce) sugar-free lemon gelatin**
- 1 **package (8 ounces) fat-free cream cheese, cubed**

Sugar substitute equivalent to 2 tablespoons sugar
- 1/2 **cup reduced-fat whipped topping**
- 1-1/2 **cups quartered fresh strawberries**
- 1-1/2 **cups sliced halved peeled kiwifruit**
- 1 **can (8 ounces) unsweetened pineapple chunks, drained**

- On a lightly floured surface, roll out pastry to a 12-in. circle. Transfer to a 14-in. pizza pan; prick with a fork. Bake at 450° for 5-6 minutes or until golden brown. Cool on a wire rack.

- In a saucepan, combine the water and pudding mix until smooth. Bring to a boil over medium heat, stirring constantly. Whisk in gelatin; cook and stir 1 minute longer or until thickened. Remove from the heat and let cool.

- In a small bowl, beat cream cheese and sugar substitute until smooth; fold in whipped topping. Spread cream cheese mixture over crust to within 1/2 in. of edges. Spread gelatin mixture evenly over cream cheese mixture. Arrange fruit over top. Refrigerate 1 hour or until chilled. Refrigerate leftovers.

YIELD: 8 servings.

EDITOR'S NOTE: This recipe was tested with Splenda no-calorie sweetener.

NUTRITION FACTS: 1 piece equals 216 calories, 8 g fat (4 g saturated fat), 7 mg cholesterol, 303 mg sodium, 29 g carbohydrate, 2 g fiber, 6 g protein. **DIABETIC EXCHANGES:** 1-1/2 starch, 1-1/2 fat, 1/2 fruit.

235 CALORIES

TRIPLE-BERRY COBBLER

triple-berry cobbler

PREP: 20 minutes | **BAKE:** 25 minutes

Edna Woodard | FREDERICKSBURG, TEXAS
I combined several recipes to come up with this one, and it's very versatile. Sometimes I use other fruits depending on what is in season or on hand.

- 1/2 cup sugar
-   3 tablespoons cornstarch
- 1/4 teaspoon ground cinnamon
-   1 cup water
-   1 cup fresh *or* frozen cranberries, thawed
-   1 cup fresh blueberries
-   1 cup fresh blackberries

TOPPING:
- 1/4 cup sugar
-   2 tablespoons butter, softened
- 1/3 cup fat-free milk
- 1/4 teaspoon vanilla extract
- 2/3 cup all-purpose flour
- 3/4 teaspoon baking powder
- 1/4 teaspoon salt

- In a small heavy saucepan, combine the sugar, cornstarch, cinnamon and water until smooth. Bring to a boil; cook and stir for 2 minutes or until thickened. Remove from the heat; stir in berries. Transfer to an 8-in. square baking dish coated with cooking spray.

- For topping, in a small bowl, beat sugar and butter until crumbly, about 2 minutes. Beat in milk and vanilla. Combine the flour, baking powder and salt; stir into butter mixture just until blended. Drop by tablespoonfuls over fruit mixture.

- Bake at 375° for 25-30 minutes or until filling is bubbly and a toothpick inserted in topping comes out clean. Serve warm.

YIELD: 6 servings.

NUTRITION FACTS: 1 serving equals 235 calories, 4 g fat (2 g saturated fat), 10 mg cholesterol, 195 mg sodium, 49 g carbohydrate, 3 g fiber, 2 g protein.

banana split cheesecake

PREP: 35 minutes + freezing

Cherie Sweet | EVANSVILLE, INDIANA
This fun dessert makes a festive treat that's sure to dazzle friends and family at the end of any meal. I top the tempting sweet with chocolate, caramel and pecans for a fantastic look and mouthwatering taste.

-     1 can (8 ounces) unsweetened crushed pineapple, *divided*
-     2 medium firm bananas, sliced
-     1 reduced-fat graham cracker crust (8 inches)
-     1 package (8 ounces) fat-free cream cheese
- 1-1/2 cups pineapple sherbet, softened
-     1 package (1 ounce) sugar-free instant vanilla pudding mix
-     1 carton (8 ounces) frozen reduced-fat whipped topping, thawed, *divided*
-     4 maraschino cherries, *divided*
-     1 tablespoon chocolate syrup
-     1 tablespoon caramel ice cream topping
-     1 tablespoon chopped pecans

- Drain pineapple, reserving juice. In a small bowl, combine bananas and 2 tablespoons reserved juice; let stand for 5 minutes. Drain bananas, discarding juice. Arrange bananas over bottom of crust; set aside.

- In a large bowl, beat cream cheese and 2 tablespoons reserved pineapple juice. Gradually beat in sherbet. Gradually beat in pudding mix; beat 2 minutes longer. Refrigerate 1/3 cup pineapple until serving; fold remaining pineapple into cream cheese mixture. Fold in 2 cups whipped topping; spread evenly over banana slices. Cover and freeze until firm.

- Remove from the freezer 10-15 minutes before serving. Chop three maraschino cherries and pat dry; arrange cherries and reserved pineapple around edge of pie. Drizzle with chocolate syrup and caramel topping.

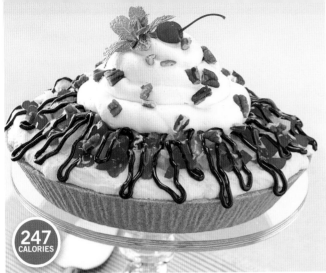

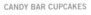
247 CALORIES

BANANA SPLIT CHEESECAKE

- Dollop remaining whipped topping onto center of pie. Sprinkle with pecans; top with remaining cherry.

YIELD: 10 servings.

NUTRITION FACTS: 1 piece equals 247 calories, 6 g fat (4 g saturated fat), 3 mg cholesterol, 336 mg sodium, 41 g carbohydrate, 1 g fiber, 5 g protein.

candy bar cupcakes

PREP: 30 minutes I **BAKE:** 20 minutes + cooling

Edie DeSpain I LOGAN, UTAH

Everyone in my family loves cupcakes, so I experimented to create these mini cakes that fit my family's tastes. I also tried to make them healthier. I hope you enjoy them as much as we do!

- 1 cup sugar
- 1 cup buttermilk
- 1/4 cup canola oil
- 1 teaspoon vanilla extract
- 1-1/2 cups all-purpose flour
- 1/3 cup baking cocoa
- 1 teaspoon baking soda
- 1/2 teaspoon salt

FILLING:
- 6 ounces fat-free cream cheese
- 2 tablespoons confectioners' sugar
- 1 egg
- 2 Snickers candy bars (2.07 ounces *each*), finely chopped

FROSTING:
- 1/3 cup butter, cubed
- 1/3 cup packed brown sugar
- 3 tablespoons fat-free milk
- 1-1/2 cups confectioners' sugar

- In a large bowl, beat the sugar, buttermilk, oil and vanilla until well blended. Combine the flour, cocoa, baking soda and salt; gradually beat into sugar mixture until blended.

- For filling, in a small bowl, beat cream cheese and confectioners' sugar until light and fluffy. Add egg; mix well. Stir in the candy bars.

- Fill paper-lined muffin cups one-third full with batter. Drop filling by tablespoonfuls into the center of each cupcake (cups will be about half full). Bake at 350° for 20-25 minutes or until a toothpick inserted in the filling comes out clean. Cool for 10 minutes before removing from pans to wire racks to cool completely.

- For frosting, in a small saucepan, melt butter. Stir in brown sugar. Bring to a boil; cook for two minutes, stirring occasionally. Remove from the heat; stir in the milk, then confectioners' sugar. Cool until frosting reaches spreading consistency. Frost cupcakes.

YIELD: 1-1/2 dozen.

NUTRITION FACTS: 1 cupcake equals 250 calories, 9 g fat (3 g saturated fat), 23 mg cholesterol, 248 mg sodium, 40 g carbohydrate, 1 g fiber, 4 g protein.

CANDY BAR CUPCAKES

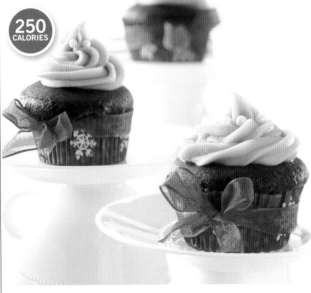
250 CALORIES

I keep chocolate with 60% or more cocoa handy. It's healthier, has a deep chocolate taste and, in small portions, is a satisfying treat. —**Barbara Menzel Jones**

tres leches cake

PREP: 35 minutes | **BAKE:** 20 minutes + chilling

Anna Yeatts | PINEHURST, NORTH CAROLINA

Finish off a fiesta with a piece of this moist and refreshing cake. Though it has been lightened, the sweet flavors of this traditional Mexican dessert aren't lost, making it the perfect end to any meal.

    5 eggs
    1 cup sugar, *divided*
    1 tablespoon butter, softened
  1/3 cup fat-free milk
    1 teaspoon vanilla extract
    1 cup all-purpose flour
    1 teaspoon baking powder

MILK SYRUP:

    1 can (14 ounces) fat-free sweetened condensed milk
    1 can (12 ounces) fat-free evaporated milk
    1 cup fat-free half-and-half
    3 teaspoons vanilla extract
   15 tablespoons frozen reduced-fat whipped topping
   15 fresh strawberries

- Place egg whites in a large bowl; let stand at room temperature for 30 minutes. Coat a 13-in. x 9-in. baking dish with cooking spray and dust with flour; set aside.

- In a large bowl, beat egg yolks on high speed for 5 minutes or until thick and lemon-colored. Gradually beat in 3/4 cup sugar and butter. Stir in milk and vanilla. Sift flour and baking powder; gradually add to yolk mixture and mix well (batter will be thick).

- With clean beaters, beat egg whites on medium speed until soft peaks form. Gradually beat in remaining sugar, 1 tablespoon at a time, on high until stiff peaks form. Gradually fold into batter.

- Spread evenly into prepared dish. Bake at 350° for 18-22 minutes or until cake springs back when lightly touched. Place on a wire rack.

- In a large saucepan, combine the condensed milk, evaporated milk and half-and-half. Bring to a boil over medium heat, stirring constantly; cook and stir for 2 minutes. Remove from the heat; stir in vanilla. Cool slightly.

- Cut cake into 15 pieces, leaving cake in the baking dish. Poke holes in cake with a skewer. Slowly pour a third of the milk syrup over cake, allowing syrup to absorb into the cake. Repeat twice. Let stand for 30 minutes.

- Cover and refrigerate for 2 hours before serving. Top each piece with whipped topping and a strawberry.

YIELD: 15 servings.

NUTRITION FACTS: 1 piece equals 233 calories, 3 g fat (2 g saturated fat), 76 mg cholesterol, 126 mg sodium, 42 g carbohydrate, 1 g fiber, 8 g protein.

TRES LECHES CAKE

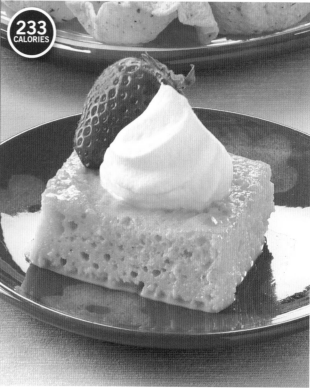

233 CALORIES

Need a light dessert? Try these hints and easy ideas for satisfying treats!

- Sift a couple of tablespoons of baking cocoa with the dry contents of an angel food cake mix before adding the liquid. It makes a light dessert that satisfies your chocolate craving.
June E., Wisconsin

- Preparing angel food cake from a boxed mix as a light dessert? Dress it up after stirring together the batter by pouring half into the pan. Then put drops of food coloring in different areas and gently swirl into the batter with a toothpick. Add the rest of the batter and repeat with more food coloring. Once you've baked, cooled and cut the cake, you'll see the colorful design. It's fun to coordinate the colors for different holidays. Use green and red for Christmas, red and blue for the Fourth of July, etc.
June B., Alabama

- Try this idea for a quick, lighter dessert. Spritz a flour tortilla with refrigerated butter-flavored spray and sprinkle with a little sugar and a couple of dashes of cinnamon. Broil 2-3 inches from the heat until browned. It's sweet and satisfying.
Kathy V., Arizona

- Like to enjoy apple pie a la mode for dessert but can't afford the calories? Try this trick. Heat up some applesauce in the microwave and pour it over a scoop of low-fat frozen yogurt. Then sprinkle it with a little cinnamon and granola.
Martha P., Iowa

- Just because you're trying to eat lighter doesn't mean you have to swear off those chocolaty desserts you've come to love. Savvy cooks learn to substitute baking cocoa for some or all of the chocolate called for in a recipe—and lighten up cakes, cookies, quick breads and frosting in the process! Baking cocoa is the powdery residue produced when cocoa beans are processed. Most of the cocoa butter (the main fat in chocolate) is removed from this powder, making it an ideal ingredient for baking light. You might replace a 1-ounce square of melted unsweetened chocolate with 3 tablespoons of cocoa plus 1 tablespoon of unsweetened applesauce and reduce the calories in a recipe by 90 and the total fat by 13 grams. Or try replacing 1/2 cup of melted semisweet chocolate chips (3 ounces) with 3 tablespoons of cocoa powder, 2 tablespoons of unsweetened applesauce and 3 tablespoons of sugar to save 222 calories and 26 grams of fat!
Taste of Home Test Kitchen

- Need a light and tasty topping for cakes and other desserts? I add a little extra flavor to reduced-fat whipped topping with different extracts, such as coconut, cherry, lemon, etc. My family thinks it's a real treat!
Dorothy F., Washington

- Sugar-free instant butterscotch pudding made with fat-free milk makes a good low-calorie fruit dip. A neighbor regularly prepared this as a low-cal treat for her husband and herself.
Fay H., Oregon

- For a refreshing treat, push a Popsicle stick through the foil cover of a small fat-free yogurt. (Be sure to remove the plastic lid first if there is one.) Pop it in the freezer until it's frozen, then remove the plastic container and enjoy your frosty fruit pop!
Dianne M., Illinois

- When you need a bite to treat yourself, try biscotti. Usually served alongside mugs of coffee or hot chocolate, most of these crunchy, twice-baked cookies are wonderful low-fat snacks. Consider scones, too. A biscuit-like quick bread, scones offer just enough sugar to satisfy a sweet tooth without being a hindrance to a healthy diet. A lighter choice than most brownies and cookies, scones are an ideal way to end breakfast or brunch and make fine accompaniments to cups of tea. Also, look into phyllo dough desserts. Thin, crispy layers of phyllo dough make this ingredient popular and versatile. Traditionally, phyllo sheets are brushed with butter before baking, but butter-flavored spray works just as well in many recipes. Phyllo dough sheets and appetizer-size tartlets are found in the freezer section of most supermarkets.
Taste of Home Test Kitchen

- To make sure my kids got plenty of calcium, I used to keep a quart jar filled with 2 cups of milk in the refrigerator. When my teens needed a snack, they selected their favorite instant pudding, added it to the jar, covered it and shook it until it turned to pudding. This wholesome treat can also be made with fat-free milk and sugar-free pudding.
Lynda H., Texas

- My husband and I are watching our weight and trying to cut fat in our diet. For a treat, I make low-sugar cupcakes and muffins. Then I top them with fat-free, sugar-free frosting. To make the frosting, I combine a package of fat-free cream cheese with a little vanilla, cornstarch and sugar substitute. This makes enough frosting to top 24 cupcakes or muffins.
Diana B., Washington

- To make sugar-free gelatin more appealing, I came up with this fun way to serve it. I found ice cube trays that are shaped like a variety of fruits at a local discount store. I spritz the trays with cooking spray. After mixing the gelatin with water according to package directions, I use a turkey baster to fill the trays. Then I place them in the refrigerator to set. The cute gelatin shapes slip right out of the trays and make a fun snack or dessert.
Anna Victoria R., New Mexico

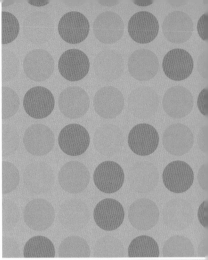

slow cooker favorites

Your slow cooker will be your new best friend on the Comfort Food Diet. Prepare your meal in the morning or at noon, pop it into the slow cooker and come home to a delicious, hot entree, side or dessert that will help you meet your 1,400 calorie goal and satisfy your family!

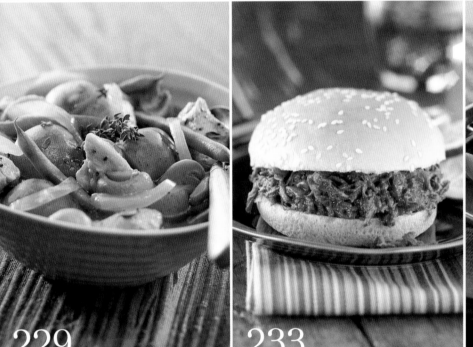

229   233   234

Using a slow cooker can take the stress out of meal planning. No more scrambling after work to find healthy options or settling for fast food. This handy bonus chapter gives you options for sandwiches, chilis, roasts and more arranged from lowest to highest calories. No matter which wonderful recipe you choose, each serving is 500 calories or less.

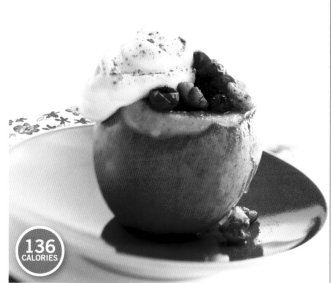

136 CALORIES

CRANBERRY-STUFFED APPLES

cranberry-stuffed apples

PREP: 10 minutes I **COOK:** 4 hours

Graciela Sandvigen I ROCHESTER, NEW YORK
Cinnamon, nutmeg and walnuts add a homey flavor to these stuffed apples, and the slow cooker does most of the work for me.

- 5 medium apples
- 1/3 cup fresh *or* frozen cranberries, thawed and chopped
- 1/4 cup packed brown sugar
- 2 tablespoons chopped walnuts
- 1/4 teaspoon ground cinnamon
- 1/8 teaspoon ground nutmeg

Whipped cream *or* vanilla ice cream, optional

- Core apples, leaving bottoms intact. Peel top third of each apple; place in a 5-qt. slow cooker. Combine the cranberries, brown sugar, walnuts, cinnamon and nutmeg; spoon into apples.

- Cover and cook on low for 4-5 hours or until apples are tender. Serve with whipped cream or ice cream if desired.

YIELD: 5 servings.

NUTRITION FACTS: 1 apple (calculated without whipped cream or ice cream) equals 136 calories, 2 g fat (trace saturated fat), 0 cholesterol, 6 mg sodium, 31 g carbohydrate, 4 g fiber, 1 g protein. **DIABETIC EXCHANGES:** 1 starch, 1 fruit.

sirloin roast with gravy

PREP: 15 minutes I **COOK:** 5-1/2 hours

Rita Clark I MONUMENT, COLORADO
This recipe is perfect for my husband, who is a meat-and-potatoes kind of guy. The peppery, fork-tender roast combined with the rich gravy creates a tasty centerpiece for any meal.

- 1 beef sirloin tip roast (3 pounds)
- 1 to 2 tablespoons coarsely ground pepper
- 1-1/2 teaspoons minced garlic
- 1/4 cup reduced-sodium soy sauce
- 3 tablespoons balsamic vinegar
- 1 tablespoon Worcestershire sauce
- 2 teaspoons ground mustard
- 2 tablespoons cornstarch
- 1/4 cup cold water

- Rub roast with pepper and garlic; cut in half and place in a 3-qt. slow cooker. Combine the soy sauce, vinegar, Worcestershire sauce and mustard; pour over beef. Cover and cook on low for 5-1/2 to 6 hours or until the meat is tender.

- Remove roast and keep warm. Strain cooking juices into a small saucepan; skim fat. Combine cornstarch and water until smooth; gradually stir into cooking juices. Bring to a boil; cook and stir for 2 minutes or until thickened. Serve with beef.

YIELD: 10 servings.

NUTRITION FACTS: 4 ounces cooked beef with 3 tablespoons gravy equals 185 calories, 6 g fat (2 g saturated fat), 72 mg cholesterol, 318 mg sodium, 4 g carbohydrate, trace fiber, 26 g protein. **DIABETIC EXCHANGE:** 4 lean meat.

SIRLOIN ROAST WITH GRAVY

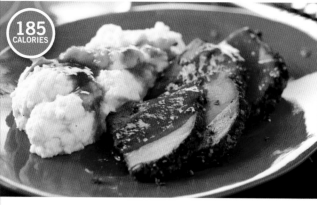

185 CALORIES

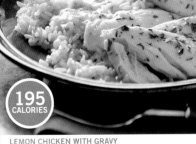

195 CALORIES

LEMON CHICKEN WITH GRAVY

lemon chicken with gravy

PREP: 25 minutes | **COOK:** 3 hours

Shona Germino | CASA GRANDE, ARIZONA
Chicken tenders are nicely seasoned with tantalizing lemon and thyme flavor in this recipe. It's especially tasty with brown rice.

      1 pound chicken tenderloins
    1/4 cup chicken broth
      3 tablespoons lemon juice
      3 tablespoons butter, cubed
      1 tablespoon grated lemon peel
      2 large garlic cloves, peeled and sliced
    1/2 teaspoon salt
    1/2 teaspoon white pepper
      2 tablespoons minced fresh parsley
         or 2 teaspoons dried parsley flakes
      2 tablespoons minced fresh thyme
         or 2 teaspoons dried thyme
      2 teaspoons cornstarch
      2 teaspoons cold water
  Hot cooked rice, optional

- In a 1-1/2-qt. slow cooker, combine the first eight ingredients. Cover and cook on low for 2-1/2 hours. Add parsley and thyme; cover and cook 30 minutes longer or until chicken is no longer pink.

- Remove chicken to a serving plate and keep warm. Transfer juices to a small saucepan. Combine cornstarch and water until smooth; add to juices. Bring to a boil; cook and stir for 2 minutes or until thickened. Serve with chicken and rice if desired.

YIELD: 4 servings.

NUTRITION FACTS: 3 ounces cooked chicken with 3 tablespoons gravy (calculated without rice) equals 195 calories, 9 g fat (5 g saturated fat), 90 mg cholesterol, 466 mg sodium, 4 g carbohydrate, 1 g fiber, 26 g protein. **DIABETIC EXCHANGES:** 3 lean meat, 2 fat.

slow-cooked sausage dressing

PREP: 20 minutes | **COOK:** 3 hours

Raquel Haggard | EDMOND, OKLAHOMA
This slow cooker dressing is so delicious that no one will know it's lower in fat. Best of all, the stove and oven are freed up for other dishes.

    1/2 pound reduced-fat bulk pork sausage
      2 celery ribs, chopped
      1 large onion, chopped
      7 cups seasoned stuffing cubes
      1 can (14-1/2 ounces) reduced-sodium chicken broth
      1 medium tart apple, chopped
    1/3 cup chopped pecans
      2 tablespoons reduced-fat butter, melted
  1-1/2 teaspoons rubbed sage
    1/2 teaspoon pepper

- In a large nonstick skillet, cook the sausage, celery and onion over medium heat until meat is no longer pink; drain. Transfer mixture to a large bowl; stir in the remaining ingredients.

SLOW-COOKED SAUSAGE DRESSING

201 CALORIES

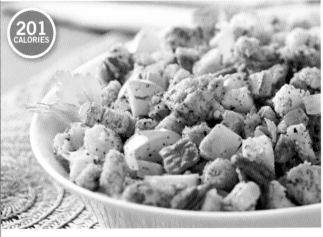

- Transfer to a 5-qt. slow cooker coated with cooking spray. Cover and cook on low for 3-4 hours or until heated through and apple is tender, stirring once.

YIELD: 8 cups.

EDITOR'S NOTE: This recipe was tested with Land O'Lakes light stick butter.

NUTRITION FACTS: 2/3 cup equals 201 calories, 8 g fat (2 g saturated fat), 17 mg cholesterol, 640 mg sodium, 26 g carbohydrate, 3 g fiber, 7 g protein.

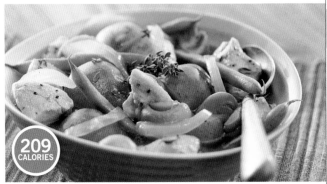

CHICKEN WITH BEANS AND POTATOES

chicken with beans and potatoes

PREP: 20 MIN. **COOK:** 4 HOURS

Have a busy afternoon? Pop this all-in-one entree into the slow cooker and come home to a hot meal. The veggies and onion soup mix give the broth lots of flavor.

- 2 pounds boneless skinless chicken breasts, cut into 1-inch cubes
- 1/2 teaspoon lemon-pepper seasoning
- 1 tablespoon canola oil
- 1 pound fresh green beans, trimmed
- 1 pound small red potatoes, quartered
- 1/2 pound medium fresh mushrooms, halved
- 1/2 cup thinly sliced sweet onion
- 2 cans (14-1/2 ounces each) chicken broth
- 2 tablespoons onion soup mix
- 2 teaspoons Worcestershire sauce
- 1 teaspoon grated lemon peel
- 1/2 teaspoon *each* salt and pepper
- 1/4 teaspoon garlic powder

- Sprinkle chicken with lemon-pepper. In a large skillet, cook chicken in oil over medium heat for 4-5 minutes or until lightly browned.

- In a 5 or 6-qt. slow cooker, layer the green beans, potatoes, mushrooms and onion. In a small bowl, combine the remaining ingredients; pour over vegetables. Top with chicken.

- Cover and cook on low for 4-5 hours or until vegetables are tender. Serve with a slotted spoon.

YIELD: 10 servings.

NUTRITION FACTS: 1-1/4 cups equals 209 calories, 5 g fat (1 g saturated fat), 63 mg cholesterol, 324 mg sodium, 15 g carbohydrate, 3 g fiber, 26 g protein.

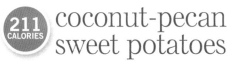

coconut-pecan sweet potatoes

PREP: 15 minutes I **COOK:** 4 hours

Raquel Haggard I EDMOND, OKLAHOMA

These delicious sweet potatoes cook effortlessly in the slow cooker so you can tend to other things. Coconut gives this classic dish a new, mouthwatering taste.

- 4 pounds sweet potatoes, peeled and cut into chunks
- 1/2 cup chopped pecans
- 1/2 cup flaked coconut
- 1/3 cup sugar
- 1/3 cup packed brown sugar
- 1/4 cup reduced-fat butter, melted
- 1/2 teaspoon ground cinnamon
- 1/4 teaspoon salt
- 1/2 teaspoon coconut extract
- 1/2 teaspoon vanilla extract

- Place sweet potatoes in a 5-qt. slow cooker coated with cooking spray. Combine the pecans, coconut, sugar, brown sugar, butter, cinnamon and salt; sprinkle over potatoes.

- Cover and cook on low for 4 hours or until potatoes are tender. Stir in extracts.

YIELD: 12 servings.

EDITOR'S NOTE: This recipe was tested with Land O'Lakes light stick butter.

NUTRITION FACTS: 2/3 cup equals 211 calories, 7 g fat (3 g saturated fat), 5 mg cholesterol, 103 mg sodium, 37 g carbohydrate, 3 g fiber, 2 g protein.

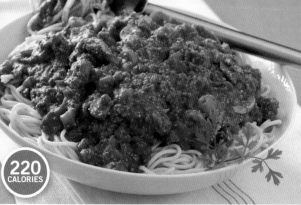

220 CALORIES

ZIPPY SPAGHETTI SAUCE

zippy spaghetti sauce

PREP: 20 minutes I **COOK:** 6 hours

Elaine Priest I DOVER, PENNSYLVANIA

If you're looking for a flavorful spaghetti sauce, give this version a try. Serve it with any kind of noodles for a fabulous dinner option.

- 2 pounds lean ground beef (90% lean)
- 1 cup chopped onion
- 1/2 cup chopped green pepper
- 2 cans (15 ounces *each*) tomato sauce
- 1 can (28 ounces) diced tomatoes, undrained
- 1 can (12 ounces) tomato paste
- 1/2 pound sliced fresh mushrooms
- 1 cup grated Parmesan cheese
- 1/2 to 3/4 cup dry red wine *or* beef broth
- 1/2 cup sliced pimiento-stuffed olives
- 1/4 cup dried parsley flakes
- 1 to 2 tablespoons dried oregano
- 2 teaspoons Italian seasoning
- 2 teaspoons minced garlic
- 1/2 teaspoon salt
- 1 teaspoon pepper

Hot cooked spaghetti

- In a large skillet, cook the beef, onion and green pepper over medium heat until meat is no longer pink; drain. Transfer to a 5-qt. slow cooker.

- Stir in the tomato sauce, tomatoes, tomato paste, mushrooms, Parmesan cheese, wine or broth, olives, parsley, oregano, Italian seasoning, garlic, salt and pepper.

- Cover and cook on low for 6-8 hours. Serve with spaghetti.

YIELD: about 3 quarts.

slow cooker favorites

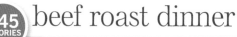

NUTRITION FACTS: 1 cup equals 220 calories, 9 g fat (3 g saturated fat), 49 mg cholesterol, 729 mg sodium, 15 g carbohydrate, 3 g fiber, 20 g protein. **DIABETIC EXCHANGES:** 2 lean meat, 1 starch, 1/2 fat.

245 CALORIES

beef roast dinner

PREP: 20 minutes I **COOK:** 8 hours

Sandra Dudley I BEMIDJI, MINNESOTA

Since this healthy dish is slow cooked, you can use less-expensive roasts and have the same mouthwatering results you would get with more costly cuts. Change up the veggies for variety, nutrition or to suit your taste!

- 1 pound red potatoes (about 4 medium), cubed
- 1/4 pound small fresh mushrooms
- 1-1/2 cups fresh baby carrots
- 1 medium green pepper, chopped
- 1 medium parsnip, chopped
- 1 small red onion, chopped
- 1 beef rump roast *or* bottom round roast (3 pounds)
- 1 can (14-1/2 ounces) beef broth
- 3/4 teaspoon salt
- 3/4 teaspoon dried oregano
- 1/4 teaspoon pepper
- 3 tablespoons cornstarch
- 1/4 cup cold water

- Place vegetables in a 5-qt. slow cooker. Cut roast in half; place in slow cooker. Combine the broth, salt, oregano and pepper; pour over meat. Cover and cook on low for 8 hours or until meat is tender.

- Remove meat and vegetables to a serving platter; keep warm. Skim fat from cooking juices; transfer to a small saucepan. Bring liquid to a boil.

- Combine cornstarch and water until smooth. Gradually stir into the pan. Bring to a boil; cook and stir for 2 minutes or until thickened. Serve with the meat and vegetables.

YIELD: 10 servings.

NUTRITION FACTS: 4 ounces cooked beef with 2/3 cup vegetables and 1/4 cup gravy equals 245 calories, 7 g fat (2 g saturated fat), 82 mg cholesterol, 427 mg sodium, 16 g carbohydrate, 2 g fiber, 29 g protein. **DIABETIC EXCHANGES:** 4 lean meat, 1 starch.

I started eating out less and cooking at home more, monitoring what went into my foods while also watching my portions. That helped me drop 40 pounds.
—Airus Copeland

turkey sloppy joes

247 CALORIES

PREP: 15 minutes | **COOK:** 4 hours

Marylou LaRue | FREELAND, MICHIGAN

At large and small gatherings, this tangy sandwich filling goes over well, and it's so easy to prepare in the slow cooker. I frequently take it to potlucks, and I'm always asked for my secret ingredient.

- 1 pound lean ground turkey
- 1 small onion, chopped
- 1/2 cup chopped celery
- 1/4 cup chopped green pepper
- 1 can (10-3/4 ounces) reduced-sodium condensed tomato soup, undiluted
- 1/2 cup ketchup
- 1 tablespoon brown sugar
- 2 tablespoons prepared mustard
- 1/4 teaspoon pepper
- 8 hamburger buns, split

- In a large saucepan coated with cooking spray, cook the turkey, onion, celery and green pepper over medium heat until meat is no longer pink; drain if necessary. Stir in the soup, ketchup, brown sugar, mustard and pepper.

- Transfer to a 3-qt. slow cooker. Cover and cook on low for 4 hours. Serve on buns.

YIELD: 8 servings.

NUTRITION FACTS: 1 sandwich equals 247 calories, 7 g fat (2 g saturated fat), 45 mg cholesterol, 553 mg sodium, 32 g carbohydrate, 2 g fiber, 14 g protein. **DIABETIC EXCHANGES:** 2 starch, 1-1/2 lean meat.

zippy slow-cooked chili

PREP: 10 minutes | **COOK:** 6 hours

Travis Skrock | STRATFORD, WISCONSIN

Invest just 10 minutes to serve steaming bowls of this spiced-up chili to warm your family on a cold day. You'll get plenty of compliments on your cooking!

- 1 pound lean ground beef (90% lean)
- 1 can (28 ounces) diced tomatoes, undrained
- 1 medium onion, chopped
- 1 medium green pepper, chopped
- 1 can (15 ounces) vegetarian chili with beans
- 1 can (8 ounces) tomato sauce
- 2 tablespoons chili powder
- 2 tablespoons minced fresh parsley
- 1 tablespoon dried basil
- 2 teaspoons ground cumin
- 4 garlic cloves, minced
- 1 teaspoon dried oregano
- 3/4 teaspoon pepper
- 1/8 teaspoon hot pepper sauce
- 6 tablespoons shredded reduced-fat cheddar cheese
- 1 tablespoon minced chives

- In a nonstick skillet, cook beef over medium heat until no longer pink; drain. Transfer to a 3-qt. slow cooker. Add the tomatoes, onion, green pepper, chili, tomato sauce, chili powder, parsley, basil, cumin, garlic, oregano, pepper and hot pepper sauce. Cover and cook on low for 6-8 hours or until the vegetables are tender. Sprinkle with cheese and chives before serving.

YIELD: 6 servings.

NUTRITION FACTS: 1-1/3 cups equals 266 calories, 8 g fat (3 g saturated fat), 42 mg cholesterol, 759 mg sodium, 27 g carbohydrate, 8 g fiber, 23 g protein. **DIABETIC EXCHANGES:** 3 lean meat, 2 starch.

ZIPPY SLOW-COOKED CHILI

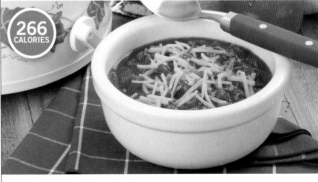

266 CALORIES

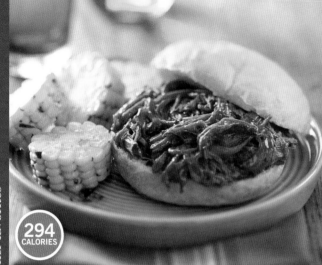

294 CALORIES

TEX-MEX BEEF BARBECUES

tex-mex beef barbecues

PREP: 20 minutes | **COOK:** 5 hours

Lynda Zuniga | CRYSTAL CITY, TEXAS

I took these easy but impressive sandwiches to a potluck recently, and everyone loved them! They also taste good made with lean ground beef.

- 1 fresh beef brisket (3-1/2 pounds)
- 1 jar (18 ounces) hickory smoke-flavored barbecue sauce
- 1/2 cup finely chopped onion
- 1 envelope chili seasoning
- 1 tablespoon Worcestershire sauce
- 1 teaspoon minced garlic
- 1 teaspoon lemon juice
- 14 hamburger buns, split

- Cut brisket in half; place in a 5-qt. slow cooker.

- In a small bowl, combine the barbecue sauce, onion, chili seasoning, Worcestershire sauce, garlic and lemon juice. Pour over beef. Cover and cook on high for 5-6 hours or until meat is tender.

- Remove beef; cool slightly. Shred and return to the slow cooker. Heat through. Serve on buns.

YIELD: 14 servings.

EDITOR'S NOTE: This is a fresh beef brisket, not corned beef.

NUTRITION FACTS: 1 sandwich equals 294 calories, 7 g fat (2 g saturated fat), 47 mg cholesterol, 732 mg sodium, 28 g carbohydrate, 2 g fiber, 28 g protein. **DIABETIC EXCHANGES:** 3 lean meat, 2 starch.

red clam sauce

PREP: 25 minutes | **COOK:** 3 hours

JoAnn Brown | LATROBE, PENNSYLVANIA

People will think you slaved over this awesome recipe all day. Instead, it cooks while you do other things. What a great way to jazz up pasta.

- 1 medium onion, chopped
- 1 tablespoon canola oil
- 2 garlic cloves, minced
- 2 cans (6-1/2 ounces *each*) chopped clams, undrained
- 1 can (14-1/2 ounces) diced tomatoes, undrained
- 1 can (6 ounces) tomato paste
- 1/4 cup minced fresh parsley
- 1 bay leaf
- 1 teaspoon sugar
- 1 teaspoon dried basil
- 1/2 teaspoon dried thyme
- 6 ounces linguine, cooked and drained

- In a small skillet, saute onion in oil until tender. Add garlic; cook 1 minute longer.

- Transfer to a 1-1/2- or 2-qt. slow cooker. Stir in the clams, tomatoes, tomato paste, parsley, bay leaf, sugar, basil and thyme. Cover and cook on low for 3-4 hours or until heated through. Discard bay leaf. Serve with linguine.

YIELD: 4 servings.

NUTRITION FACTS: 1 cup sauce with 3/4 cup cooked linguine equals 305 calories, 5 g fat (trace saturated fat), 15 mg cholesterol, 553 mg sodium, 53 g carbohydrate, 7 g fiber, 15 g protein.

RED CLAM SAUCE

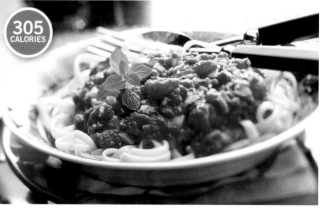

305 CALORIES

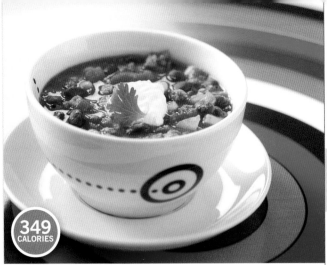

349 CALORIES

FAMILY-PLEASING TURKEY CHILI

family-pleasing turkey chili

PREP: 25 minutes | **COOK:** 4 hours

Sheila Christensen | SAN MARCOS, CALIFORNIA
My children really love this chili, and it has become one of their favorite comfort foods. It's relatively inexpensive, and leftovers are wonderful!

- 1 pound lean ground turkey
- 1 medium green pepper, finely chopped
- 1 small red onion, finely chopped
- 2 garlic cloves, minced
- 1 can (28 ounces) diced tomatoes, undrained
- 1 can (16 ounces) kidney beans, rinsed and drained
- 1 can (15 ounces) black beans, rinsed and drained
- 1 can (14-1/2 ounces) reduced-sodium chicken broth
- 1-3/4 cups frozen corn, thawed
- 1 can (6 ounces) tomato paste
- 1 tablespoon chili powder
- 1/2 teaspoon pepper
- 1/4 teaspoon ground cumin
- 1/4 teaspoon garlic powder

Optional toppings: reduced-fat sour cream and minced fresh cilantro

- In a large nonstick skillet, cook the turkey, green pepper and onion over medium heat until meat is no longer pink. Add garlic; cook 1 minute longer. Drain.

- Transfer to a 4-qt. slow cooker. Stir in the tomatoes, kidney beans, black beans, broth, corn, tomato paste, chili powder, pepper, cumin and garlic powder.

- Cover and cook on low for 4-5 hours or until heated through. Serve with optional toppings if desired.

YIELD: 6 servings (2-1/4 quarts).

NUTRITION FACTS: 1-1/2 cups (calculated without optional toppings) equals 349 calories, 7 g fat (2 g saturated fat), 60 mg cholesterol, 725 mg sodium, 47 g carbohydrate, 12 g fiber, 27 g protein. **DIABETIC EXCHANGES:** 3 lean meat, 2 starch, 2 vegetable.

354 CALORIES

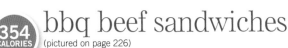

bbq beef sandwiches
(pictured on page 226)

PREP: 15 minutes | **COOK:** 8 hours

Rebecca Rohland | MEDFORD, WISCONSIN
After years of searching, I found a recipe for shredded barbecue beef that's a hit with all of my family and friends. Plus, it's easy to freeze for future meals!

- 2 cups ketchup
- 1 medium onion, chopped
- 1/4 cup cider vinegar
- 1/4 cup molasses
- 2 tablespoons Worcestershire sauce
- 2 garlic cloves, minced
- 1/2 teaspoon salt
- 1/2 teaspoon ground mustard
- 1/2 teaspoon pepper
- 1/4 teaspoon garlic powder
- 1/4 teaspoon crushed red pepper flakes
- 1 boneless beef chuck roast (3 pounds)
- 14 sesame seed hamburger buns, split

- In a large bowl, combine the first 11 ingredients. Cut roast in half; place in a 5-qt. slow cooker. Pour ketchup mixture over roast.

- Cover and cook on low for 8-9 hours or until the meat is tender.

- Remove meat and shred with two forks. Skim fat from cooking juices. Return meat to slow cooker; heat through. Using a slotted spoon, serve beef on buns.

YIELD: 14 sandwiches.

NUTRITION FACTS: 1 sandwich equals 354 calories, 12 g fat (5 g saturated fat), 63 mg cholesterol, 805 mg sodium, 37 g carbohydrate, 1 g fiber, 24 g protein.

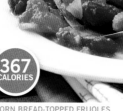

367 CALORIES

CORN BREAD-TOPPED FRIJOLES

corn bread-topped frijoles

PREP: 20 minutes | **COOK:** 3 hours

Suzanne Caldwell | ARTESIA, NEW MEXICO

My family often requests this economical slow-cooker favorite. It's loaded with fresh Southwestern flavors. One batch makes several servings, but it never lasts long at our house!

- 1 medium onion, chopped
- 1 medium green pepper, chopped
- 1 tablespoon canola oil
- 2 garlic cloves, minced
- 1 can (16 ounces) kidney beans, rinsed and drained
- 1 can (15 ounces) pinto beans, rinsed and drained
- 1 can (14-1/2 ounces) diced tomatoes, undrained
- 1 can (8 ounces) tomato sauce
- 1 teaspoon chili powder
- 1/2 teaspoon pepper
- 1/8 teaspoon hot pepper sauce

CORN BREAD TOPPING:
- 1 cup all-purpose flour
- 1 cup yellow cornmeal
- 1 tablespoon sugar
- 1-1/2 teaspoons baking powder
- 1/2 teaspoon salt
- 2 eggs, lightly beaten
- 1-1/4 cups fat-free milk
- 1 can (8-3/4 ounces) cream-style corn
- 3 tablespoons canola oil

- In a large skillet, saute the onion and green pepper in oil until tender. Add garlic; cook 1 minute longer. Transfer to a greased 5-qt. slow cooker.

- Stir in the beans, tomatoes, tomato sauce, chili powder, pepper and hot pepper sauce. Cover and cook on high for 1 hour.

- In a large bowl, combine the flour, cornmeal, sugar, baking powder and salt. Combine the eggs, milk, corn and oil; add to dry ingredients and mix well. Spoon evenly over bean mixture.

- Cover and cook on high 2 hours longer or until a toothpick inserted near the center of corn bread comes out clean.

YIELD: 8 servings.

NUTRITION FACTS: 1 serving equals 367 calories, 9 g fat (1 g saturated fat), 54 mg cholesterol, 708 mg sodium, 59 g carbohydrate, 9 g fiber, 14 g protein.

burgundy beef stew

PREP: 25 minutes | **COOK:** 8 hours

Mindy Ilar | ST ALBANS, WEST VIRGINIA

Here's a stew that's brimming with home-cooked comfort. I dress up the dish with sirloin, turkey bacon and herbs, making it special enough for company.

- 1/2 cup all-purpose flour
- 1 pound beef top sirloin steak, cut into 1/2-inch pieces

BURGUNDY BEEF STEW

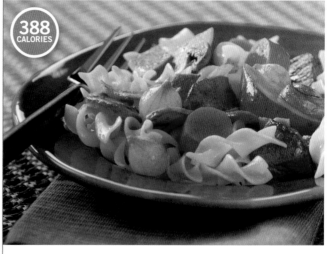

388 CALORIES

3 turkey bacon strips, diced

8 small red potatoes, halved

2 medium carrots, cut into 1-inch pieces

1 cup sliced fresh mushrooms

3/4 cup frozen pearl onions, thawed

3 garlic cloves, minced

1 bay leaf

1 teaspoon dried marjoram

1/2 teaspoon salt

1/2 teaspoon dried thyme

1/4 teaspoon pepper

1/2 cup reduced-sodium beef broth

1 cup Burgundy wine *or* additional reduced-sodium beef broth

6 cups hot cooked egg noodles

- Place flour in a large resealable plastic bag. Add beef, a few pieces at a time, and shake to coat.

- In a large skillet coated with cooking spray, brown beef and bacon in batches on all sides.

- Place beef and bacon in a 5-qt. slow cooker. Stir in the vegetables, garlic, seasonings, broth and wine or additional broth.

- Cover and cook on low for 8-9 hours or until the meat is tender.

- Discard bay leaf. Thicken cooking juices if desired. Serve with noodles.

YIELD: 6 servings.

NUTRITION FACTS: 1 cup stew with 1 cup noodles equals 388 calories, 7 g fat (2 g saturated fat), 70 mg cholesterol, 434 mg sodium, 49 g carbohydrate, 4 g fiber, 26 g protein. **DIABETIC EXCHANGES:** 3 starch, 3 lean meat.

cranberry-apricot pork roast with potatoes

PREP: 15 minutes I **COOK:** 5 hours

Pat Barnes I PANAMA CITY, FLORIDA

Why not try this delightful meal-in-one? It makes weeknight dining a snap. The apricots blend well with whole-berry cranberry sauce for a popular sweet-and-tart taste. Cayenne pepper adds just the right touch of zing to this meat-and-potatoes meal.

1 boneless whole pork loin roast (3 pounds)

4 medium potatoes, peeled and quartered

1 can (14 ounces) whole-berry cranberry sauce

1 can (15 ounces) apricot halves, drained

1 medium onion, quartered

1/2 cup chopped dried apricots

1 tablespoon sugar

1/2 teaspoon ground mustard

1/4 teaspoon cayenne pepper

- Cut roast in half. Place potatoes in a 5-qt. slow cooker. Add the pork.

- In a blender, combine the cranberry sauce, apricots, onion, dried apricots, sugar, mustard, and cayenne. Cover and process for 30 seconds or until almost smooth. Pour over pork. Cover and cook on low for 5-6 hours or until a meat thermometer reads 160° and pork is tender.

- Remove pork and potatoes to a serving platter and bowl. Pour cooking juices into a pitcher; serve with meat and potatoes.

YIELD: 8 servings.

NUTRITION FACTS: 1 serving equals 433 calories, 8 g fat (3 g saturated fat), 85 mg cholesterol, 71 mg sodium, 56 g carbohydrate, 4 g fiber, 35 g protein.

CRANBERRY-APRICOT PORK ROAST WITH POTATOES

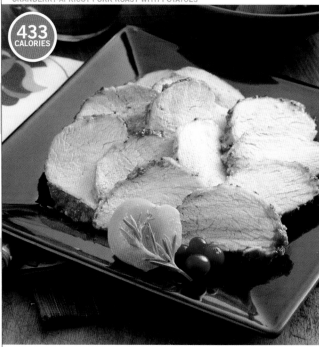

433 CALORIES

8-ingredient or less recipes

Preparing healthy recipes can be quick and easy when you reach for recipes with short ingredient lists. The delicious choices in this section all have 8 or fewer ingredients. We've included short, light recipes for breakfast, lunch, dinner and even dessert.

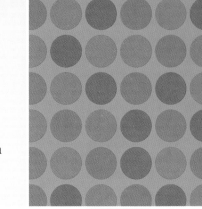

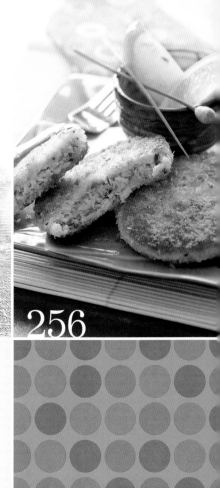

250

241

256

Looking for an easy, healthy recipe? Consider the great recipes here, which are arranged in calorie order from the lowest to the highest. Every one has 8 ingredients or less (not including salt, pepper or water), so you can get done preparing meals fast and have more time to work some exercise or other fun activities into your busy days! Check out the exercise-related tips from readers sprinkled throughout this special bonus chapter.

winter vegetables

PREP: 25 minutes | **COOK:** 20 minutes

Charlene Augustyn | GRAND RAPIDS, MICHIGAN
The flavor of thyme shines through in this recipe. Its colorful array of vegetables is so appealing on the table.

- 3 medium turnips, peeled and cut into 2-inch julienne strips
- 1 large rutabaga, peeled and cut into 2-inch julienne strips
- 4 medium carrots, cut into 2-inch julienne strips
- 3 fresh broccoli spears
- 1 tablespoon butter
- 1 tablespoon minced fresh parsley
- 1/2 teaspoon salt
- 1/2 teaspoon dried thyme

Pepper to taste

- Place the turnips, rutabaga and carrots in a large saucepan and cover with water. Bring to a boil. Reduce heat; cover and cook for 10 minutes.

- Meanwhile, cut florets from broccoli and save for another use. Cut broccoli stalks into 2-in. julienne strips; add to saucepan. Cover and cook 5 minutes longer or until vegetables are crisp-tender; drain well.

- In a large skillet, saute vegetables in butter. Stir in the parsley, salt, thyme and pepper.

YIELD: 12 servings.

NUTRITION FACTS: 3/4 cup equals 51 calories, 1 g fat (1 g saturated fat), 3 mg cholesterol, 151 mg sodium, 10 g carbohydrate, 3 g fiber, 2 g protein. **DIABETIC EXCHANGE:** 2 vegetable.

WINTER VEGETABLES

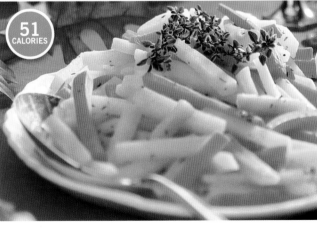

51 CALORIES

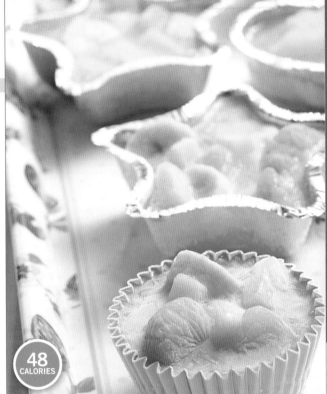

48 CALORIES

FROZEN FRUIT CUPS

frozen fruit cups

PREP: 30 minutes + freezing

Sue Ross | CASA GRANDE, ARIZONA
These refreshing citrus treats burst with color and flavor. Keep a supply in the freezer for a frosty treat anytime.

- 5 packages (3 ounces *each*) lemon gelatin
- 10 cups boiling water
- 5 cans (20 ounces *each*) unsweetened pineapple tidbits, undrained
- 5 cans (11 ounces *each*) mandarin oranges, drained
- 5 cans (6 ounces *each*) frozen orange juice concentrate, partially thawed
- 5 large firm bananas, sliced

- In a very large bowl, dissolve gelatin in boiling water; cool for 10 minutes. Stir in the remaining ingredients.

- Spoon into foil cups. Freeze until firm. Remove from the freezer 30 minutes before serving.

YIELD: 9-1/2 dozen.

NUTRITION FACTS: 1 fruit cup equals 48 calories, trace fat (trace saturated fat), 0 cholesterol, 11 mg sodium, 12 g carbohydrate, 1 g fiber, 1 g protein. **DIABETIC EXCHANGE:** 1 fruit.

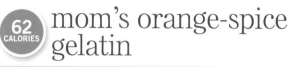

8-ingredient or less recipes

NUTRITION FACTS: 1/2 cup equals 70 calories, trace fat (trace saturated fat), 0 cholesterol, 42 mg sodium, 16 g carbohydrate, 2 g fiber, 1 g protein. **DIABETIC EXCHANGE:** 1 fruit.

62 CALORIES

mom's orange-spice gelatin

PREP: 25 minutes + chilling

Karen Grimes I STEPHENS CITY, VIRGINIA

I remember my mom making this tangy gelatin salad frequently when I was growing up. The cinnamon and cloves make it extra special. It was always one of our favorite light treats.

- 1 can (15 ounces) sliced peaches in extra-light syrup
- 2 tablespoons cider vinegar
- 3 cinnamon sticks (3 inches)
- 12 whole cloves
- 3 cups boiling water
- 4 packages (.3 ounce *each*) sugar-free orange gelatin
- 2 cups cold water

Sugar substitute equivalent to 1/3 cup sugar
- 1/4 cup finely chopped pecans

- Drain peaches, reserving syrup; set peaches aside. In a small saucepan, combine the vinegar, cinnamon sticks, cloves and reserved syrup. Bring to a boil; cook until reduced to about 1/2 cup. Strain, discarding cinnamon and cloves.

- Add boiling water to syrup mixture; stir in gelatin until dissolved. Stir in the cold water and sugar substitute. Refrigerate until slightly thickened, about 35 minutes.

- Coarsely chop the peaches. Stir peaches and pecans into gelatin mixture. Transfer to a 6-cup ring mold coated with cooking spray (mold will be full). Refrigerate for 3-4 hours or until firm. Unmold onto a serving plate.

YIELD: 10 servings.

EDITOR'S NOTE: This recipe was tested with Splenda no-calorie sweetener.

NUTRITION FACTS: 2/3 cup equals 62 calories, 2 g fat (trace saturated fat), 0 cholesterol, 91 mg sodium, 8 g carbohydrate, 1 g fiber, 2 g protein. **DIABETIC EXCHANGES:** 1/2 starch, 1/2 fat.

70 CALORIES

APPLE CRANBERRY DELIGHT

apple cranberry delight

PREP: 25 minutes + chilling

Beverly Koester I APPLETON, WISCONSIN

My husband and I went to a cranberry festival, and I came home with 5 pounds of the berries! Luckily they freeze well and taste great in this simple dish.

- 1-1/2 cups fresh *or* frozen cranberries
- 1-3/4 cups unsweetened apple juice, *divided*
- 1 package (.3 ounce) sugar-free cranberry gelatin
- 2 cups chopped peeled Golden Delicious apples

- In a small saucepan, combine cranberries and 1 cup apple juice. Bring to a boil. Reduce heat; cover and simmer for 10-15 minutes or until the berries pop. Stir in gelatin until dissolved. Remove from the heat; stir in apples and remaining apple juice.

- Pour into a 4-cup mold coated with cooking spray. Refrigerate for 4 hours or until firm. Unmold onto a serving plate.

YIELD: 6 servings.

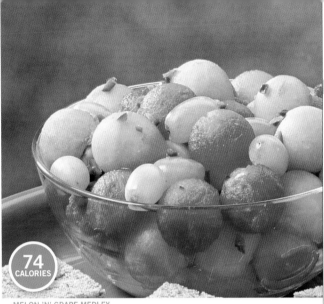

74 CALORIES

MELON 'N' GRAPE MEDLEY

melon 'n' grape medley

PREP: 15 minutes + chilling

Taste of Home Test Kitchen
This colorful fruit salad has a zesty honey-orange dressing with a surprising twist.

1-1/2 cups cantaloupe balls
1-1/2 cups watermelon balls
1-1/2 cups green grapes
DRESSING:
   1/4 cup orange juice
     1 tablespoon honey
     1 tablespoon lime juice
     2 teaspoons chopped seeded jalapeno pepper
   1/2 teaspoon grated lime peel

- In a resealable plastic bag, combine the cantaloupe, watermelon and grapes. In a small bowl, whisk the orange juice, honey and lime juice. Stir in the jalapeno and lime peel.

- Pour over fruit. Seal bag, removing as much air as possible, and turn to coat; refrigerate for at least 1 hour. Serve with a slotted spoon.

YIELD: 6 servings.

EDITOR'S NOTE: We recommend wearing disposable gloves when cutting hot peppers. Avoid touching your face.

NUTRITION FACTS: 3/4 cup equals 74 calories, 1 g fat (trace saturated fat), 0 cholesterol, 6 mg sodium, 18 g carbohydrate, 1 g fiber, 1 g protein.

hard-cooked eggs

PREP: 20 minutes + cooling

Taste of Home Test Kitchen
Our home economists share this recipe for hard-cooked eggs that can be eaten plain as part of a meal or used in various recipes.

  12 eggs
Cold water

- Place eggs in a single layer on a large saucepan; add enough cold water to cover by 1 in. Cover and quickly bring to a boil. Remove from the heat. Let stand for 15 minutes for large eggs, 18 minutes for extra-large eggs or 12 minutes for medium eggs.

- Rinse eggs in cold water and place in ice water until completely cooled. Drain and refrigerate.

YIELD: 12 servings.

NUTRITION FACTS: 1 egg equals 75 calories, 5 g fat (2 g saturated fat), 213 mg cholesterol, 63 mg sodium, 1 g carbohydrate, 0 fiber, 6 g protein.

HARD-COOKED EGGS

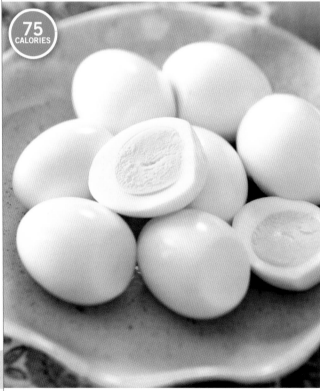

75 CALORIES

8-ingredient or less recipes

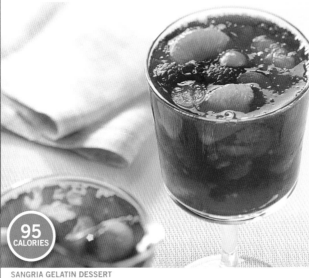

95 CALORIES

SANGRIA GELATIN DESSERT

sangria gelatin dessert

PREP: 15 minutes + chilling

Taste of Home Test Kitchen
You'll love this light yet festive finale. White wine gives it a refreshing twist, and the vibrant color dresses up a special occasion dinner.

    1 package (.3 ounce) sugar-free lemon gelatin
    1 package (.3 ounce) sugar-free raspberry gelatin
1-1/2 cups boiling water
    1 cup cold water
    1 cup white wine
    1 can (11 ounces) mandarin oranges, drained
    1 cup fresh raspberries
    1 cup green grapes, halved

- In a large bowl, dissolve gelatins in boiling water. Let stand for 10 minutes. Stir in cold water and the wine; refrigerate for 45 minutes or until partially set.

- Fold in the oranges, raspberries and grapes. Transfer to six large wine glasses, 1 cup in each. Refrigerate for 4 hours or until set.

YIELD: 6 servings.

NUTRITION FACTS: 1 serving equals 95 calories, trace fat (trace saturated fat), 0 cholesterol, 83 mg sodium, 13 g carbohydrate, 2 g fiber, 2 g protein. **DIABETIC EXCHANGE:** 1 fruit.

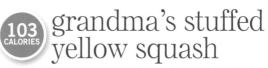

103 CALORIES

grandma's stuffed yellow squash

PREP: 25 minutes | **BAKE:** 25 minutes

Janie McGraw | SALLISAW, OKLAHOMA
My grandma, who raised me, was an awesome cook. This is a recipe she fixed every summer when our garden overflowed with yellow squash. This side dish for lunch or dinner is a simple but tasty way to use this abundant crop.

    1 medium yellow summer squash
  1/4 cup egg substitute
    2 tablespoons finely chopped onion
  1/4 teaspoon salt
  1/8 teaspoon pepper
    2 slices bread, toasted and diced

- Place squash in a large saucepan; cover with water. Bring to a boil; cover and cook for 7-9 minutes or until crisp-tender. Drain.

- When cool enough to handle, cut the squash in half lengthwise; scoop out and reserve the pulp, leaving a 3/8-in. shell. Invert the shells on paper towel.

- In a small bowl, combine the egg substitute, onion, salt and pepper. Stir in toasted bread cubes and squash pulp. Spoon into squash shells.

- Place the squash in an 8-in. square baking dish coated with cooking spray. Cover and bake at 375° for 20 minutes. Uncover; bake 5-10 minutes longer or until lightly browned.

YIELD: 2 servings.

NUTRITION FACTS: 1/2 squash equals 103 calories, 1 g fat (trace saturated fat), trace cholesterol, 490 mg sodium, 18 g carbohydrate, 3 g fiber, 6 g protein. **DIABETIC EXCHANGES:** 1 starch, 1 vegetable.

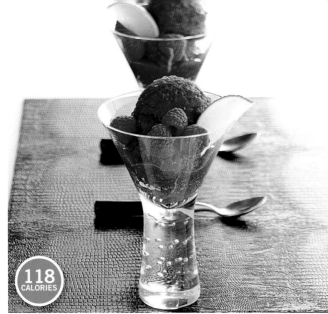

STRAWBERRY-RASPBERRY ICE

strawberry-raspberry ice

PREP: 10 minutes + freezing

Sandra Sakaitis | ST. LOUIS, MISSOURI

What's more refreshing on a hot day than lovely berry ice? The bright color and flavor will please everyone!

- 2 packages (10 ounces *each*) frozen sweetened sliced strawberries, partially thawed
- 2 cups frozen unsweetened raspberries, partially thawed
- 1/3 cup sugar
- 3 tablespoons lime juice
- 2 tablespoons orange juice

Fresh raspberries and lime wedges, optional

- Place the strawberries, raspberries, sugar and juices in a blender. Cover and process for 2-3 minutes or until smooth. Transfer to a 13-in. x 9-in. dish. Freeze for 1 hour or until edges begin to firm.

- Stir and return to freezer. Freeze 2 hours longer or until firm.

- Just before serving, transfer to a food processor; cover and process for 2-3 minutes or until smooth.

- Scoop into individual dishes; garnish with raspberries and lime wedges if desired.

YIELD: 3-1/2 cups.

NUTRITION FACTS: 1/2 cup equals 118 calories, trace fat (trace saturated fat), 0 cholesterol, 3 mg sodium, 31 g carbohydrate, 2 g fiber, 1 g protein. **DIABETIC EXCHANGES:** 1 starch, 1/2 fruit.

lemon-soy roughy

PREP: 5 minutes + marinating | **BAKE:** 15 minutes

Anne Powers | MUNFORD, ALABAMA

I enjoy fish very much, and I especially like it fried. But my doctor has said that's a no-no! So this is a very tasty way to prepare fish without adding lots of extra calories.

- 1/4 cup lemon juice
- 1/4 cup reduced-sodium soy sauce
- 1 tablespoon sugar
- 1/2 teaspoon ground ginger
- 4 orange roughy fillets (6 ounces *each*)
- 1/2 teaspoon salt-free lemon-pepper seasoning

- In a large resealable plastic bag, combine the lemon juice, soy sauce, sugar and ginger; add fish. Seal bag and turn to coat; refrigerate for 30 minutes.

- Drain and discard marinade. Arrange the fillets in a 15-in. x 10-in. x 1-in. baking pan coated with cooking spray; sprinkle with lemon pepper. Bake, uncovered, at 350° for 12-15 minutes or until fish flakes easily with a fork.

YIELD: 4 servings.

NUTRITION FACTS: 1 fillet equals 124 calories, 1 g fat (trace saturated fat), 34 mg cholesterol, 258 mg sodium, 1 g carbohydrate, trace fiber, 25 g protein. **DIABETIC EXCHANGE:** 4 lean meat.

LEMON-SOY ROUGHY

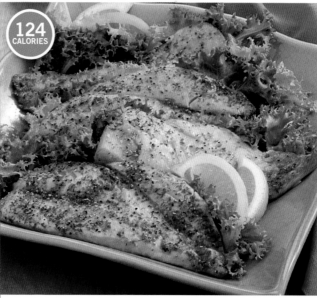

131 CALORIES hawaiian breakfast cups

PREP: 15 minutes | **BAKE:** 20 minutes

Judy Reagan | HANNIBAL, MISSOURI

In Hawaii, this dish is called Hua Moa Pua'a Ipu, meaning flower, cup and egg. This sweet and savory ham cup has a nice surprise inside with just a touch of mild salsa and sharp cheddar cheese.

- 6 thin slices deli ham
- 1/4 cup shredded cheddar cheese
- 2 tablespoons mild salsa
- 6 canned pineapple slices
- 6 eggs
- 1/2 teaspoon salt-free seasoning blend

- Line six greased 8-oz. ramekins with ham. Layer each with cheese, salsa and pineapple. Crack an egg into the center of each cup; sprinkle with seasoning blend.

- Place ramekins on a baking sheet. Bake at 350° for 20-25 minutes or until egg whites are completely set and yolks are still soft.

YIELD: 6 servings.

NUTRITION FACTS: 1 breakfast cup equals 131 calories, 7 g fat (3 g saturated fat), 226 mg cholesterol, 320 mg sodium, 6 g carbohydrate, trace fiber, 11 g protein. **DIABETIC EXCHANGES:** 2 medium-fat meat, 1/2 starch.

133 CALORIES vanilla tapioca pudding

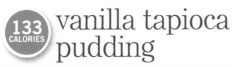

PREP: 10 minutes + chilling

Robert Daggit | SHOREVIEW, MINNESOTA

As a widower, I've recently started learning how to cook. I created this tapioca pudding that's not only low in fat, but it's easy to make, too. I love that it's so simple yet has such wonderful old-fashioned goodness.

- 3-1/4 cups fat-free milk
- 2 tablespoons quick-cooking tapioca
- 2 tablespoons sugar
- 1 package (.8 ounce) cook-and-serve vanilla pudding mix
- 1/4 teaspoon vanilla extract

- In a large saucepan, combine the milk, tapioca, sugar and pudding mix. Bring to a boil, stirring constantly. Remove from the heat; stir in vanilla.

- Spoon into four dessert dishes. Cover and refrigerate for 2 hours before serving.

YIELD: 4 servings.

NUTRITION FACTS: 3/4 cup equals 133 calories, trace fat (trace saturated fat), 4 mg cholesterol, 118 mg sodium, 26 g carbohydrate, trace fiber, 7 g protein. **DIABETIC EXCHANGES:** 1 starch, 1 fat-free milk.

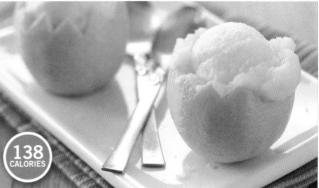

LEMON SORBET

lemon sorbet

PREP: 15 minutes + cooling | **PROCESS:** 20 minutes + freezing

Goldene Petersen | BRIGHAM CITY, UTAH

Served in chilled bowls or scooped into cut lemon halves, this creamy sorbet is both sweet and tart.

- 1 cup sugar
- 1 cup water
- 3/4 cup lemon juice
- 3 tablespoons grated lemon peel

- In a small saucepan over medium heat, cook and stir sugar and water until mixture comes to a boil. Reduce heat; simmer, uncovered, for 2 minutes. Remove from the heat; cool to room temperature.

- Stir in lemon juice and lemon peel. Freeze in an ice cream freezer according to manufacturer's directions. Transfer to a freezer container; freeze for at least 4 hours before serving.

YIELD: 2 cups.

NUTRITION FACTS: 1/3 cup equals 138 calories, trace fat (trace saturated fat), 0 cholesterol, 1 mg sodium, 36 g carbohydrate, trace fiber, trace protein. **DIABETIC EXCHANGES:** 2 starch.

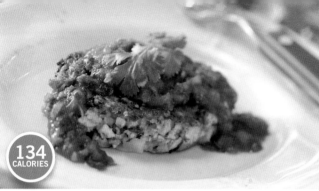

134 CALORIES

CHICKEN PATTIES WITH ROASTED TOMATO SALSA

chicken patties with roasted tomato salsa

PREP: 30 minutes | **COOK:** 45 minutes

Mary Relyea | CANASTOTA, NEW YORK

Bold and zesty tomato salsa perks up these moist and tender chicken patties. Great for lunch or dinner, this recipe ranks high among my Southwestern specialties.

 6 plum tomatoes
 3 teaspoons olive oil, *divided*
 3/4 teaspoon salt, *divided*
1-1/2 cups fresh cilantro leaves, *divided*
 1 teaspoon adobo sauce
 2 cups cubed cooked chicken breast, *divided*
 1 small zucchini, cut into 3/4-inch chunks
 1/3 cup dry bread crumbs
 1/3 cup reduced-fat mayonnaise
 1/4 teaspoon pepper

- Core tomatoes and cut in half lengthwise. Place cut side up on a broiler pan coated with cooking spray; brush with 2 teaspoons oil and sprinkle with 1/4 teaspoon salt. Turn tomatoes cut side down. Bake at 425° for 30-40 minutes or until edges are well browned. Cool slightly. Remove and discard tomato peels.

- Place cilantro in a food processor; cover and process until coarsely chopped. Set aside 1/4 cup cilantro for chicken patties. Add the roasted tomatoes, adobo sauce and 1/4 teaspoon salt to the food processor; cover and process just until chunky. Place salsa in a bowl; set aside.

- For chicken patties, in same food processor, combine 1-1/2 cups chicken and zucchini. Cover and process just until chicken is coarsely chopped. Add the bread crumbs, mayonnaise, pepper, reserved cilantro and remaining chicken and salt. Cover and process just until mixture is chunky.

- Shape into eight 3-in. patties. In a nonstick skillet coated with cooking spray, cook patties in remaining oil for 4 minutes on each side or until golden brown. Serve with salsa.

YIELD: 8 servings.

NUTRITION FACTS: 1 chicken patty with 1-1/2 tablespoons salsa equals 134 calories, 7 g fat (1 g saturated fat), 30 mg cholesterol, 373 mg sodium, 7 g carbohydrate, 1 g fiber, 12 g protein. **DIABETIC EXCHANGES:** 2 lean meat, 1 fat, 1/2 starch.

135 CALORIES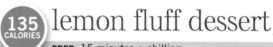

lemon fluff dessert

PREP: 15 minutes + chilling

Nancy Brown | DAHINDA, ILLINOIS

I occasionally slice fresh strawberries over the top of this light and fluffy dessert.

 1 can (12 ounces) evaporated milk
1-1/2 cups graham cracker crumbs
 1/3 cup butter, melted
 1 package (.3 ounce) sugar-free lemon gelatin
 1 cup boiling water
 3 tablespoons lemon juice
 1 package (8 ounces) reduced-fat cream cheese
 3/4 cup sugar
 1 teaspoon vanilla extract

- Pour milk into a large metal bowl; place mixer beaters in the bowl. Cover and refrigerate for at least 2 hours.

- In a small bowl, combine graham cracker crumbs and butter; set aside 1 tablespoon for topping. Press remaining crumb mixture into a 13-in. x 9-in. baking dish. Chill until set.

- Meanwhile, in a small bowl, dissolve gelatin in boiling water. Stir in lemon juice; cool.

- In another bowl, beat the cream cheese, sugar and vanilla until smooth. Add gelatin mixture and mix well. Beat evaporated milk until soft peaks form; fold into cream cheese mixture. Pour over crust. Sprinkle with reserved crumbs. Refrigerate for at least 2 hours before serving. Refrigerate leftovers.

YIELD: 20 servings.

NUTRITION FACTS: 1 piece equals 135 calories, 7 g fat (4 g saturated fat), 21 mg cholesterol, 136 mg sodium, 15 g carbohydrate, trace fiber, 3 g protein. **DIABETIC EXCHANGES:** 1 starch, 1 fat.

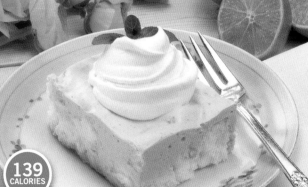

139 CALORIES

LUSCIOUS LIME ANGEL SQUARES

luscious lime angel squares

PREP: 15 minutes + chilling

Beverly Marshall | ORTING, WASHINGTON

A creamy lime topping turns angel food cake into these yummy squares that are perfect for potlucks or picnics.

- 1 package (.3 ounce) sugar-free lime gelatin
- 1 cup boiling water
- 1 prepared angel food cake (8 inches), cut into 1-inch cubes
- 1 package (8 ounces) reduced-fat cream cheese, cubed
- 1/2 cup sugar
- 2 teaspoons lemon juice
- 1-1/2 teaspoons grated lemon peel
- 1 carton (8 ounces) reduced-fat whipped topping, thawed, *divided*

- In a small bowl, dissolve gelatin in boiling water. Refrigerate until mixture just begins to thicken, about 35 minutes. Place cake cubes in a 13-in. x 9-in. dish coated with cooking spray; set aside.

- In a small bowl, beat cream cheese until smooth. Beat in the sugar, lemon juice and peel. Add gelatin mixture; beat until combined. Fold in 1-1/2 cups whipped topping.

- Spread over top of cake, covering completely. Refrigerate for at least 2 hours or until firm. Cut into squares; top with remaining whipped topping.

YIELD: 15 servings.

NUTRITION FACTS: 1 piece equals 139 calories, 4 g fat (3 g saturated fat), 8 mg cholesterol, 145 mg sodium, 21 g carbohydrate, trace fiber, 3 g protein. **DIABETIC EXCHANGES:** 1-1/2 starch, 1 fat.

cherry chocolate parfaits

PREP: 15 minutes + chilling

Taste of Home Test Kitchen

Families will love this budget-friendly blend of chocolate cookies, cherry gelatin and creamy topping.

- 1 package (.3 ounce) sugar-free cherry gelatin
- 1 cup boiling water
- 1/2 cup reduced-fat sour cream
- 1/4 teaspoon almond extract
- 1/2 cup diet lemon-lime soda
- 8 reduced-fat cream-filled chocolate sandwich cookies, crushed
- 1/4 cup reduced-fat whipped topping

- In a small bowl, dissolve gelatin in boiling water. Transfer 1/2 cup to another bowl; stir in sour cream and extract. Divide among four parfait glasses or dessert dishes. Refrigerate until firm, about 35 minutes. Stir soda into the remaining gelatin; cover and refrigerate until partially set.

- To assemble, sprinkle half of the cookies over cherry layer. Top with soda mixture and remaining cookies. Refrigerate until firm. Just before serving, dollop with whipped topping.

YIELD: 4 servings.

NUTRITION FACTS: 1 parfait equals 146 calories, 5 g fat (3 g saturated fat), 10 mg cholesterol, 207 mg sodium, 20 g carbohydrate, 1 g fiber, 4 g protein. **DIABETIC EXCHANGES:** 1 starch, 1 fat.

CHERRY CHOCOLATE PARFAITS

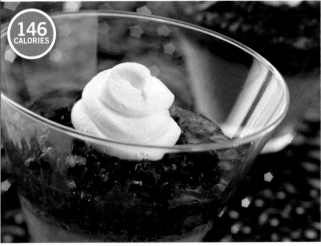

146 CALORIES

I make frequent trips up and down the stairs. And instead of asking my kids to bring me things, I get them myself. Remember to keep moving. Each step is burning more calories. —**Pam Richardson**

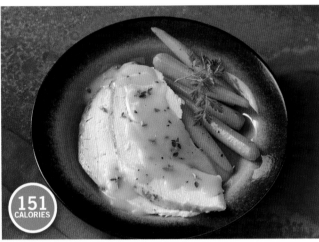

151 CALORIES

ROAST TURKEY BREAST WITH ROSEMARY GRAVY

roast turkey breast with rosemary gravy

PREP: 20 minutes | **BAKE:** 1-3/4 hours + standing

Rebecca Clark | WARRIOR, ALABAMA
A velvety gravy coats this remarkably tender and juicy turkey breast that's perfect for a holiday get-together.

- 2 medium apples, sliced
- 1-1/2 cups sliced leeks (white portion only)
- 2-1/4 cups reduced-sodium chicken broth, *divided*
- 1 bone-in turkey breast (6 pounds)
- 1 tablespoon canola oil
- 2 teaspoons minced fresh rosemary, *divided*
- 3 tablespoons reduced-fat butter
- 1/4 cup all-purpose flour

- Arrange apples and leeks in a roasting pan; add 1 cup broth. Place turkey over apples. In a bowl, combine oil and 1-1/2 teaspoons rosemary. With fingers, loosen turkey skin; rub rosemary mixture under the skin. Secure skin to underside of breast with toothpicks.

- Bake, uncovered, at 325° for 1-3/4 to 2-1/4 hours or until a meat thermometer reads 170°, basting every 30 minutes. Cover loosely with foil if turkey browns too

quickly. Cover; let stand for 15 minutes before carving, reserving 1/4 cup pan juices. Discard apples and leeks.

- In a small saucepan, melt butter; add flour and remaining rosemary until blended, stirring constantly. Skim fat from pan juices. Gradually add pan juices and remaining broth to saucepan. Bring to a boil. Cook and stir for 1 minute or until thickened. Serve with turkey.

YIELD: 18 servings (1-1/3 cups gravy).

EDITOR'S NOTE: This recipe was tested with Land O'Lakes light stick butter.

NUTRITION FACTS: 4 ounces cooked turkey with 1 tablespoon gravy equals 151 calories, 3 g fat (1 g saturated fat), 81 mg cholesterol, 136 mg sodium, 2 g carbohydrate, trace fiber, 29 g protein. **DIABETIC EXCHANGE:** 4 lean meat.

154 CALORIES # mushroom quiche

PREP: 10 minutes | **BAKE:** 30 minutes

Marian Wright | ENON, OHIO
This simple egg dish becomes a tasty meal and the recipe is easily doubled to serve two.

- 1/3 cup chopped fresh mushrooms
- 1 teaspoon butter
- 1/4 cup egg substitute
- 3 tablespoons fat-free milk
- 1/8 teaspoon pepper

 for 2

Dash ground nutmeg
- 1/4 cup shredded reduced-fat Swiss cheese
- 1 teaspoon *each* real bacon bits and minced chives

- In a skillet, saute the mushrooms in butter until softened. In a bowl, beat egg, milk, pepper and nutmeg. Stir in the mushrooms, cheese, bacon and chives.

- Pour into a 5-in. pie plate coated with cooking spray. Bake at 350° for 30 minutes or until set. Let stand for 5 minutes before serving.

YIELD: 1 serving.

NUTRITION FACTS: 1 each equals 154 calories, 6 g fat (4 g saturated fat), 24 mg cholesterol, 333 mg sodium, 6 g carbohydrate, trace fiber, 19 g protein.

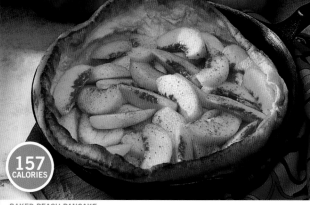

157 CALORIES

BAKED PEACH PANCAKE

baked peach pancake

PREP: 10 minutes I **BAKE:** 25 minutes

Nancy Wilkinson I PRINCETON, NEW JERSEY

This dish makes for a dramatic presentation. I usually take it right from the oven to the table, fill it with peaches and sour cream and serve it with bacon or ham. Whenever I go home, my mom—the best cook I know—asks me to make this.

> 2 cups fresh *or* frozen sliced peeled peaches
> 4 teaspoons sugar
> 1 teaspoon lemon juice
> 3 eggs
> 1/2 cup all-purpose flour
> 1/2 cup milk
> 1/2 teaspoon salt
> 2 tablespoons butter

Ground nutmeg

Sour cream, optional

- In a small bowl, combine peaches with sugar and lemon juice; set aside. In a large bowl, beat eggs until fluffy. Add the flour, milk and salt; beat until smooth.

- Place butter in a 10-in. skillet; bake at 400° for 3 to 5 minutes or until melted. Immediately pour batter into hot skillet. Bake for 20 to 25 minutes or until pancake has risen and puffed all over.

- Fill with peach slices and sprinkle with nutmeg. Serve immediately with sour cream if desired.

YIELD: 6 servings.

NUTRITION FACTS: 1 piece equals 157 calories, 7 g fat (4 g saturated fat), 119 mg cholesterol, 277 mg sodium, 18 g carbohydrate, 1 g fiber, 5 g protein.

best-ever lamb chops

PREP: 10 minutes + marinating I **Broil:** 10 minutes

Kim Mundy I VISALIA, CALIFORNIA

My mother just loved a good lamb chop, and this easy recipe was her favorite way to have them. I've also grilled these chops with great results.

> 1 teaspoon *each* dried basil, marjoram and thyme
> 1/2 teaspoon salt
> 8 lamb loin chops (3 ounces *each*)

Mint jelly, optional

- Combine herbs and salt; rub over lamb chops. Cover and refrigerate for 1 hour.

- Broil 4-6 in. from the heat for 5-8 minutes on each side or until meat reaches desired doneness (for medium-rare, a meat thermometer should read 145°; medium, 160°; well-done, 170°). Serve with mint jelly if desired.

YIELD: 4 servings.

NUTRITION FACTS: 2 lamb chops (calculated without jelly) equals 157 calories, 7 g fat (2 g saturated fat), 68 mg cholesterol, 355 mg sodium, trace carbohydrate, trace fiber, 22 g protein. **DIABETIC EXCHANGE:** 3 lean meat.

BEST-EVER LAMB CHOPS

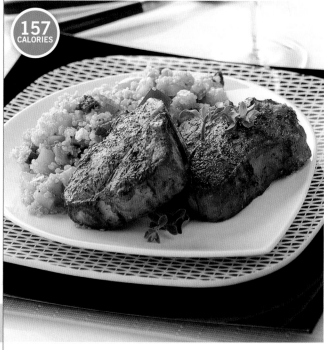

157 CALORIES

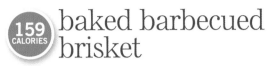

baked barbecued brisket

159 CALORIES

PREP: 20 minutes | **BAKE:** 3-1/2 hours

Joan Hallford | NORTH RICHLAND HILLS, TEXAS

For a never-fail recipe, try this simple brisket. I always hope there will be a few slices left over for sandwiches the next day.

- 1 tablespoon all-purpose flour
- 1 fresh beef brisket (5 pounds)
- 2 to 4 teaspoons Liquid Smoke, optional
- 1/2 teaspoon celery seed
- 1/4 teaspoon pepper
- 1 cup chili sauce
- 1/4 cup barbecue sauce

- Place flour in a large oven roasting bag; shake to coat bag. Rub brisket with Liquid Smoke if desired, celery seed and pepper; place in bag. Place in a roasting pan. Combine chili sauce and barbecue sauce; pour over brisket. Seal bag.

- With a knife, cut six 1/2-in. slits in top of bag. Bake at 325° for 3-1/2 to 4 hours or until meat is tender. Let stand for 5 minutes. Carefully remove brisket from bag. Thinly slice meat across the grain.

YIELD: 16-20 servings.

EDITOR'S NOTE: This is a fresh beef brisket, not corned beef.

NUTRITION FACTS: 3 ounces cooked beef equals 159 calories, 5 g fat (2 g saturated fat), 48 mg cholesterol, 250 mg sodium, 4 g carbohydrate, trace fiber, 23 g protein.
DIABETIC EXCHANGE: 3 lean meat.

tarragon-lemon turkey breast

PREP: 10 minutes | **BAKE:** 1-1/2 hours + standing

Taste of Home Test Kitchen

If you enjoy the flavors of tarragon and lemon pepper, consider this wet rub. It's so delicious with turkey or even chicken.

- 1/4 cup minced fresh tarragon
- 2 tablespoons olive oil
- 1 teaspoon lemon-pepper seasoning
- 1/2 teaspoon seasoned salt
- 1 bone-in turkey breast (4 pounds)

- In a small dish, combine the first four ingredients. With your fingers, carefully loosen the skin from both sides of turkey breast. Spread half of the tarragon mixture over the meat under the skin. Smooth skin over meat and secure to underside of breast with wooden toothpicks. Spread remaining tarragon mixture over turkey skin.

- Place turkey breast on a rack in a shallow roasting pan. Bake, uncovered, at 325° for 1-1/2 to 2 hours or until a meat thermometer reads 170°. Let stand for 10-15 minutes. Remove and discard skin and toothpicks before carving.

YIELD: 11 servings.

NUTRITION FACTS: 4 ounces cooked turkey equals 162 calories, 3 g fat (1 g saturated fat), 85 mg cholesterol, 165 mg sodium, trace carbohydrate, trace fiber, 31 g protein.
DIABETIC EXCHANGES: 4 lean meat, 1/2 fat.

TARRAGON-LEMON TURKEY BREAST

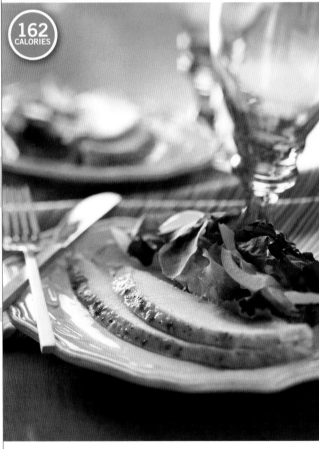

162 CALORIES

I get home after work and either immediately kick the kids off the TV to do a workout video or change clothes and leave for a jog. If I don't do it right away, sadly, I'm less likely to do it. —Vickie Southland

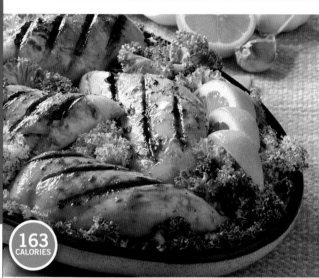

MUSTARD-HERB CHICKEN BREASTS

mustard-herb chicken breasts

PREP: 10 minutes + marinating | **GRILL:** 15 minutes

Terri Weme I SMITHERS, BRITISH COLUMBIA

The Dijon mayonnaise makes this grilled chicken moist and flavorful. Even though I learned to cook when I was young and helped make supper for our family, I didn't really enjoy it until now. My husband appreciates my new interest in finding and trying new recipes.

- 1/4 **cup chopped green onions**
- 1/4 **cup Dijon-mayonnaise blend**
- 2 **tablespoons lemon juice**
- 1 **garlic clove, minced**
- 1/2 **teaspoon salt**
- 1/2 **teaspoon dried thyme**
- 1/4 **teaspoon pepper**
- 4 **boneless skinless chicken breast halves (4 ounces *each*)**

- In a large resealable plastic bag, combine the first seven ingredients; add chicken. Seal bag and turn to coat. Refrigerate for 2 hours, turning once.

- Grill chicken, covered, over medium heat for 6-8 minutes on each side or until a meat thermometer reads 170°.

YIELD: 4 servings.

NUTRITION FACTS: 1 chicken breast half equals 163 calories, 3 g fat (1 g saturated fat), 73 mg cholesterol, 720 mg sodium, 2 g carbohydrate, trace fiber, 27 g protein. **DIABETIC EXCHANGES:** 3 lean meat, 1/2 fat.

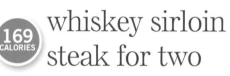

whiskey sirloin steak for two

PREP: 10 minutes + marinating | **Broil:** 15 minutes

Taste of Home Test Kitchen

Juicy, tender and slightly sweet from the marinade, this steak boasts wonderful flavor and oh-so-easy preparation. Serve with potatoes and a green vegetable for a complete meal.

- 2 **tablespoons whiskey *or* apple cider**
- 2 **tablespoons reduced-sodium soy sauce**
- 1-1/2 **teaspoons sugar**
- 1 **garlic clove, thinly sliced**
- 1/4 **teaspoon ground ginger**
- 1/2 **pound beef top sirloin steak (1 inch thick)**

- In a large resealable plastic bag, combine the first five ingredients; add the beef. Seal bag and turn to coat; refrigerate for 8 hours or overnight.

- Drain and discard marinade. Place beef on a broiler pan coated with cooking spray. Broil 4-6 in. from the heat for 7-8 minutes on each side or until meat reaches desired doneness (for medium-rare, a meat thermometer should read 145°; medium, 160°; well-done, 170°).

YIELD: 2 servings.

NUTRITION FACTS: 3 ounces cooked beef equals 169 calories, 5 g fat (2 g saturated fat), 46 mg cholesterol, 353 mg sodium, 2 g carbohydrate, trace fiber, 25 g protein. **DIABETIC EXCHANGE:** 3 lean meat.

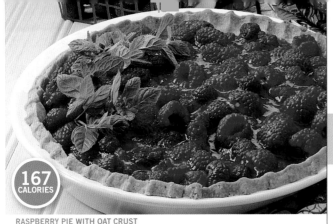

RASPBERRY PIE WITH OAT CRUST

167 CALORIES

raspberry pie with oat crust

PREP: 25 minutes + chilling

Ginny Arandas I GREENSBURG, PENNSYLVANIA
A diabetic for 30 years, I adapted this recipe to fit my needs. When I serve this pie, no one can believe it's sugarless. The oatmeal crust is so tender, and the filling is berry delicious.

- 3/4 cup all-purpose flour
- 1/2 cup quick-cooking oats
- 1/2 teaspoon salt
- 1/4 cup canola oil
- 3 to 4 tablespoons cold water

FILLING:

- 2 cups water
- 1 package (.8 ounces) sugar-free cook-and-serve vanilla pudding mix
- 1 package (.3 ounce) sugar-free raspberry gelatin
- 4 cups fresh raspberries

- In a food processor, combine the flour, oats and salt. While processing, slowly drizzle in oil. Gradually add water until a ball forms. Roll out dough between two sheets of waxed paper. Remove top sheet of waxed paper; invert dough onto a 9-in. pie plate. Remove remaining waxed paper.

- Trim, seal and flute edges. Line unpricked pastry with a double thickness of heavy-duty foil. Bake at 450° for 8 minutes. Remove foil; bake 5-7 minutes longer or until golden brown. Cool on a wire rack.

- In a large saucepan, heat water over medium heat. Whisk in pudding mix. Cook and stir for 5 minutes or until thickened and bubbly. Whisk in gelatin until

completely dissolved. Remove from the heat; cool slightly. Fold in raspberries. Spoon into crust. Chill for at least 3 hours or overnight. Refrigerate leftovers.

YIELD: 8 servings.

NUTRITION FACTS: 1 piece equals 167 calories, 8 g fat (1 g saturated fat), 0 cholesterol, 238 mg sodium, 22 g carbohydrate, 5 g fiber, 3 g protein. **DIABETIC EXCHANGES:** 1-1/2 fat, 1 starch, 1/2 fruit.

170 CALORIES

bacon-broccoli quiche cups

PREP: 10 minutes I **BAKE:** 25 minutes

Irene Steinmeyer I DENVER, COLORADO
Chock-full of veggies and melted cheese, this comforting and colorful egg bake has become a special occasion brunch classic.

- 4 bacon strips, diced
- 1/4 cup fresh broccoli florets
- 1/4 cup chopped onion
- 1 garlic clove, minced
- 3/4 cup egg substitute
- 1 tablespoon dried parsley flakes
- 1/8 teaspoon seasoned salt, optional

Dash pepper

- 1/4 cup shredded reduced-fat cheddar cheese
- 2 tablespoons chopped tomato

for 2

- In a large skillet, cook bacon over medium heat until crisp. Using a slotted spoon, remove to paper towels; drain, reserving 1 tablespoon drippings. In the drippings, cook broccoli and onion over medium heat for 2-3 minutes or until vegetables are tender. Add garlic; cook 1 minute longer.

- In a small bowl, beat the eggs, parsley, seasoned salt if desired and pepper. Stir in bacon and broccoli mixture; add cheese and tomato.

- Pour into two 10-oz. ramekins or custard cups coated with cooking spray. Bake at 400° for 22-25 minutes or until a knife inserted near the center comes out clean.

YIELD: 2 servings.

NUTRITION FACTS: 1 quiche equals 170 calories, 8 g fat (4 g saturated fat), 24 mg cholesterol, 576 mg sodium, 6 g carbohydrate, 1 g fiber, 18 g protein.

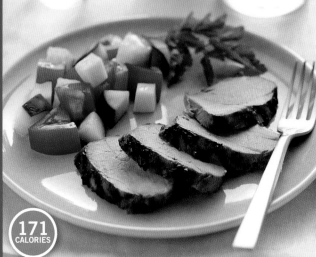

(171 CALORIES)

GRILLED PORK TENDERLOIN

grilled pork tenderloin

PREP: 10 minutes + marinating I **GRILL:** 25 minutes

Debbie Wigle I **WILLIAMSON, NEW YORK**
We've been making this simple yet tasty dish for years, and everyone who tries it requests the recipe. We often double it and serve the leftovers on a mixed green salad.

- 1/2 cup Italian salad dressing
- 1/4 cup reduced-sodium soy sauce
- 1 pork tenderloin (1 pound)
- 1/2 teaspoon steak seasoning

- In a large resealable plastic bag, combine salad dressing and soy sauce; add pork. Seal bag and turn to coat; refrigerate for up to 4 hours.

- Drain and discard marinade. Rub pork with steak seasoning. Using long-handled tongs, moisten a paper towel with cooking oil and lightly coat the grill rack.

- Prepare grill using a drip pan for indirect heat. Place pork over drip pan and grill, covered, over indirect medium-hot heat for 25-40 minutes or until a meat thermometer reads 160°. Let stand for 5 minutes before slicing.

YIELD: 4 servings.

EDITOR'S NOTE: This recipe was tested with McCormick's Montreal Steak Seasoning. Look for it in the spice aisle.

NUTRITION FACTS: 3 ounces cooked pork equals 171 calories, 8 g fat (2 g saturated fat), 63 mg cholesterol, 500 mg sodium, 1 g carbohydrate, trace fiber, 23 g protein. **DIABETIC EXCHANGES:** 3 lean meat, 1/2 fat.

pina colada pudding cups

PREP: 15 minutes + chilling

Betty May I **TOPEKA, KANSAS**
This dessert is so easy but it's chock-full of refreshing pineapple and coconut flavor. It is a nice, light treat after a big meal with make-ahead convenience for busy cooks.

- 3 cups fat-free milk
- 2 envelopes whipped topping mix (Dream Whip)
- 2 packages (1 ounce *each*) sugar-free instant vanilla pudding mix
- 2 cans (8 ounces *each*) unsweetened crushed pineapple, undrained
- 1/2 teaspoon coconut extract
- 1/4 cup flaked coconut, toasted
- 8 maraschino cherries

- In a bowl, whisk the milk, whipped topping and pudding mixes for 2 minutes. Stir in the pineapple and extract.

- Spoon 3/4 cup pudding mixture into eight dessert dishes. Cover and refrigerate for 30 minutes or until chilled.

- Sprinkle each serving with 1-1/2 teaspoons coconut and top each with a cherry.

YIELD: 8 servings.

NUTRITION FACTS: 1 pudding cup equals 171 calories, 3 g fat (3 g saturated fat), 2 mg cholesterol, 350 mg sodium, 31 g carbohydrate, 1 g fiber, 4 g protein. **DIABETIC EXCHANGES:** 1-1/2 starch, 1/2 fruit.

PINA COLADA PUDDING CUPS

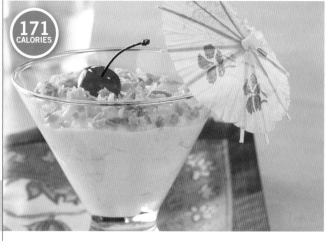

(171 CALORIES)

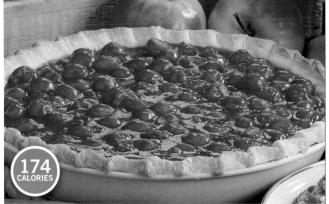

174 CALORIES

TART CHERRY PIE

tart cherry pie

PREP: 15 minutes + cooling

Bonnie Johnson | DEKALB, ILLINOIS
My aunt and I are diabetic. We both enjoy this yummy, fruity pie, and our friends always request this dessert when they come to visit.

- 2 cans (14-1/2 ounces *each*) pitted tart cherries
- 1 package (3 ounces) cook-and-serve vanilla pudding mix
- 1 package (.3 ounce) sugar-free cherry gelatin

Sugar substitute equivalent to 4 teaspoons sugar

- 1 pastry shell (9 inches), baked

- Drain cherries, reserving juice; set cherries aside. In a large saucepan, combine cherry juice and dry pudding mix. Cook and stir until mixture comes to a boil and is thickened and bubbly. Remove from the heat; stir in gelatin powder and sweetener until dissolved. Stir in cherries; transfer to pastry shell. Cool completely. Store in the refrigerator.

YIELD: 8 servings.

NUTRITION FACTS: 1 piece equals 174 calories, 7 g fat (3 g saturated fat), 5 mg cholesterol, 162 mg sodium, 25 g carbohydrate, 1 g fiber, 2 g protein. **DIABETIC EXCHANGES:** 1 starch, 1 fat, 1/2 fruit.

zippy tomato-topped snapper *for 2*

PREP: 10 minutes | **BAKE:** 25 minutes

Mary Anne Zimmerman | SILVER SPRINGS, FLORIDA
Seafood fans will be more than satisfied with this pleasantly zesty entree for two. Serve the fish fillets with a salad and baked potato, and it's a whole meal.

- 1 red snapper fillet (3/4 pound), cut in half
- 3/4 teaspoon lemon-pepper seasoning
- 1/8 teaspoon salt
- 1/2 cup canned diced tomatoes and green chilies
- 2 tablespoons chopped onion
- 2 tablespoons chopped celery
- 1 tablespoon minced fresh parsley
- 1/8 teaspoon celery seed

- Sprinkle both sides of red snapper with lemon pepper and salt. Place in a greased 11-in. x 7-in. baking dish.

- Combine the tomatoes, onion, celery, parsley and celery seed; spoon over snapper.

- Cover and bake at 350° for 25-30 minutes or until fish flakes easily with a fork.

YIELD: 2 servings.

NUTRITION FACTS: 1 serving equals 179 calories, 2 g fat (trace saturated fat), 60 mg cholesterol, 643 mg sodium, 4 g carbohydrate, 1 g fiber, 34 g protein. **DIABETIC EXCHANGE:** 5 lean meat.

ZIPPY TOMATO-TOPPED SNAPPER

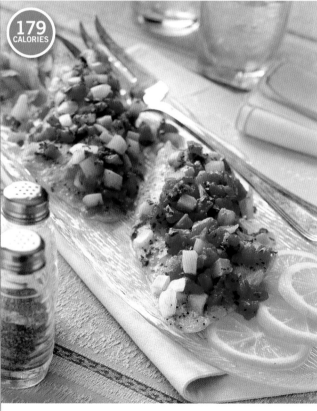

179 CALORIES

194 CALORIES

SAUSAGE KALE SOUP

sausage kale soup

PREP: 10 minutes | **COOK:** 25 minutes

Susan Pursell | FOUNTAIN VALLEY, CALIFORNIA

The hearty sausage slices, white kidney beans and kale in this soup will have your crew asking for seconds.

- 3/4 cup chopped onion
- 1 tablespoon olive oil
- 2 garlic cloves, minced
- 4 cups reduced-sodium chicken broth
- 2 medium potatoes, peeled and cubed
- 1/4 teaspoon salt
- 1/4 teaspoon pepper
- 1 bunch kale, trimmed and chopped
- 1 can (15 ounces) white kidney or cannellini beans, rinsed and drained
- 1/2 pound reduced-fat fully cooked Polish sausage or turkey kielbasa, sliced

- In a large saucepan or Dutch oven, saute onion in oil until tender. Add garlic; cook 1 minute longer. Add the broth, potatoes, salt and pepper. Bring to a boil. Reduce heat; cover and simmer for 10-15 minutes or until potatoes are tender.

- Using a potato masher, mash potatoes slightly. Add the kale, beans and sausage; cook over medium-low heat until kale is tender.

YIELD: 7 servings.

NUTRITION FACTS: 1 cup equals 194 calories, 4 g fat (1 g saturated fat), 14 mg cholesterol, 823 mg sodium, 28 g carbohydrate, 50 g fiber, 11 g protein. **DIABETIC EXCHANGES:** 1-1/2 starch, 1 lean meat, 1 vegetable.

honey-lime roasted chicken

PREP: 10 minutes | **BAKE:** 2-1/2 hours + standing

Lori Carbonell | SPRINGFIELD, VERMONT

It's hard to believe this finger-licking main course has only five ingredients. The chicken is also easy and tasty prepared outside on the grill.

- 1 whole roasting chicken (5 to 6 pounds)
- 1/2 cup lime juice
- 1/4 cup honey
- 1 tablespoon stone-ground mustard or spicy brown mustard
- 1 teaspoon ground cumin

- Carefully loosen the skin from the entire chicken. Place breast side up on a rack in a roasting pan. In a small bowl, whisk the lime juice, honey, mustard and cumin.

- Using a turkey baster, baste under the chicken skin with 1/3 cup lime juice mixture. Tie drumsticks together. Pour the remaining lime juice mixture over chicken.

- Bake, uncovered, at 350° for 2-1/2 to 3 hours or until a meat thermometer reads 180°, basting every 30 minutes with drippings (cover loosely with foil after 1 to 1-1/2 hours or when golden brown). Let stand for 10 minutes before carving. Remove and discard skin before serving.

YIELD: 10 servings.

NUTRITION FACTS: 3 ounces cooked chicken equals 197 calories, 7 g fat (2 g saturated fat), 77 mg cholesterol, 95 mg sodium, 8 g carbohydrate, trace fiber, 25 g protein.

HONEY-LIME ROASTED CHICKEN

197 CALORIES

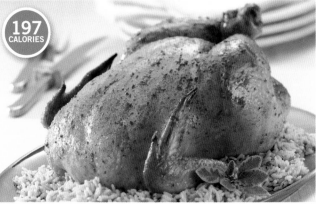

I pack my gym bag the night before so I can just grab it in the morning and go to the gym right after work. —**Neo Senkge**

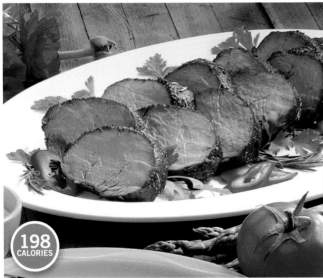

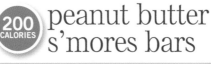

198 CALORIES

HERBED BEEF TENDERLOIN

herbed beef tenderloin

PREP: 5 minutes I **BAKE:** 40 minutes + standing

Ruth Andrewson I LEAVENWORTH, WASHINGTON
You don't need much seasoning to add flavor to this tender beef roast. The mild blending of rosemary, basil and garlic does the trick.

1	beef tenderloin roast (3 pounds)
2	teaspoons olive oil
2	garlic cloves, minced
1-1/2	teaspoons dried basil
1-1/2	teaspoons dried rosemary, crushed
1	teaspoon salt
1	teaspoon pepper

• Tie tenderloin at 2-in. intervals with kitchen string. Combine oil and garlic; brush over meat. Combine the basil, rosemary, salt and pepper; sprinkle evenly over meat. Place on a rack in a shallow roasting pan.

• Bake, uncovered, at 425° for 40-50 minutes or until meat reaches desired doneness (for medium-rare, a meat thermometer should read 145°; medium,

160°; well-done, 170°). Let stand for 10 minutes before slicing.

YIELD: 12 servings.

NUTRITION FACTS: 3 ounces cooked beef equals 198 calories, 10 g fat (4 g saturated fat), 78 mg cholesterol, 249 mg sodium, 1 g carbohydrate, trace fiber, 25 g protein. **DIABETIC EXCHANGE:** 3 lean meat.

200 CALORIES

peanut butter s'mores bars

PREP: 10 minutes I **BAKE:** 20 minutes + chilling

Julie Wischmeier I BROWNSTOWN, INDIANA
I make these ahead when it's convenient for me because they freeze well. You can use M&Ms in different color combinations for holidays year-round.

1	tube (16-1/2 ounces) refrigerated peanut butter cookie dough
3-1/2	cups miniature marshmallows
3/4	cup milk chocolate chips
2	teaspoons shortening
1-1/2	cups milk chocolate M&M's

• Let dough stand at room temperature for 5-10 minutes to soften. Cut into 24 slices; arrange side by side in an ungreased 13-in. x 9-in. baking pan. Pat together to close gaps.

• Bake at 350° for 18-20 minutes or until lightly browned and edges are firm. Sprinkle with marshmallows; bake 2-3 minutes longer or until marshmallows are puffy.

• In a microwave, melt chocolate chips and shortening; stir until smooth. Sprinkle M&M's over marshmallow layer; drizzle with melted chocolate. Chill until set before cutting.

YIELD: 2 dozen.

NUTRITION FACTS: 1 bar equals 200 calories, 9 g fat (4 g saturated fat), 5 mg cholesterol, 105 mg sodium, 29 g carbohydrate, 1 g fiber, 2 g protein.

fork. Brush with reserved vinaigrette and sprinkle with remaining basil.

YIELD: 2 servings.

NUTRITION FACTS: 1 fillet equals 206 calories, 8 g fat (2 g saturated fat), 83 mg cholesterol, 398 mg sodium, 2 g carbohydrate, trace fiber, 32 g protein. **DIABETIC EXCHANGES:** 5 lean meat, 1-1/2 fat.

(214 CALORIES) coconut custard pie

PREP: 25 minutes + cooling | **BAKE:** 40 minutes + cooling

Eva Wright | GRANT, ALABAMA

We really appreciate desserts such as this creamy custard pie. Coconut extract in the filling and a toasted coconut topping make this low-sugar creation delicious.

- 1/2 cup flaked coconut
- 1 refrigerated pastry shell (9 inches)
- 4 eggs
- 1/2 teaspoon salt
- 1-3/4 cups fat-free milk

Sugar substitute equivalent to 1/2 cup sugar

- 1-1/2 teaspoons coconut extract
- 1/2 teaspoon vanilla extract

- Place coconut in an ungreased 9-in. pie plate. Bake at 350° for 4 minutes, stirring several times; set aside. (Coconut will not be fully toasted.)

- Line unpricked pastry shell with a double thickness of heavy-duty foil. Bake at 450° for 8 minutes. Remove foil; bake 4-6 minutes longer. Cool.

- In a bowl, beat the eggs and salt for 5 minutes. (Mixture will be lemon-colored and slightly thickened.) Add the milk, sugar substitute, coconut extract and vanilla. Transfer to crust. (Crust will be full.)

- Bake at 350° for 30 minutes. Sprinkle with coconut. Bake 8-10 minutes longer or until a knife inserted near the center comes out clean and coconut is lightly browned. Cool on a wire rack for 1 hour. Cover and refrigerate.

YIELD: 8 servings.

EDITOR'S NOTE: This recipe was tested with Splenda no-calorie sweetener.

NUTRITION FACTS: 1 piece equals 214 calories, 12 g fat (6 g saturated fat), 112 mg cholesterol, 320 mg sodium, 20 g carbohydrate, trace fiber, 6 g protein.

GRILLED TILAPIA WITH LEMON BASIL VINAIGRETTE FOR TWO

grilled tilapia with lemon basil vinaigrette for two

PREP/TOTAL TIME: 25 minutes

Beth Cooper | COLUMBUS, OHIO

A friend made this for us, and we couldn't believe how wonderful it was! Now we eat it regularly. It is simple, looks lovely and tastes restaurant-worthy.

- 4-1/2 teaspoons lemon juice
- 4-1/2 teaspoons minced fresh basil, *divided*
- 1 tablespoon olive oil
- 1 garlic clove, minced
- 1 teaspoon capers, drained
- 1/4 teaspoon grated lemon peel
- 2 tilapia fillets (6 ounces *each*)
- 1/4 teaspoon salt
- 1/8 teaspoon pepper

for 2

- For vinaigrette, in a small bowl, whisk the lemon juice, 3 teaspoons basil, olive oil, garlic, capers and lemon peel; set aside 1 tablespoon for sauce. Sprinkle fillets with salt and pepper. Brush both sides of fillets with remaining vinaigrette.

- Using long-handled tongs, moisten a paper towel with cooking oil and lightly coat the grill rack. Grill, covered, over medium heat or broil 4 in. from the heat for 3-4 minutes on each side or until fish flakes easily with a

frozen yogurt cookie dessert

PREP: 20 minutes + freezing

Ellen Thompson | SPRINGFIELD, OHIO
We often prepare this yummy dessert for company. Just five ingredients are all that's needed for the creamy chocolate- and peanut-flavored sensation. It's easy to take just the portion you want and freeze the rest for later.

- 12 reduced-fat cream-filled chocolate sandwich cookies, crushed
- 1 quart low-fat vanilla frozen yogurt, softened
- 1/3 cup chocolate syrup
- 1/2 cup dry roasted peanuts
- 1 carton (8 ounces) frozen fat-free whipped topping, thawed

- Set aside 1 tablespoon cookie crumbs. Sprinkle the remaining crumbs into an 11-in. x 7-in. dish coated with cooking spray. Freeze for 10 minutes.

- Carefully spread frozen yogurt over crumbs. Drizzle with chocolate syrup and sprinkle with peanuts. Spread with whipped topping; sprinkle with reserved crumbs.

- Cover and freeze for at least 2 hours. Remove from the freezer 10 minutes before serving.

YIELD: 12 servings.

NUTRITION FACTS: 1 piece equals 220 calories, 7 g fat (2 g saturated fat), 3 mg cholesterol, 193 mg sodium, 34 g carbohydrate, 1 g fiber, 6 g protein. **DIABETIC EXCHANGES:** 2 starch, 1 fat.

FROZEN YOGURT COOKIE DESSERT

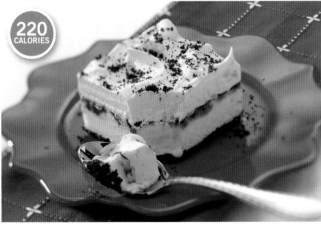

220 CALORIES

224 CALORIES chipotle sweet potato and spiced apple purees

PREP: 30 minutes | **BAKE:** 35 minutes

Shannon Abdollmohammadi | WOODINVILLE, WASHINGTON
I used to make this dish with lots of butter, brown sugar and cream. I slimmed it down and this low-fat version is just as scrumptious.

- 2 large tart apples, peeled and quartered
- 1/4 cup lemon juice
- 1/4 cup honey
- 2 tablespoons butter, melted
- 1-1/2 teaspoons salt, *divided*
- 1/4 teaspoon Chinese five-spice powder
- 4 pounds sweet potatoes (about 6 large), peeled and quartered
- 1/4 cup fat-free milk, warmed
- 2 teaspoons minced chipotle peppers in adobo sauce
- 1/4 teaspoon pepper

- In an ungreased 11-in. x 7-in. baking dish, toss the apples, lemon juice, honey, butter, 1/2 teaspoon salt and five-spice powder. Bake, uncovered, at 400° for 35-40 minutes or until apples are tender, turning once.

- Meanwhile, place sweet potatoes in a Dutch oven and cover with water. Bring to a boil. Reduce heat; cover and cook for 15-20 minutes or until tender. Drain well. Over very low heat, stir potatoes for 1-2 minutes or until steam has evaporated.

- Place potatoes in a food processor; add the milk, chipotle peppers, pepper and remaining salt. Cover and process until smooth. Transfer to a serving bowl; keep warm.

- Place apples and cooking juices in a clean food processor; cover and process until smooth. Spoon over sweet potato puree.

YIELD: 8 servings.

NUTRITION FACTS: 3/4 cup sweet potato puree with 4 teaspoons apple puree equals 224 calories, 3 g fat (2 g saturated fat), 8 mg cholesterol, 498 mg sodium, 49 g carbohydrate, 5 g fiber, 3 g protein.

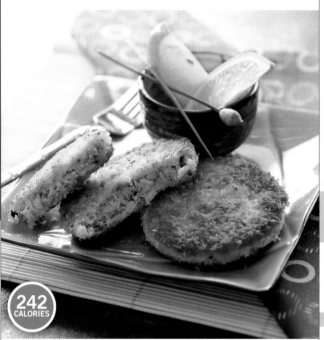

CHIVE CRAB CAKES

242 CALORIES

chive crab cakes

PREP: 20 minutes + chilling | **COOK:** 10 minutes/batch

Cindy Worth | LAPWAI, IDAHO
These tasty crab cakes are perfect for appetizers, or try them with a salad for a light meal.

- 4 egg whites
- 1 egg
- 6 tablespoons minced chives
- 3 tablespoons all-purpose flour
- 1 to 2 teaspoons hot pepper sauce
- 1 teaspoon baking powder
- 1/2 teaspoon salt
- 1/4 teaspoon pepper
- 4 cans (6 ounces *each*) crabmeat, drained, flaked and cartilage removed
- 2 cups panko (Japanese) bread crumbs
- 2 tablespoons canola oil

- In a large bowl, lightly beat the egg whites and egg. Add the chives, flour, pepper sauce, baking powder, salt and pepper; mix well. Fold in crab. Cover and refrigerate for at least 2 hours.

- Place bread crumbs in a shallow bowl. Drop crab mixture by 1/4 cupfuls into crumbs. Gently coat and shape into 3/4-in.-thick patties.

- In a large nonstick skillet, cook crab cakes in oil in batches over medium-high heat for 3-4 minutes on each side or until golden brown.

YIELD: 6 servings.

NUTRITION FACTS: 2 crab cakes equals 242 calories, 7 g fat (1 g saturated fat), 136 mg cholesterol, 731 mg sodium, 12 g carbohydrate, 1 g fiber, 29 g protein. **DIABETIC EXCHANGES:** 3 lean meat, 1 starch, 1/2 fat.

glazed pork chops

PREP: 10 minutes + marinating | **GRILL:** 10 minutes

Louise Gilbert | QUESNEL, BRITISH COLUMBIA
Rosemary adds a special touch to these beautifully glazed chops that are just right for any weeknight meal.

- 1/2 cup ketchup
- 1/4 cup packed brown sugar
- 1/4 cup white vinegar
- 1/4 cup orange juice
- 1/4 cup Worcestershire sauce
- 2 garlic cloves, minced
- 1/2 teaspoon dried rosemary, crushed
- 8 bone-in pork loin chops (1/2 inch thick and 7 ounces *each*)

- In a small bowl, combine the first seven ingredients. Pour 3/4 cup into a large resealable plastic bag; add the pork chops. Seal bag and turn to coat; refrigerate for 8 hours or overnight. Cover and refrigerate remaining marinade for basting.

- Drain and discard marinade. Using long-handled tongs, moisten a paper towel with cooking oil and lightly coat the grill rack. Grill pork, covered, over medium heat or broil 4 in. from the heat for 4-6 minutes on each side or until a meat thermometer reads 160°, basting occasionally with reserved marinade.

YIELD: 8 servings.

NUTRITION FACTS: 1 pork chop equals 246 calories, 8 g fat (3 g saturated fat), 86 mg cholesterol, 284 mg sodium, 11 g carbohydrate, trace fiber, 30 g protein. **DIABETIC EXCHANGES:** 4 lean meat, 1 starch.

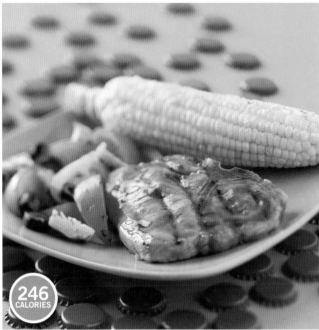

GLAZED PORK CHOPS

beef kabobs with chutney sauce

PREP: 15 minutes + marinating I **GRILL:** 5 minutes

Judy Thompson I ANKENY, IOWA
I created this speedy entree for our daughter, who is a fan of Indian food. The mango chutney and subtle curry give the beef a sweet and spicy flavor. Once you marinate the beef overnight, these grill up in a snap.

- 1/2 cup plain yogurt
- 3 tablespoons mango chutney
- 1 teaspoon lemon juice
- 1/2 teaspoon curry powder
- 1/4 teaspoon ground cumin
- 1/8 teaspoon cayenne pepper

MARINATED BEEF:
- 1/4 cup mango chutney
- 1 tablespoon cider vinegar
- 1 tablespoon water
- 1 teaspoon curry powder
- 1/4 teaspoon cayenne pepper
- 1 pound beef top sirloin steak, cut into 1/4-inch strips

- For sauce, in a small bowl, combine the first six ingredients. Cover and refrigerate until serving.

- For marinade, in a large resealable plastic bag, combine the chutney, vinegar, water, curry and cayenne; add beef. Seal bag and turn to coat; refrigerate overnight.

- Drain and discard marinade. Thread beef onto eight metal or soaked wooden skewers.

- Using long-handled tongs, moisten a paper towel with cooking oil and lightly coat the grill rack. Grill kabobs, covered, over medium heat or broil 4 in. from the heat for 4-6 minutes or until meat reaches desired doneness, turning occasionally. Serve with dipping sauce.

YIELD: 8 kabobs (about 1/2 cup sauce).

NUTRITION FACTS: 2 skewers with 2 tablespoons sauce equals 258 calories, 6 g fat (2 g saturated fat), 50 mg cholesterol, 321 mg sodium, 23 g carbohydrate, trace fiber, 25 g protein. **DIABETIC EXCHANGES:** 3 lean meat, 1-1/2 starch.

BEEF KABOBS WITH CHUTNEY SAUCE

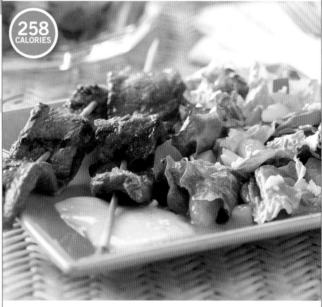

279 CALORIES

BRUNCH RISOTTO

brunch risotto

PREP: 10 minutes | **COOK:** 30 minutes

Jennifer Dines | BRIGHTON, MASSACHUSETTS

This light, flavorful and inexpensive risotto makes a surprising addition to a traditional brunch menu. It has received lots of compliments from my friends.

5-1/4 to 5-3/4 cups reduced-sodium chicken broth
3/4 pound Italian turkey sausage links, casings removed
2 cups uncooked arborio rice
1 garlic clove, minced
1/4 teaspoon pepper
1 tablespoon olive oil
1 medium tomato, chopped

• In a large saucepan, heat broth and keep warm. In a large nonstick skillet, cook sausage until no longer pink; drain and set aside.

• In the same skillet, saute the rice, garlic and pepper in oil for 2-3 minutes. Return sausage to skillet. Carefully stir in 1 cup heated broth. Cook and stir until all of the liquid is absorbed.

• Add remaining broth, 1/2 cup at a time, stirring constantly. Allow liquid to absorb between additions. Cook just until risotto is creamy and rice is almost tender. Total cooking time is about 20 minutes. Add tomato; cook and stir until heated through. Serve immediately.

YIELD: 8 servings.

NUTRITION FACTS: 2/3 cup equals 279 calories, 6 g fat (2 g saturated fat), 23 mg cholesterol, 653 mg sodium, 42 g carbohydrate, 1 g fiber, 12 g protein. **DIABETIC EXCHANGES:** 2-1/2 starch, 1 lean meat, 1/2 fat.

crunchy onion barbecue chicken

PREP: 10 minutes | **BAKE:** 25 minutes

Jane Holey | CLAYTON, MICHIGAN

I threw this recipe together one night when I had chicken breasts to use up. After adding french-fried onions and baked-on barbecue sauce, I was thrilled with how moist and tasty the chicken turned out. My husband was, too!

1/2 cup barbecue sauce
1-1/3 cups french-fried onions, crushed
1/4 cup grated Parmesan cheese
1/2 teaspoon pepper
4 boneless skinless chicken breast halves (6 ounces *each*)

• Place barbecue sauce in a shallow bowl. In another shallow bowl, combine the onions, cheese and pepper. Dip both sides of chicken in barbecue sauce, then one side in onion mixture.

• Place chicken, crumb side up, on a baking sheet coated with cooking spray. Bake at 400° for 22-27 minutes or until a meat thermometer reads 170°.

YIELD: 4 servings.

NUTRITION FACTS: 1 chicken breast half equals 286 calories, 10 g fat (3 g saturated fat), 97 mg cholesterol, 498 mg sodium, 9 g carbohydrate, trace fiber, 36 g protein. **DIABETIC EXCHANGES:** 5 lean meat, 1 fat, 1/2 starch.

CRUNCHY ONION BARBECUE CHICKEN

286 CALORIES

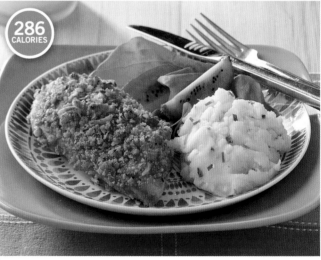

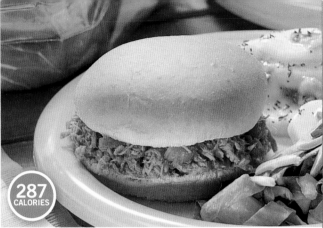

287 CALORIES

BARBECUED PORK SANDWICHES

barbecued pork sandwiches

PREP: 15 minutes I **COOK:** 4 hours

Karla Labby I OTSEGO, MICHIGAN
When our office held a bridal shower, we presented the future bride with a collection of our favorite recipes. I included this one. I like serving this savory pork as an alternative to a typical ground beef barbecue.

    2 boneless pork loin roasts (3 pounds *each*)
    1 cup water
    2 teaspoons salt
    2 cups ketchup
    2 cups diced celery
  1/3 cup steak sauce
  1/4 cup packed brown sugar
  1/4 cup white vinegar
    2 teaspoons lemon juice
   25 hamburger buns, split

- Place roasts in an 8-qt. Dutch oven; add water and salt. Cover and cook on medium-low heat for 2-1/2 hours or until meat is tender.

- Remove roasts and shred with a fork; set aside. Skim fat from cooking liquid and discard. Drain all but 1 cup cooking liquid. Add meat, ketchup, celery, steak sauce, brown sugar, vinegar and lemon juice. Cover and cook over medium-low heat for 1-1/2 hours. Serve on buns.

YIELD: 25 servings.

NUTRITION FACTS: 1 sandwich equals 287 calories, 7 g fat (2 g saturated fat), 54 mg cholesterol, 737 mg sodium, 29 g carbohydrate, 1 g fiber, 25 g protein. **DIABETIC EXCHANGES:** 3 lean meat, 2 starch.

applesauce-glazed pork chops

PREP/TOTAL TIME: 30 minutes

Brenda Campbell I OLYMPIA, WASHINGTON
These tasty, tender chops are glazed with a sweet, smoky, apple-flavored sauce. They're on the table in no time at all, so they're perfect for hectic weeknights.

    4 bone-in pork loin chops (7 ounces *each*)
    1 cup unsweetened applesauce
  1/4 cup packed brown sugar
    1 tablespoon barbecue sauce
    1 tablespoon Worcestershire sauce
    1 garlic clove, minced
  1/2 teaspoon salt
  1/2 teaspoon pepper

- Place pork chops in a 13-in. x 9-in. baking dish coated with cooking spray. In a small bowl, combine the remaining ingredients; spoon over chops.

- Bake, uncovered, at 350° for 20-25 minutes or until a meat thermometer reads 160°.

YIELD: 4 servings.

NUTRITION FACTS: 1 pork chop with 1/3 cup sauce equals 291 calories, 9 g fat (3 g saturated fat), 86 mg cholesterol, 442 mg sodium, 22 g carbohydrate, 1 g fiber, 30 g protein. **DIABETIC EXCHANGES:** 4 lean meat, 1 starch, 1/2 fruit.

APPLESAUCE-GLAZED PORK CHOPS

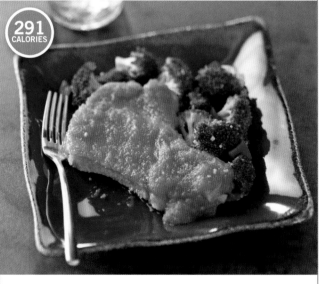

291 CALORIES

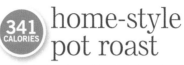

8-ingredient or less recipes

honey-grilled pork tenderloin

298 CALORIES

HONEY-GRILLED PORK TENDERLOIN

PREP: 10 minutes + marinating | **GRILL:** 20 minutes + standing

Milton Nicholas | BEAUMONT, TEXAS

I received this recipe from my daughter. We were having guests for dinner one night and I thought this entree would be the perfect start in planning the menu.

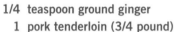

- 3 tablespoons reduced-sodium soy sauce
- 2 garlic cloves, minced
- 1/4 teaspoon ground ginger
- 1 pork tenderloin (3/4 pound)
- 4-1/2 teaspoons honey
- 1 tablespoon brown sugar
- 1 teaspoon sesame oil

for 2

- In a large resealable plastic bag, combine the soy sauce, garlic and ginger; add the pork. Seal bag and turn to coat; refrigerate for at least 8 hours or overnight.

- In a small saucepan, combine the honey, brown sugar and oil. Cook and stir over low heat until sugar is dissolved. Remove from the heat; set aside.

- Drain and discard marinade. Using long-handled tongs, moisten a paper towel with cooking oil and lightly coat the grill rack. Prepare grill for indirect heat using a drip pan.

- Place pork over drip pan and grill, covered, over indirect medium-hot heat for 20-25 minutes or until a meat thermometer reads 160°, basting frequently with honey mixture. Let stand for 5 minutes before slicing.

YIELD: 2 servings.

home-style pot roast

341 CALORIES

PREP: 15 minutes | **COOK:** 3-1/4 hours

Olga Montecorboli | MANCHESTER, CONNECTICUT

Tender meat, lots of vegetables and a pleasant gravy make this meal-in-one satisfying and filling.

- 1 beef eye round roast (2-1/2 pounds)
- 6 tablespoons all-purpose flour, *divided*
- 1 tablespoon canola oil
- 1-1/2 cups plus 1/3 cup water, *divided*
- 1-1/2 cups dry red wine *or* reduced-sodium beef broth
- 2 teaspoons beef bouillon granules
- 1/4 teaspoon pepper
- 16 small red potatoes (2 pounds), halved
- 4 medium carrots (3/4 pound), halved lengthwise and cut into 2-inch pieces
- 2 medium onions, quartered
- 1/2 teaspoon salt
- 1/2 teaspoon browning sauce, optional

- Coat the roast with 2 tablespoons flour. In a large nonstick skillet, brown roast on all sides in oil over medium-high heat; drain. Add 1-1/2 cups water, wine, bouillon and pepper. Bring to a boil. Reduce heat; cover and simmer for 2 hours.

- Add the potatoes, carrots and onions; cover and simmer for 45 minutes or until meat and vegetables are tender. Remove meat and vegetables; keep warm.

- Pour pan juices into a measuring cup; skim fat. Add enough water to measure 2 cups. In a small saucepan, combine remaining flour and water until smooth. Stir in salt and browning sauce if desired. Gradually stir in the 2 cups pan juices. Bring to a boil; cook and stir for 2 minutes or until thickened. Serve with roast and vegetables.

YIELD: 8 servings.

I jump on my treadmill while I watch the evening news. That way I kill two birds with one stone. —**Elaine Vindas Berberian**

super flatbread wraps

PREP: 40 minutes + rising | **GRILL:** 15 minutes

Fay Strait | WAUKEE, IOWA

These are my family's favorite! My kids will eat anything we roll up in this. The original recipe called for all white flour and a lot of salt. I added whole wheat flour to make it healthier and cut back on the salt. I know you'll enjoy these delicious wraps, too.

- 1/2 teaspoon active dry yeast
- 1/2 cup warm water (110° to 115°)
- 1 teaspoon olive oil
- 1/2 teaspoon salt
- 1/3 cup whole wheat flour
- 1 cup all-purpose flour

FILLING:

- 1 beef flank steak (1 pound)
- 1/2 teaspoon salt
- 1/4 teaspoon pepper
- 1 cup shredded lettuce
- 1/4 cup sliced ripe olives
- 2 tablespoons crumbled feta cheese

- In a small bowl, dissolve yeast in warm water. Add the oil, salt, whole wheat flour and 3/4 cup all-purpose flour; beat on medium speed for 3 minutes. Stir in enough remaining flour to form a firm dough.

- Turn onto a lightly floured surface; knead until smooth and elastic, about 6-8 minutes. Place in a large bowl coated with cooking spray, turning once to coat the top. Cover and let rise in a warm place until doubled, about 45 minutes.

- Punch dough down. Turn onto a lightly floured surface; divide into four portions. Roll each into an 8-in. circle.

- Heat a large nonstick skillet coated with cooking spray over medium heat; add a portion of dough. Cook for 30-60 seconds or until bubbles form on top. Turn and cook until the second side is golden brown. Remove and keep warm. Repeat with remaining dough, adding cooking spray as needed.

- Using long-handled tongs, moisten a paper towel with cooking oil and lightly coat the grill rack. Sprinkle steak with salt and pepper. Grill, covered, over medium-high heat or broil 4 in. from the heat for 6-8 minutes on each side or until meat reaches desired doneness (for medium-rare, a meat thermometer should read 145°; medium, 160°; well-done, 170°).

- Let stand for 5 minutes before cutting steak thinly across the grain. Serve on warm flatbreads with lettuce, olives and cheese.

YIELD: 4 servings.

NUTRITION FACTS: 1 wrap equals 348 calories, 11 g fat (4 g saturated fat), 56 mg cholesterol, 770 mg sodium, 32 g carbohydrate, 3 g fiber, 28 g protein. **DIABETIC EXCHANGES:** 3 lean meat, 2 starch, 1/2 fat.

SUPER FLATBREAD WRAPS

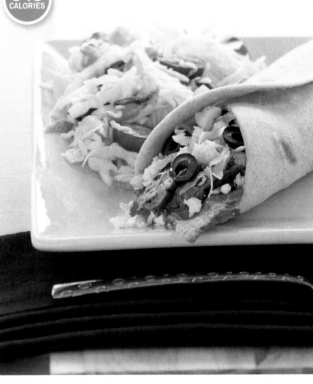

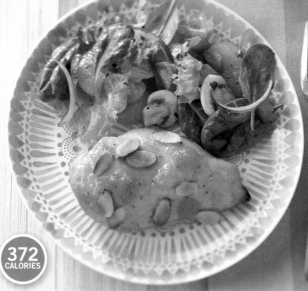

372 CALORIES

APRICOT-ALMOND CHICKEN BREASTS

apricot-almond chicken breasts

PREP: 10 minutes | **BAKE:** 30 minutes

Trisha Kruse | EAGLE, IDAHO

This chicken dish is delicious, and I constantly get asked for the recipe. It's so simple to prepare.

- 4 boneless skinless chicken breast halves (6 ounces *each*)
- 1/2 teaspoon salt
- 1/4 teaspoon pepper
- 3/4 cup apricot preserves
- 1/4 cup reduced-sodium chicken broth
- 1 tablespoon honey mustard
- 1/4 cup sliced almonds

- Sprinkle chicken with salt and pepper. Place in a 13-in. x 9-in. baking dish coated with cooking spray. Bake, uncovered, at 350° for 15 minutes.

- In a small bowl, combine the preserves, broth and mustard. Pour over chicken; sprinkle with almonds. Bake 15-20 minutes longer or until chicken juices run clear.

YIELD: 4 servings.

NUTRITION FACTS: 1 chicken breast half equals 372 calories, 7 g fat (1 g saturated fat), 94 mg cholesterol, 468 mg sodium, 42 g carbohydrate, 1 g fiber, 36 g protein. **DIABETIC EXCHANGES:** 5 lean meat, 3 starch, 1/2 fat.

italian beef and shells

PREP/TOTAL TIME: 30 minutes

Mike Tchou | PEPPER PIKE, OHIO

A hearty entree comes easy tonight with this veggie and pasta combo. Wine lends an extra touch of flavor to the sauce and makes this main dish a winner.

- 1-1/2 cups uncooked medium pasta shells
- 1 pound lean ground beef (90% lean)
- 1 small onion, chopped
- 1 garlic clove, minced
- 1 jar (23 ounces) marinara sauce
- 1 *each* small yellow summer squash and small zucchini, quartered and sliced
- 1/4 cup dry red wine *or* reduced-sodium beef broth
- 1/2 teaspoon salt
- 1/2 teaspoon Italian seasoning
- 1/2 teaspoon pepper

- Cook pasta according to package directions.

- Meanwhile, in a Dutch oven, cook the beef, onion and garlic over medium heat until meat is no longer pink; drain. Stir in the marinara sauce, squash, zucchini, wine and seasonings. Bring to a boil. Reduce heat; simmer, uncovered, for 10-15 minutes or until thickened. Drain pasta; stir into beef mixture and heat through.

YIELD: 4 servings.

NUTRITION FACTS: 1-3/4 cups equals 396 calories, 10 g fat (4 g saturated fat), 71 mg cholesterol, 644 mg sodium, 45 g carbohydrate, 5 g fiber, 29 g protein. **Diabetic Exchanges:** 3 starch, 3 lean meat.

ITALIAN BEEF AND SHELLS

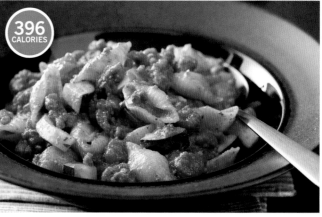

396 CALORIES

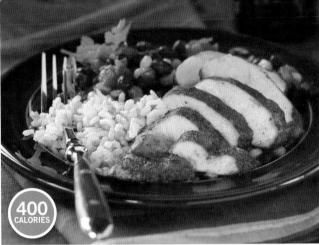

BLACK BEAN CHICKEN WITH RICE

black bean chicken with rice

PREP/TOTAL: 25 minutes

Molly Newman | PORTLAND, OREGON
This family favorite only requires a few ingredients, so it's easy to fix on a busy weeknight.

- 3 teaspoons chili powder
- 1 teaspoon ground cumin
- 1 teaspoon pepper
- 1/4 teaspoon salt
- 4 boneless skinless chicken breast halves (4 ounces each)
- 2 teaspoons canola oil
- 1 can (15 ounces) black beans, rinsed and drained
- 1 cup frozen corn
- 1 cup salsa
- 2 cups cooked brown rice

- Combine the chili powder, cumin, pepper and salt; rub over chicken. In a large nonstick skillet coated with cooking spray, brown chicken in oil on both sides. Stir in the beans, corn and salsa. Cover and cook over medium heat for 10-15 minutes or until a meat thermometer reads 170°.

- Slice chicken; serve with rice and bean mixture.

YIELD: 4 servings.

NUTRITION FACTS: 1 chicken breast half with 3/4 cup bean mixture and 1/2 cup rice equals 400 calories, 7 g fat (1 g saturated fat), 63 mg cholesterol, 670 mg sodium, 52 g carbohydrate, 8 g fiber, 32 g protein.

barley beef skillet

PREP: 20 minutes | **COOK:** 1 hour

Kit Tunstall | BOISE, IDAHO
Even my 3-year-old loves this tasty meal-in-one dish. It's very filling, inexpensive and full of vegetables. It's also really good spiced up with chili powder, cayenne or a dash of hot pepper sauce.

- 1 pound lean ground beef (90% lean)
- 1/4 cup chopped onion
- 1 garlic clove, minced
- 1 can (14-1/2 ounces) reduced-sodium beef broth
- 1 can (8 ounces) tomato sauce
- 1 cup water
- 2 small carrots and 1 *each* small tomato and zucchini, chopped
- 1 cup medium pearl barley
- 2 teaspoons Italian seasoning
- 1/4 teaspoon salt
- 1/8 teaspoon pepper

- In a large skillet, cook beef and onion over medium heat until meat is no longer pink. Add garlic; cook 1 minute longer. Drain. Add the broth, tomato sauce and water; bring to a boil. Stir in the remaining ingredients. Reduce heat; cover and simmer for 45-50 minutes or until barley is tender.

YIELD: 4 servings.

NUTRITION FACTS: 1-1/2 cups equals 400 calories, 10 g fat (4 g saturated fat), 73 mg cholesterol, 682 mg sodium, 48 g carbohydrate, 10 g fiber, 30 g protein.

BARLEY BEEF SKILLET

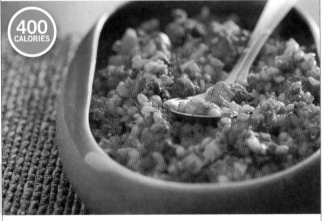

20-minute or less prep recipes

In the time it takes to pick up items in the fast-food drive-thru, you can put together delicious, healthy recipes at home (and save cash, too). All the dishes in this special bonus chapter can be prepped to cook in 20 minutes or less. It can be speedy to eat light!

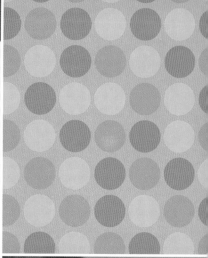

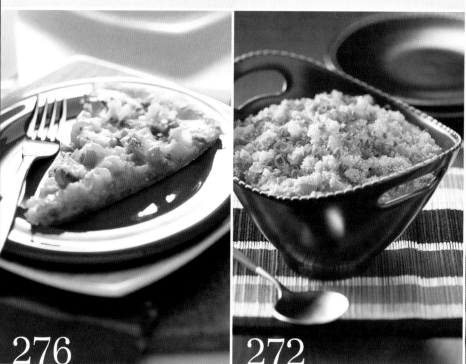

276

272

275

Looking for a quick, healthy recipe? Consider the great recipes here, which are arranged in calorie order from the lowest to the highest. Every one preps in no time, so you can get out of the kitchen and on with your day! And all will help you meet your 1,400 calorie goal. Get inspired by some of our readers' tips on how to fit exercise into even a busy day!

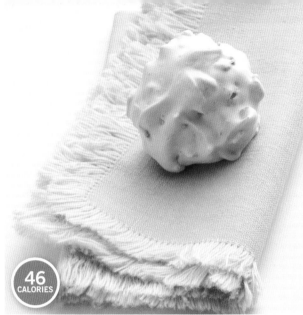

46 CALORIES

PECAN KISSES

pecan kisses

PREP: 15 minutes I **BAKE:** 15 minutes/batch

Norlene Razak I KYLE, TEXAS

These lighter-than-air treats make for a sweet snack kids of all ages will love. They're made with just six ingredients and melt in your mouth.

2	egg whites
1	teaspoon vanilla extract
1/4	teaspoon vinegar
1/8	teaspoon salt
2	cups confectioners' sugar
1-1/2	cups chopped pecans

- In a large bowl, beat the egg whites, vanilla, vinegar and salt on medium speed until soft peaks form. Gradually add confectioners' sugar, 1 tablespoon at a time, beating on high until stiff glossy peaks form and sugar is dissolved. Fold in pecans.

- Drop by rounded teaspoonfuls 1 in. apart onto greased baking sheets.

- Bake at 300° for 15-20 minutes or until firm to the touch and lightly browned. Remove to wire racks to cool. Store in an airtight container.

YIELD: 4 dozen.

NUTRITION FACTS: 1 cookie equals 46 calories, 3 g fat (trace saturated fat), 0 cholesterol, 8 mg sodium, 6 g carbohydrate, trace fiber, trace protein. **DIABETIC EXCHANGES:** 1/2 starch, 1/2 fat.

apple skewers

PREP: 15 minutes I **COOK:** 15 minutes

Doris Sowers I HUTCHINSON, KANSAS

We enjoy these flavorful grilled apples with a lightly spiced coating all year. Best of all, they're a cinch to grill, and cleanup's a breeze.

4	medium apples, peeled and quartered
4	teaspoons sugar
1-1/4	teaspoons ground cinnamon

- Thread apples on four metal or soaked wooden skewers. Lightly spray with cooking spray. Combine sugar and cinnamon; sprinkle over apples.

- Using long-handled tongs, moisten a paper towel with cooking oil and lightly coat the grill rack. Grill, covered, over medium heat or broil 4 in. from the heat for 6-8 minutes or until golden. Turn; cook 8-10 minutes longer or until golden and tender. Serve warm.

YIELD: 4 servings.

NUTRITION FACTS: 1 skewer equals 80 calories, trace fat (trace saturated fat), 0 cholesterol, trace sodium, 21 g carbohydrate, 2 g fiber, trace protein. **DIABETIC EXCHANGE:** 1 fruit.

APPLE SKEWERS

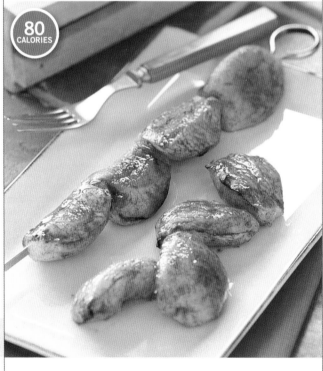

80 CALORIES

cafe mocha mini muffins

81 CALORIES

PREP: 15 minutes | BAKE: 15 minutes + cooling

Tina Sawchuk | ARDMORE, ALBERTA

It's easy to keep these muffins on hand since they freeze well. They're just the right size for breakfast or snacking.

2	teaspoons instant coffee granules
1/3	cup boiling water
1/4	cup quick-cooking oats
3	tablespoons butter, softened
1/4	cup sugar
3	tablespoons brown sugar
1	egg yolk
1/2	teaspoon vanilla extract
1/2	cup all-purpose flour
1	tablespoon baking cocoa
1/2	teaspoon baking powder
1/8	teaspoon baking soda
1/8	teaspoon salt
1/2	cup miniature semisweet chocolate chips, *divided*

• In a small bowl, dissolve coffee granules in water. Stir in the oats; set aside. In a small bowl, cream butter and sugars. Beat in egg yolk and vanilla. Beat in reserved oat mixture. Combine the flour, cocoa, baking powder, baking soda and salt; add to oat mixture. Stir in 1/3 cup chocolate chips.

• Fill greased miniature muffin cups three-fourths full. Sprinkle with remaining chips. Bake at 350° for 12-15 minutes or until a toothpick inserted near the center comes out clean. Cool for 5 minutes before removing from pans to wire racks.

YIELD: 1-1/2 dozen.

NUTRITION FACTS: 1 muffin equals 81 calories, 4 g fat (2 g saturated fat), 17 mg cholesterol, 53 mg sodium, 12 g carbohydrate, 1 g fiber, 1 g protein. **DIABETIC EXCHANGES:** 1 starch, 1/2 fat.

zucchini parmesan

PREP: 15 minutes | COOK: 15 minutes

Sandi Guettler | BAY CITY, MICHIGAN

You'll knock their socks off with this easy-to-prep side that's absolutely delicious. My favorite time to make it is when the zucchini is fresh out of the garden.

1/2 to 1	teaspoon minced garlic
1	tablespoon olive oil
4	medium zucchini, cut into 1/4-inch slices
1	can (14-1/2 ounces) Italian diced tomatoes, undrained
1	teaspoon seasoned salt
1/4	teaspoon pepper
1/4	cup grated Parmesan cheese

• In a large skillet, saute garlic in oil. Add zucchini; cook and stir for 4-5 minutes or until crisp-tender.

• Stir in the tomatoes, seasoned salt and pepper. Simmer, uncovered, for 9-10 minutes or until liquid is absorbed and mixture is heated through. Sprinkle with Parmesan cheese. Serve with a slotted spoon.

YIELD: 6 servings.

NUTRITION FACTS: 1/2 cup equals 81 calories, 3 g fat (1 g saturated fat), 3 mg cholesterol, 581 mg sodium, 10 g carbohydrate, 2 g fiber, 3 g protein. **DIABETIC EXCHANGES:** 2 vegetable, 1/2 fat.

ZUCCHINI PARMESAN

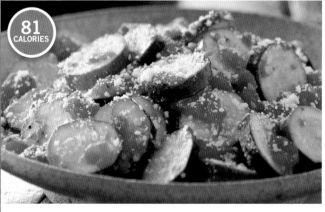

81 CALORIES

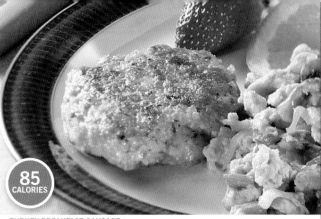

85 CALORIES

TURKEY BREAKFAST SAUSAGE

turkey breakfast sausage

PREP: 10 minutes | **COOK:** 15 minutes

Judy Culbertson | DANSVILLE, NEW YORK
These hearty patties are loaded with savory flavor but contain a fraction of the sodium and fat of commercial breakfast sausages.

> 1 pound lean ground turkey
> 3/4 teaspoon salt
> 1/2 teaspoon rubbed sage
> 1/2 teaspoon pepper
> 1/4 teaspoon ground ginger

- Crumble turkey into a large bowl. Add the salt, sage, pepper and ginger. Shape into eight 2-in. patties.

- In a nonstick skillet coated with cooking spray, cook patties over medium heat for 6-8 minutes on each side or until no longer pink and a meat thermometer reads 165°.

YIELD: 8 servings.

NUTRITION FACTS: 1 patty equals 85 calories, 5 g fat (1 g saturated fat), 45 mg cholesterol, 275 mg sodium, trace carbohydrate, trace fiber, 10 g protein. **DIABETIC EXCHANGES:** 1 lean meat, 1/2 fat.

baked eggs with cheddar and bacon `for 2`

PREP: 15 minutes | **BAKE:** 15 minutes

Catherine Wilkinson | DEWEY, ARIZONA
Smoky cheese and bacon elevate eggs to another level with this recipe! It's super easy to make and perfect for a special day. These eggs are also very nice for a casual dinner.

> 2 eggs
> 2 tablespoons fat-free milk, *divided*
> 1 tablespoon shredded smoked cheddar cheese
> 1 teaspoon minced fresh parsley
> 1/8 teaspoon salt
> Dash pepper
> 1 bacon strip

- Coat two 4-oz. ramekins with cooking spray; break an egg into each dish. Spoon 1 tablespoon milk over each egg. Combine the cheese, parsley, salt and pepper; sprinkle over tops.

- Bake, uncovered, at 325° for 12-15 minutes or until whites are completely set and yolks begin to thicken but are not firm.

- Meanwhile, in a small skillet, cook bacon over medium heat until crisp. Remove to paper towels to drain. Crumble bacon and sprinkle over eggs.

YIELD: 2 servings.

NUTRITION FACTS: 1 serving equals 107 calories, 7 g fat (3 g saturated fat), 219 mg cholesterol, 319 mg sodium, 1 g carbohydrate, trace fiber, 9 g protein.

BAKED EGGS WITH CHEDDAR AND BACON

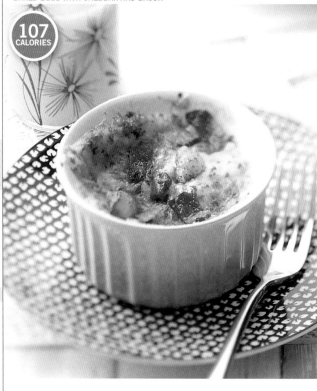
107 CALORIES

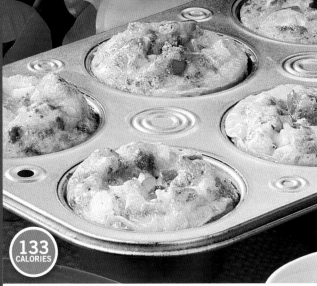

133 CALORIES

SCRAMBLED EGG MUFFINS

scrambled egg muffins

PREP: 5 minutes | **BAKE:** 25 minutes

Cathy Larkins | MARSHFIELD, MISSOURI

After enjoying scrambled egg muffins at a local restaurant, I came up with this savory version that my husband likes even better. Freeze the extras to reheat on busy mornings.

- 1/2 pound bulk pork sausage
- 12 eggs
- 1/2 cup chopped onion
- 1/4 cup chopped green pepper
- 1/2 teaspoon salt
- 1/4 teaspoon pepper
- 1/4 teaspoon garlic powder
- 1/2 cup shredded cheddar cheese

- In a large skillet, cook the sausage over medium heat until no longer pink; drain.

- In a large bowl, beat the eggs. Add the onion, green pepper, salt, pepper and garlic powder. Stir in sausage and cheese.

- Spoon by 1/3 cupfuls into greased muffin cups. Bake at 350° for 20-25 minutes or until a knife inserted near the center comes out clean.

YIELD: 1 dozen.

NUTRITION FACTS: 1 muffin equals 133 calories, 10 g fat (4 g saturated fat), 224 mg cholesterol, 268 mg sodium, 2 g carbohydrate, trace fiber, 9 g protein.

quick crisp snack bars

PREP/TOTAL TIME: 20 minutes

Ursula Maurer | WAUWATOSA, WISCONSIN

My daughters have loved these nutritious snacks since they were in grade school. Now, both are adults and still make these bars when they want a quick treat.

- 1/2 cup honey
- 1/2 cup reduced-fat chunky peanut butter
- 1/2 cup nonfat dry milk powder
- 4 cups crisp rice cereal

- In a large saucepan, combine honey, peanut butter and milk powder. Cook and stir over low heat until blended.

- Remove from the heat; stir in cereal. Press into an 8-in. square dish coated with cooking spray. Let stand until set. Cut into bars.

YIELD: 1 dozen.

NUTRITION FACTS: 1 bar equals 144 calories, 4 g fat (1 g saturated fat), 1 mg cholesterol, 144 mg sodium, 25 g carbohydrate, 1 g fiber, 5 g protein. **DIABETIC EXCHANGES:** 1-1/2 starch, 1/2 fat.

QUICK CRISP SNACK BARS

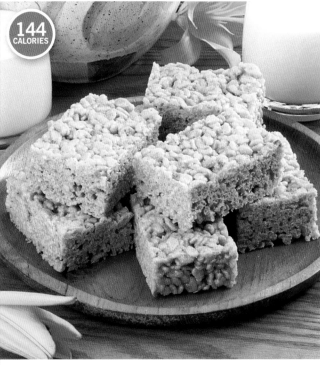

144 CALORIES

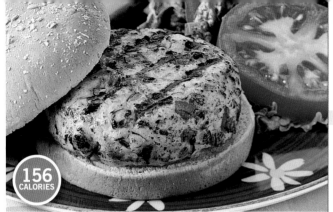

156 CALORIES

GARDEN TURKEY BURGERS

garden turkey burgers

PREP: 15 minutes | **COOK:** 15 minutes

Sandy Kitzmiller | UNITYVILLE, PENNSYLVANIA

These moist burgers get plenty of color and flavor from onion, zucchini and red pepper. I often make the mixture ahead of time and put it in the refrigerator. Later, after helping my husband with farm chores, I can put the burgers on the grill while whipping up a salad or side dish.

- 1 cup old-fashioned oats
- 3/4 cup chopped onion
- 3/4 cup finely chopped sweet red *or* green pepper
- 1/2 cup shredded zucchini
- 1/4 cup ketchup
- 2 garlic cloves, minced
- 1/4 teaspoon salt, optional
- 1 pound ground turkey
- 6 whole wheat hamburger buns, split and toasted

- In a large bowl, combine the first seven ingredients. Crumble turkey over mixture and mix well. Shape into six 1/2-in.-thick patties.

- Using long-handled tongs, moisten a paper towel with cooking oil and lightly coat the grill rack. Prepare grill for indirect heat, using a drip pan.

- Place burgers over drip pan and grill, covered, over indirect medium heat or broil 4 in. from the heat for 6 minutes on each side or until a meat thermometer reads 165° and juices run clear. Serve on buns.

YIELD: 6 servings.

NUTRITION FACTS: 1 burger (prepared with lean ground turkey and without salt; calculated without the bun) equals 156 calories, 2 g fat (0 saturated fat), 37 mg cholesterol, 174 mg sodium, 15 g carbohydrate, 0 fiber, 21 g protein. **DIABETIC EXCHANGES:** 2 lean meat, 1 starch.

dijon-crusted chicken breasts

PREP: 15 minutes | **COOK:** 15 minutes

Jacqueline Correa | LANDING, NEW JERSEY

If you're craving fried chicken, this dish will hit the spot! A crisp and flavorful coating makes this easy entree feel special and indulgent.

- 1/3 cup dry bread crumbs
- 1 tablespoon grated Parmesan cheese
- 1 teaspoon Italian seasoning
- 1/2 teaspoon dried thyme
- 1/4 teaspoon salt
- 1/4 teaspoon pepper
- 4 boneless skinless chicken breast halves (4 ounces *each*)
- 2 tablespoons Dijon mustard
- 1 teaspoon olive oil
- 1 teaspoon reduced-fat margarine

- Place the first six ingredients in a shallow bowl. Brush chicken with mustard; roll in crumb mixture.

- In a large nonstick skillet, cook chicken in oil and margarine over medium heat for 5-6 minutes on each side or until a meat thermometer reads 170°.

YIELD: 4 servings.

EDITOR'S NOTE: This recipe was tested with Parkay Light stick margarine.

NUTRITION FACTS: 1 chicken breast half equals 169 calories, 5 g fat (1 g saturated fat), 63 mg cholesterol, 380 mg sodium, 6 g carbohydrate, trace fiber, 24 g protein. **DIABETIC EXCHANGES:** 3 lean meat, 1/2 starch, 1/2 fat.

DIJON-CRUSTED CHICKEN BREASTS

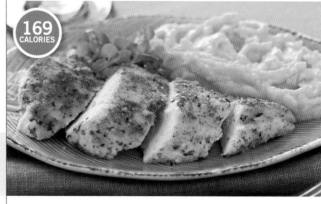

169 CALORIES

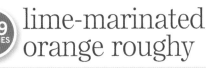

lime-marinated orange roughy

169 CALORIES

PREP: 10 minutes + marinating | **Broil:** 10 minutes

Pam Corder | MONROE, LOUISIANA
This dish is simple, tasty and not fattening at all. And since it's so quick, you can have company over and spend all your time visiting.

    4 orange roughy fillets (6 ounces *each*)
  1/3 cup water
  1/3 cup lime juice
    2 tablespoons honey
    1 tablespoon canola oil
  1/2 teaspoon dill weed

- Place fillets in a 13-in. x 9-in. baking dish. In a small bowl, combine the remaining ingredients; set aside 3 tablespoons marinade. Pour remaining marinade over fillets; turn to coat. Cover and refrigerate for 1 hour.

- Drain and discard marinade. Transfer fillets to a broiler pan coated with cooking spray. Broil 4-6 in. from the heat for 4-6 minutes on each side or until fish flakes easily with a fork, basting frequently with reserved marinade.

YIELD: 4 servings.

NUTRITION FACTS: 1 fillet equals 169 calories, 3 g fat (trace saturated fat), 102 mg cholesterol, 123 mg sodium, 6 g carbohydrate, trace fiber, 28 g protein. **DIABETIC EXCHANGES:** 4 lean meat, 1/2 starch, 1/2 fat.

blueberry oatmeal pancakes

PREP: 20 minutes | **COOK:** 5 minutes/batch

Amy Spainhoward | BOWLING GREEN, KENTUCKY
Wonderful blueberry flavor abounds in these thick and moist pancakes. They are very nutritious, easy and inexpensive—and my kids love them!

    2 cups all-purpose flour
    2 packets (1.51 ounces *each*) instant maple and brown sugar oatmeal mix
    2 tablespoons sugar
    2 teaspoons baking powder
  1/8 teaspoon salt

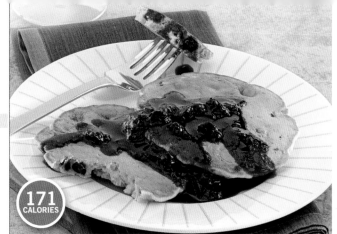

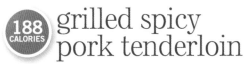
BLUEBERRY OATMEAL PANCAKES

171 CALORIES

    2 egg whites
    1 egg
1-1/2 cups fat-free milk
  1/2 cup reduced-fat sour cream
    2 cups fresh *or* frozen blueberries
BLUEBERRY SYRUP:
1-1/2 cups fresh *or* frozen blueberries
  1/2 cup sugar

- In a large bowl, combine the first five ingredients. In another bowl, whisk the egg whites, egg, milk and sour cream. Stir into dry ingredients just until moistened. Fold in blueberries.

- Spoon batter by 1/4 cupfuls onto a hot griddle coated with cooking spray. Turn when bubbles form on top of pancake; cook until the second side is golden brown.

- In a microwave-safe bowl, combine the syrup ingredients. Microwave, uncovered, on high for 1 minute; stir. Microwave 1-2 minutes longer or until hot and bubbly. Serve warm with pancakes.

YIELD: 14 pancakes (1-1/4 cups syrup).

NUTRITION FACTS: 1 pancake with 1 tablespoon syrup equals 171 calories, 2 g fat (1 g saturated fat), 19 mg cholesterol, 145 mg sodium, 34 g carbohydrate, 2 g fiber, 5 g protein.

grilled spicy pork tenderloin

188 CALORIES

PREP: 15 minutes + marinating | **GRILL:** 25 minutes

Mary Ann Lee | CLIFTON PARK, NEW YORK
Prep this tender and delicious pork the night before, marinate during the day, then grill when you get home.

The only time I could run today was at 4 o'clock this morning, so that's what I did. It starts the day off right and helps me feel good. I would rather get up insanely early and work out than not work out at all! —**Michelle Smith Jarc**

2 tablespoons brown sugar

3/4 teaspoon salt

3/4 teaspoon dried thyme

1/4 teaspoon onion powder

1/4 teaspoon garlic powder

1/4 teaspoon ground mustard

1/4 teaspoon ground cumin

1/4 teaspoon dried oregano

1/4 teaspoon ground allspice

1/4 teaspoon pepper

1 pork tenderloin (1 pound)

SAUCE:

1/2 cup cola

1 tablespoon brown sugar

1/4 teaspoon ground cinnamon

1/4 teaspoon chili powder

- In a small bowl, combine the first 10 ingredients; rub over pork. Cover and refrigerate for 8 hours or overnight.

- In a small bowl, combine sauce ingredients. Using long-handled tongs, moisten a paper towel with cooking oil and lightly coat the grill rack. Prepare sauce ingredients; set aside.

- Prepare grill for indirect heat using a drip pan. Place pork over drip pan and grill, covered, over indirect medium-hot heat for 25-30 minutes or until a meat thermometer reads 160°, basting occasionally with reserved sauce. Let stand for 5 minutes before slicing.

YIELD: 4 servings.

NUTRITION FACTS: 3 ounces cooked pork equals 188 calories, 4 g fat (1 g saturated fat), 63 mg cholesterol, 495 mg sodium, 14 g carbohydrate, 1 g fiber, 23 g protein. **DIABETIC EXCHANGES:** 3 lean meat, 1 starch.

ratatouille with polenta

PREP: 20 minutes I **COOK:** 15 minutes

Taste of Home Test Kitchen
Created in the Provence region of France, the dish features seasoned veggies sauteed in oil.

1/2 pound small fresh mushrooms, halved

1 medium sweet red pepper, chopped

1 small onion, chopped

4 teaspoons olive oil, *divided*

4 cups cubed peeled eggplant

1 small zucchini, chopped

1 cup cherry tomatoes

2 garlic cloves, minced

1-1/2 teaspoons Italian seasoning

1/2 teaspoon salt

1 tube (1 pound) polenta, cut into 1/2-inch slices

Grated Parmesan cheese, optional

- In a large skillet, saute the mushrooms, pepper and onion in 2 teaspoons oil until almost tender. Add the eggplant, zucchini, tomatoes, garlic, Italian seasoning and salt. Saute for 8-10 minutes or until vegetables are tender.

- In another skillet, cook polenta slices in remaining oil over medium-high heat for 3-4 minutes on each side or until lightly browned. Serve with ratatouille; sprinkle with cheese if desired.

YIELD: 4 servings.

NUTRITION FACTS: 1-1/2 cups ratatouille with 3 pieces of polenta equals 195 calories, 5 g fat (1 g saturated fat), 0 cholesterol, 689 mg sodium, 34 g carbohydrate, 6 g fiber, 6 g protein. **DIABETIC EXCHANGES:** 2 starch, 1 fat.

RATATOUILLE WITH POLENTA

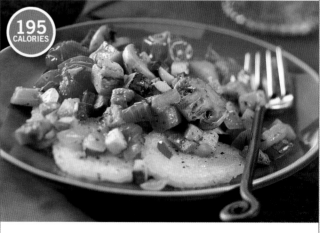

195 CALORIES

198 CALORIES

QUINOA PILAF

quinoa pilaf

PREP: 10 minutes I **COOK:** 20 minutes

Sonya Fox I PEYTON, COLORADO

I created this recipe after tasting quinoa at a local restaurant. I really enjoy rice pilaf, but I don't usually have time to make it. This quick-cooking side is a tasty and speedy alternative.

- 1 medium onion, chopped
- 1 medium carrot, finely chopped
- 1 teaspoon olive oil
- 1 garlic clove, minced
- 1 can (14-1/2 ounces) reduced-sodium chicken broth *or* vegetable broth
- 1/4 cup water
- 1/4 teaspoon salt
- 1 cup quinoa, rinsed

- In a small nonstick saucepan coated with cooking spray, cook onion and carrot in oil for 2-3 minutes or until crisp-tender. Add garlic; cook 1 minute longer. Stir in the broth, water and salt; bring to a boil.

- Add quinoa. Reduce heat; cover and simmer for 12-15 minutes or until liquid is absorbed. Remove from the heat. Fluff with a fork.

YIELD: 4 servings.

EDITOR'S NOTE: Look for quinoa in the cereal, rice or organic food aisle.

NUTRITION FACTS: 3/4 cup equals 198 calories, 4 g fat (trace saturated fat), 0 cholesterol, 434 mg sodium, 35 g carbohydrate, 4 g fiber, 8 g protein. **DIABETIC EXCHANGES:** 2 starch, 1/2 fat.

savory baked chicken

PREP: 10 minutes I **BAKE:** 20 minutes

Bonnie Baumgardner I SYLVA, NORTH CAROLINA

Crispy golden breading with robust mustard and lemon flavors make this easy main dish deliciously different.

- 2 tablespoons spicy brown mustard
- 1 teaspoon lemon juice
- 1/8 teaspoon dried savory
- 1/8 teaspoon grated lemon peel   **for 2**
- 1/8 teaspoon salt
- 1/8 teaspoon pepper
- 2/3 cup crushed seasoned stuffing
- 2 boneless skinless chicken breast halves (4 ounces *each*)

Nonstick cooking spray

- In a shallow bowl, combine the first six ingredients. Place the stuffing in another bowl. Dip chicken in mustard mixture, then coat with stuffing.

- Place chicken in an 11-in. x 7-in. baking dish coated with cooking spray. Spritz chicken with cooking spray. Bake, uncovered, at 350° for 15-20 minutes or until a meat thermometer reads 170°.

YIELD: 2 servings.

NUTRITION FACTS: 1 chicken breast half equals 210 calories, 3 g fat (1 g saturated fat), 63 mg cholesterol, 664 mg sodium, 15 g carbohydrate, 1 g fiber, 25 g protein. **DIABETIC EXCHANGES:** 3 lean meat, 1 starch.

SAVORY BAKED CHICKEN

210 CALORIES

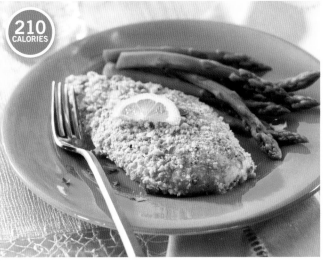

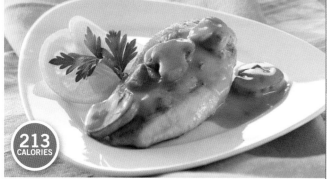

213 CALORIES

LEMON MUSHROOM CHICKEN

lemon mushroom chicken

PREP: 10 minutes I **COOK:** 20 minutes

Carrie Palmquist I CANOVA, SOUTH DAKOTA

There's a lot of flavor in this chicken. And the best part? It doesn't seem light at all!

- 4 boneless skinless chicken breast halves (4 ounces *each*)
- 1/4 cup plus 2 teaspoons all-purpose flour, *divided*
- 1/2 teaspoon salt
- 1/4 teaspoon pepper
- 2 tablespoons butter
- 1/3 cup plus 3 tablespoons reduced-sodium chicken broth, *divided*
- 1/2 pound sliced fresh mushrooms
- 1 tablespoon lemon juice

- Flatten chicken to 1/2-in. thickness. In a large resealable plastic bag, combine 1/4 cup flour, salt and pepper. Add chicken, one piece at a time; shake to coat.

- In a large nonstick skillet over medium heat, cook chicken in butter for 5-6 minutes on each side or until no longer pink. Remove and keep warm.

- Add 1/3 cup broth to the pan, stirring to loosen browned bits. Bring to a boil. Add mushrooms; cook and stir for 3-5 minutes or until tender.

- Combine the remaining flour and broth until smooth; stir into the mushroom mixture. Bring to a boil; cook and stir for 2 minutes or until thickened. Stir in lemon juice. Serve with chicken.

YIELD: 4 servings.

NUTRITION FACTS: 1 chicken breast half with 1/4 cup sauce equals 213 calories, 9 g fat (4 g saturated fat), 78 mg cholesterol, 368 mg sodium, 8 g carbohydrate, 1 g fiber, 26 g protein. **DIABETIC EXCHANGES:** 3 lean meat, 1-1/2 fat, 1/2 starch.

presto chicken tacos

PREP: 20 minutes I **COOK:** 25 minutes

Nanette Hilton I LAS VEGAS, NEVADA

Slowly cooking the chicken with the seasonings is the key to perfection with this dish. The chicken mixture also makes a great salad topping.

- 3 pounds boneless skinless chicken breasts, cut into strips
- 2 tablespoons canola oil
- 1 garlic clove, minced
- 2 cans (14-1/2 ounces *each*) diced tomatoes, undrained
- 1 teaspoon ground cumin
- 1 teaspoon chili powder
- 12 corn tortillas (6 inches), warmed

Optional toppings: shredded lettuce, shredded cheddar cheese, diced tomatoes, fresh cilantro leaves, sour cream and cubed avocado

- In a Dutch oven, brown chicken in oil in batches. Add garlic; cook 1 minute longer. Add the tomatoes, cumin and chili powder. Bring to a boil. Reduce heat; cover and simmer for 15-20 minutes or until chicken is no longer pink, stirring occasionally. Fill each tortilla with about 1/2 cup chicken mixture. Serve with toppings of your choice.

YIELD: 12 servings.

NUTRITION FACTS: 1 taco (calculated without toppings) equals 215 calories, 6 g fat (1 g saturated fat), 63 mg cholesterol, 186 mg sodium, 16 g carbohydrate, 3 g fiber, 25 g protein. **DIABETIC EXCHANGES:** 3 lean meat, 1 starch.

PRESTO CHICKEN TACOS

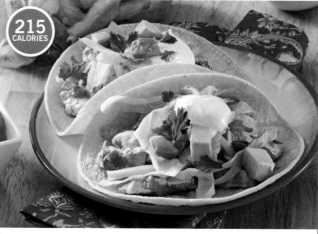

215 CALORIES

I make breakfast for my 3-year-old and let him eat and watch cartoons while I work out. He's distracted by the TV, so there are no interruptions for Mommy!
— **Evelyn Copeland**

tuscan chicken for two

PREP/TOTAL TIME: 15 minutes

Debra Legrand | PORT ORCHARD, WASHINGTON
This moist and savory entree is ready in an unbelievable 15 minutes flat! Eating light and healthy has never been quicker!

- 2 boneless skinless chicken breast halves (5 ounces *each*)
- 1/4 teaspoon salt
- 1/4 teaspoon pepper
- 1 garlic clove, sliced
- 1 teaspoon dried rosemary, crushed
- 1/4 teaspoon rubbed sage
- 1/4 teaspoon dried thyme
- 1 tablespoon olive oil

- Flatten chicken to 1/2-in. thickness; sprinkle with salt and pepper.

- In a large skillet over medium heat, cook and stir the garlic, rosemary, sage and thyme in oil for 1 minute. Add chicken; cook for 5-7 minutes on each side or until chicken juices run clear.

YIELD: 2 servings.

TUSCAN CHICKEN FOR TWO

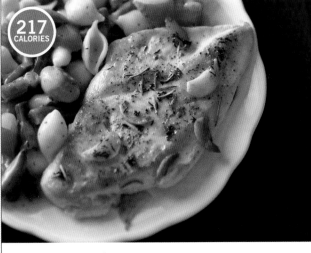

217 CALORIES

NUTRITION FACTS: 1 chicken breast half equals 217 calories, 10 g fat (2 g saturated fat), 78 mg cholesterol, 364 mg sodium, 1 g carbohydrate, 1 g fiber, 29 g protein. **DIABETIC EXCHANGES:** 4 lean meat, 1 fat.

231 CALORIES grilled veggie sandwiches

PREP: 15 minutes | **COOK:** 15 minutes

Melissa Wilbanks | MEMPHIS, TENNESSEE
Here's a fun recipe for using up those garden veggies. You won't miss the meat in these hefty grilled sandwiches.

- 1 small zucchini
- 1 small yellow summer squash
- 1 small eggplant
- Cooking spray
- 1 medium onion, sliced
- 1 large sweet red pepper, cut into rings
- 4 whole wheat hamburger buns, split
- 3 ounces fat-free cream cheese
- 1/4 cup crumbled goat cheese
- 1 garlic clove, minced
- 1/8 teaspoon salt
- 1/8 teaspoon pepper

- Cut the zucchini, squash and eggplant into 1/4-in.-thick strips; spritz with cooking spray. Spritz onion and red pepper with cooking spray.

- Grill vegetables, covered, over medium heat for 4-5 minutes on each side or until crisp-tender. Remove and keep warm. Grill buns, cut side down, over medium heat for 30-60 seconds or until toasted.

- In a small bowl, combine the cheeses, garlic, salt and pepper; spread over bun bottoms. Top with vegetables. Replace bun tops.

YIELD: 4 servings.

NUTRITION FACTS: 1 sandwich equals 231 calories, 6 g fat (2 g saturated fat), 10 mg cholesterol, 438 mg sodium, 39 g carbohydrate, 10 g fiber, 11 g protein. **DIABETIC EXCHANGES:** 2-1/2 starch, 1 fat.

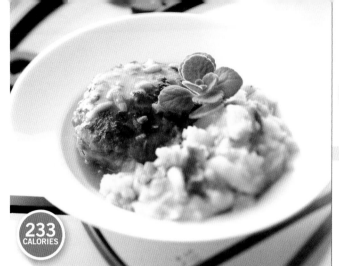

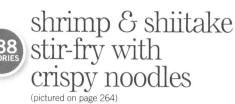

238 CALORIES

shrimp & shiitake stir-fry with crispy noodles

(pictured on page 264)

PREP: 20 minutes | **COOK:** 15 minutes

Wolfgang Hanau | WEST PALM BEACH, FLORIDA
We love the crispy noodles on top of this time-saving Thai dish, but roasted cashews are a wonderful complement as well.

1-1/2	teaspoons cornstarch
1/2	cup chicken broth
2	tablespoons reduced-sodium soy sauce
1	small head bok choy
1	pound uncooked medium shrimp, peeled and deveined
2	tablespoons canola oil, *divided*
2	tablespoons minced fresh gingerroot
1	garlic clove, thinly sliced
1/2	teaspoon crushed red pepper flakes
1	large onion, halved and thinly sliced
2	cups sliced fresh shiitake mushrooms

Hot cooked brown rice, optional
    1/4 cup chow mein noodles

- In a small bowl, combine the cornstarch, broth and soy sauce until smooth; set aside. Cut off and discard root end of bok choy, leaving stalks with leaves. Cut leaves from stalks. Slice leaves; set aside. Slice stalks.

- In a large skillet or wok, stir-fry shrimp in 1 tablespoon oil until shrimp turn pink. Remove and keep warm.

- Stir-fry the ginger, garlic and pepper flakes in remaining oil for 1 minute. Add the onion, mushrooms and bok choy stalks; stir-fry for 4 minutes. Add bok choy leaves; stir-fry 2-4 minutes longer or until the vegetables are crisp-tender.

- Stir cornstarch mixture and add to the pan. Bring to a boil; cook and stir for 2 minutes or until thickened. Add shrimp; heat through. Serve with rice if desired. Sprinkle with chow mein noodles.

YIELD: 4 servings.

NUTRITION FACTS: 1 cup stir-fry with 1 tablespoon chow mein noodles (calculated without rice) equals 238 calories, 10 g fat (1 g saturated fat), 139 mg cholesterol, 710 mg sodium, 15 g carbohydrate, 3 g fiber, 24 g protein. **DIABETIC EXCHANGES:** 3 lean meat, 2 vegetable, 1 fat.

---

233 CALORIES

HEARTY SALISBURY STEAKS

hearty salisbury steaks

PREP: 10 minutes | **COOK:** 15 minutes

Dorothy Bayes | SARDIS, OHIO
I serve this down-home main dish with mashed potatoes. With its classic taste, it will disappear fast!

1/4	cup egg substitute
1	medium onion, finely chopped
1/2	cup crushed saltines (about 15 crackers)
1/2	teaspoon pepper
1	pound lean ground beef (90% lean)
1	tablespoon canola oil
1	envelope reduced-sodium onion soup mix
2	tablespoons all-purpose flour
2	cups water

- In a large bowl, combine the egg substitute, onion, saltines and pepper. Crumble beef over mixture and mix well. Shape into five patties.

- In a large skillet, cook patties in oil over medium heat for 3 minutes on each side or until lightly browned. Remove patties and keep warm; drain drippings.

- In a small bowl combine the soup mix, flour and water; stir into skillet. Bring to a boil. Return patties to skillet. Reduce heat; cover and simmer for 5-7 minutes or until meat is no longer pink.

YIELD: 5 servings.

NUTRITION FACTS: 1 patty with 1/4 cup gravy equals 233 calories, 10 g fat (3 g saturated fat), 45 mg cholesterol, 418 mg sodium, 14 g carbohydrate, 1 g fiber, 20 g protein.
DIABETIC EXCHANGES: 2 lean meat, 1 starch, 1 fat.

241 CALORIES
grilled fish sandwiches

PREP: 15 minutes | **COOK:** 15 minutes

Violet Beard | MARSHALL, ILLINOIS

These fish fillets are seasoned with lime juice and lemon pepper before grilling. A simple mayonnaise and mustard sauce puts the sandwiches ahead of the rest.

4 cod fillets (4 ounces *each*)
1 tablespoon lime juice
1/2 teaspoon lemon-pepper seasoning
1/4 cup mayonnaise
2 teaspoons Dijon mustard
1 teaspoon honey
4 hamburger buns, split
4 lettuce leaves
4 tomato slices

- Brush both sides of fillets with lime juice; sprinkle with lemon pepper. Using long-handled tongs, moisten a paper towel with cooking oil and lightly coat the grill rack. Grill fillets, covered, over medium heat or broil 4 in. from the heat for 5-6 minutes on each side or until fish flakes easily with a fork.

- In a small bowl, combine the mayonnaise, mustard and honey. Spread over the bottom of each bun. Top with a fillet, lettuce and tomato; replace bun tops.

YIELD: 4 servings.

NUTRITION FACTS: 1 sandwich (prepared with fat-free mayonnaise) equals 241 calories, 3 g fat (1 g saturated fat), 49 mg cholesterol, 528 mg sodium, 28 g carbohydrate, 2 g fiber, 24 g protein. **DIABETIC EXCHANGES:** 3 lean meat, 2 starch.

sausage and egg pizza

PREP: 10 minutes | **COOK/BAKE:** 20 minutes

Vicki Meyers | CASTALIA, OHIO

Using turkey sausage, fat-free cheddar cheese, egg substitute and reduced-fat crescent rolls really helped cut calories and fat in this delicious recipe.

1 tube (8 ounces) refrigerated reduced-fat crescent rolls
1/2 pound Italian turkey sausage links, casings removed
1-3/4 cups sliced fresh mushrooms
1-1/4 cups frozen shredded hash brown potatoes
1/4 teaspoon garlic salt
1/4 teaspoon pepper
2 green onions, chopped
2 tablespoons finely chopped sweet red pepper
1/2 cup shredded fat-free cheddar cheese
3/4 cup egg substitute

- Separate crescent dough into eight triangles; place on an ungreased 12-in. pizza pan with points toward the center. Press onto the bottom and up the sides of pan to form a crust; seal perforations. Bake at 375° for 8 minutes.

- Meanwhile, crumble sausage into a large nonstick skillet coated with cooking spray. Add mushrooms; cook and stir over medium heat until meat is no longer pink. Drain and set aside. In the same skillet, cook the potatoes, garlic salt and pepper over medium heat until browned.

- Sprinkle the sausage mixture over crust. Layer with the potatoes, onions, red pepper and cheese; pour egg substitute over the top. Bake for 10-12 minutes or until egg is set and cheese is melted.

YIELD: 6 slices.

NUTRITION FACTS: 1 slice equals 241 calories, 10 g fat (2 g saturated fat), 24 mg cholesterol, 744 mg sodium, 22 g carbohydrate, 1 g fiber, 16 g protein. **DIABETIC EXCHANGES:** 2 lean meat, 1-1/2 starch, 1/2 fat.

SAUSAGE AND EGG PIZZA

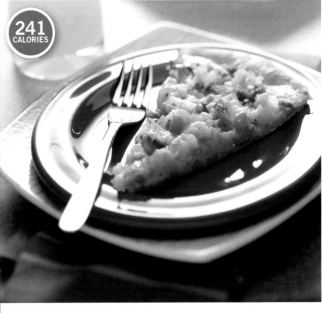

241 CALORIES

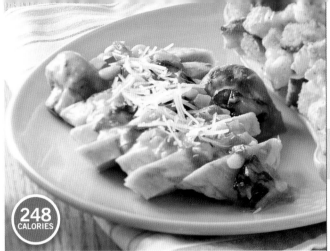

248 CALORIES

ITALIAN SKILLET SUPPER

italian skillet supper

PREP: 15 minutes | **COOK:** 15 minutes

Barbara Lento | HOUSTON, PENNSYLVANIA

You'll love this saucy chicken dinner! Romano cheese, sliced vegetables and pine nuts really jazz it up.

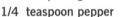

 for 2

- 2 boneless skinless chicken breast halves (4 ounces *each*)
- 1/4 teaspoon garlic salt
- 1/4 teaspoon pepper
- 2 teaspoons reduced-fat butter
- 1 teaspoon olive oil
- 1/4 pound small fresh mushrooms
- 1/2 medium onion, chopped
- 1/4 cup chopped sweet red pepper
- 1 tablespoon pine nuts
- 2 cups fresh baby spinach
- 1 tablespoon all-purpose flour
- 1/2 cup reduced-sodium chicken broth
- 1-1/2 teaspoons spicy brown mustard
- 2 teaspoons shredded Romano cheese

- Flatten chicken slightly; sprinkle with garlic salt and pepper. In a large nonstick skillet, cook chicken in butter and oil over medium heat for 3-4 minutes on each side or until no longer pink. Remove and keep warm.

- In the same skillet, saute the mushrooms, onion, red pepper and pine nuts until vegetables are tender. Add spinach; cook and stir for 2-3 minutes or until wilted. Stir in flour. Gradually stir in broth and mustard. Bring to a boil. Reduce heat; cook and stir for 2 minutes or until thickened.

- Return chicken to the pan; heat through. Sprinkle with the cheese.

YIELD: 2 servings.

EDITOR'S NOTE: This recipe was tested with Land O'Lakes light stick butter.

NUTRITION FACTS: 1 chicken breast half with 1/2 cup vegetable mixture equals 248 calories, 10 g fat (3 g saturated fat), 70 mg cholesterol, 548 mg sodium, 12 g carbohydrate, 3 g fiber, 29 g protein. **DIABETIC EXCHANGES:** 3 lean meat, 2 vegetable, 1-1/2 fat.

249 CALORIES

puffy apple omelet

PREP: 15 minutes | **BAKE:** 15 minutes

Melissa Davenport | CAMPBELL, MINNESOTA

Because of its unique and delicious flavors, you won't soon forget this fluffy oven omelet!

- 3 tablespoons all-purpose flour
- 1/4 teaspoon baking powder
- 2 eggs, *separated*
- 3 tablespoons fat-free milk
- 1 tablespoon lemon juice
- 3 tablespoons sugar

for 2

TOPPING:
- 1 large tart apple, peeled and thinly sliced
- 1 teaspoon sugar
- 1/4 teaspoon ground cinnamon

- In a small bowl, combine flour and baking powder. In a small bowl, whisk the egg yolks, milk and lemon juice. Stir into dry ingredients and mix well; set aside.

- In another small bowl, beat egg whites on medium speed until soft peaks form. Gradually beat in sugar, 1 tablespoon as a time, on high until stiff peaks form. Fold into yolk mixture.

- Pour into a shallow 1-1/2-qt. baking dish coated with cooking spray. Arrange apple slices on top. Combine sugar and cinnamon; sprinkle over apples.

- Bake, uncovered, at 375° for 18-20 minutes or until a knife inserted near the center comes out clean. Serve immediately.

YIELD: 2 servings.

NUTRITION FACTS: 1 serving equals 249 calories, 5 g fat (2 g saturated fat), 212 mg cholesterol, 130 mg sodium, 44 g carbohydrate, 2 g fiber, 9 g protein. **DIABETIC EXCHANGES:** 2 starch, 1 lean meat, 1 fruit.

261 CALORIES

ONION-DIJON PORK CHOPS

onion-dijon pork chops

PREP: 5 minutes | **COOK:** 20 minutes

Taste of Home Test Kitchen
Coated in a flavorful sauce, these chops are cooked to tender perfection. Serve them with rice and carrots for a full meal.

- 4 boneless pork loin chops (5 ounces *each*)
- 1/4 teaspoon salt
- 1/4 teaspoon pepper
- 3/4 cup thinly sliced red onion
- 1/4 cup water
- 1/4 cup cider vinegar
- 3 tablespoons brown sugar
- 2 tablespoons honey Dijon mustard

- Sprinkle pork chops with salt and pepper. In a large nonstick skillet coated with cooking spray, cook pork over medium heat for 4-6 minutes on each side or until lightly browned. Remove and keep warm.

- Add the remaining ingredients to the skillet; stir to loosen browned bits. Bring to a boil; cook and stir for 2 minutes or until thickened. Return chops to the pan. Reduce heat; cover and simmer for 4-5 minutes or until a meat thermometer reads 160°.

YIELD: 4 servings.

NUTRITION FACTS: 1 pork chop with 2 tablespoons onion mixture equals 261 calories, 9 g fat (3 g saturated fat), 69 mg cholesterol, 257 mg sodium, 17 g carbohydrate, 1 g fiber, 28 g protein. **DIABETIC EXCHANGES:** 4 lean meat, 1 starch.

274 CALORIES

country chicken with gravy

PREP: 15 minutes | **COOK:** 15 minutes

Ruth Helmuth | ABBEVILLE, SOUTH CAROLINA
This lightened-up chicken is comforting yet so quick and simple! It's always a hit when guests first try it!

- 3/4 cup crushed cornflakes
- 1/2 teaspoon poultry seasoning
- 1/2 teaspoon paprika
- 1/4 teaspoon salt
- 1/4 teaspoon dried thyme
- 1/4 teaspoon pepper
- 2 tablespoons fat-free evaporated milk
- 4 boneless skinless chicken breast halves (4 ounces *each*)
- 2 teaspoons canola oil

GRAVY:
- 1 tablespoon butter
- 1 tablespoon all-purpose flour
- 1/4 teaspoon pepper
- 1/8 teaspoon salt
- 1/2 cup fat-free evaporated milk
- 1/4 cup condensed chicken broth, undiluted
- 1 teaspoon sherry *or* additional condensed chicken broth
- 2 tablespoons minced chives

- In a shallow bowl, combine the first six ingredients. Place milk in another shallow bowl. Dip chicken in milk, then roll in cornflake mixture.

- In a large nonstick skillet coated with cooking spray, cook chicken in oil over medium heat for 6-8 minutes on each side or until a meat thermometer reads 170°.

- Meanwhile, in a small saucepan, melt butter. Stir in the flour, pepper and salt until smooth. Gradually stir in the milk, broth and sherry. Bring to a boil; cook and stir for 1-2 minutes or until thickened. Stir in chives. Serve with chicken.

YIELD: 4 servings.

NUTRITION FACTS: 1 chicken breast half with 2 tablespoons gravy equals 274 calories, 8 g fat (3 g saturated fat), 72 mg cholesterol, 569 mg sodium, 20 g carbohydrate, trace fiber, 28 g protein. **DIABETIC EXCHANGES:** 3 lean meat, 1 starch, 1/2 fat.

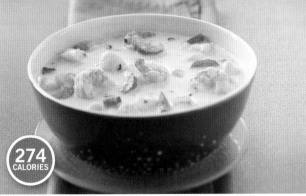

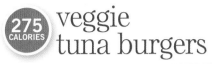

MAKEOVER CREAMY SEAFOOD SOUP

274 CALORIES

makeover creamy seafood soup

PREP: 15 minutes | **COOK:** 15 minutes

Mildred Fasig | STEPHENS CITY, VIRGINIA
With a rich and creamy texture and wonderful flavor, you won't miss the extra calories in the original recipe!

- 1/2 pound uncooked medium shrimp, peeled and deveined
- 1/2 pound bay scallops
- 2 tablespoons butter, *divided*
- 2 celery ribs, thinly sliced
- 1 medium sweet red pepper, finely chopped
- 1 medium onion, finely chopped
- 1/4 cup all-purpose flour
- 2 cups fat-free milk
- 2 cups half-and-half cream
- 1/4 cup sherry or reduced-sodium chicken broth
- 1 tablespoon minced fresh thyme *or* 1 teaspoon dried thyme
- 1/2 teaspoon salt
- 1/4 teaspoon cayenne pepper
- 1/8 teaspoon ground nutmeg

- In a Dutch oven, saute the shrimp and scallops in 1 tablespoon butter until shrimp turn pink. Remove and set aside.

- In the same pan, saute the celery, red pepper and onion in remaining butter until tender. Sprinkle with flour; stir until blended. Gradually stir in remaining ingredients. Bring to a boil; cook and stir for 2 minutes or until thickened. Return seafood to the pan; heat through.

YIELD: 6 servings.

NUTRITION FACTS: 1 cup equals 274 calories, 13 g fat (8 g saturated fat), 120 mg cholesterol, 436 mg sodium, 16 g carbohydrate, 1 g fiber, 19 g protein.

275 CALORIES

veggie tuna burgers

PREP: 15 minutes | **COOK:** 15 minutes

Laura Davis | RUSTON, LOUISIANA
You don't have to be a health nut to enjoy the taste of these moist and nutritious burgers. They're an easy way to get my children to eat their vegetables and a fun way to serve tuna.

- 1/4 cup finely chopped onion
- 1 garlic clove, minced
- 1 cup *each* shredded zucchini, yellow summer squash and carrots
- 1 egg, lightly beaten
- 2 cups soft whole wheat bread crumbs
- 1 can (6 ounces) light water-packed tuna, drained and flaked
- 1/4 teaspoon salt
- 1/4 teaspoon pepper
- 1 teaspoon butter
- 6 hamburger buns, split
- 6 slices reduced-fat cheddar cheese
- 6 lettuce leaves
- 6 slices tomato

- In a large nonstick skillet coated with cooking spray, saute onion and garlic for 1 minute. Add the zucchini, yellow squash and carrots; saute until tender. Drain and cool to room temperature.

- In a large bowl, combine the egg, bread crumbs, tuna, salt and pepper. Add vegetable mixture. Shape into six 3-1/2-in. patties.

- Coat the same skillet again with cooking spray; cook the patties in butter for 3-5 minutes on each side or until lightly browned. Serve on buns with cheese, lettuce and tomato.

YIELD: 6 servings.

NUTRITION FACTS: 1 burger equals 275 calories, 8 g fat (4 g saturated fat), 58 mg cholesterol, 643 mg sodium, 32 g carbohydrate, 3 g fiber, 20 g protein. **DIABETIC EXCHANGES:** 2 starch, 2 lean meat, 1 vegetable.

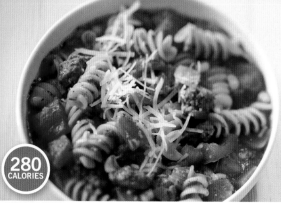

280 CALORIES

LASAGNA SOUP

lasagna soup

PREP: 10 minutes I **COOK:** 20 minutes

Sheryl Olenick I DEMAREST, NEW JERSEY

All the traditional flavors of lasagna come together in this heartwarming meal-in-a-bowl.

- 1 pound lean ground beef (90% lean)
- 1 large green pepper, chopped
- 1 medium onion, chopped
- 2 garlic cloves, minced
- 2 cans (14-1/2 ounces *each*) reduced-sodium beef broth
- 2 cans (14-1/2 ounces *each*) diced tomatoes
- 1 can (8 ounces) tomato sauce
- 1 cup frozen corn
- 1/4 cup tomato paste
- 2 teaspoons Italian seasoning
- 1/4 teaspoon pepper
- 2-1/2 cups uncooked spiral pasta
- 1/2 cup shredded Parmesan cheese

- In a large saucepan, cook the beef, green pepper and onion over medium heat until meat is no longer pink. Add garlic; cook 1 minute longer. Drain.

- Stir in the broth, tomatoes, tomato sauce, corn, tomato paste, Italian seasoning and pepper. Bring to a boil. Stir in pasta. Return to a boil. Reduce heat; cover and simmer for 10-12 minutes or until pasta is tender. Sprinkle with cheese.

YIELD: 8 servings.

NUTRITION FACTS: 1-1/3 cups equals 280 calories, 7 g fat (3 g saturated fat), 41 mg cholesterol, 572 mg sodium, 35 g carbohydrate, 4 g fiber, 20 g protein. **DIABETIC EXCHANGES:** 2 lean meat, 2 vegetable, 1-1/2 starch.

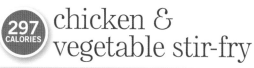

297 CALORIES

chicken & vegetable stir-fry

PREP: 20 minutes I **COOK:** 15 minutes

Samuel Onizuk I ELKTON, MARYLAND

You can't beat a stir-fry when you want a light entree that's both filling and delicious. Pepper flakes give this classic combination of chicken and veggies a palate-pleasing zip.

- 4 teaspoons cornstarch
- 1 cup reduced-sodium chicken broth
- 2 tablespoons reduced-sodium soy sauce
- 1 pound boneless skinless chicken breasts, cut into 1/4-inch strips
- 2 tablespoons olive oil, *divided*
- 1-1/2 cups fresh cauliflowerets
- 1-1/2 cups fresh broccoli florets
- 2 medium carrots, sliced
- 1 small sweet red pepper, julienned
- 1 small onion, halved and sliced
- 1 garlic clove, minced
- 1/2 teaspoon salt
- 1/2 teaspoon pepper
- 1/4 to 1/2 teaspoon crushed red pepper flakes
- 2-1/2 cups hot cooked rice

Minced fresh cilantro

- Combine the cornstarch, broth and soy sauce until smooth; set aside.

- In a large nonstick skillet or wok, stir-fry the chicken in 1 tablespoon of oil until no longer pink. Remove and keep warm.

- Stir-fry the cauliflower, broccoli, carrots, red pepper and onion in remaining oil until crisp-tender. Add the garlic, salt, pepper and pepper flakes; cook 1 minute longer.

- Stir cornstarch mixture and add to the pan. Bring to a boil; cook and stir for 2 minutes or until thickened. Add chicken; heat through. Serve with rice. Sprinkle each serving with cilantro.

YIELD: 5 servings.

NUTRITION FACTS: 1 cup stir-fry with 1/2 cup rice equals 297 calories, 8 g fat (1 g saturated fat), 50 mg cholesterol, 670 mg sodium, 32 g carbohydrate, 3 g fiber, 23 g protein. **DIABETIC EXCHANGES:** 2 lean meat, 1-1/2 starch, 1 vegetable, 1 fat.

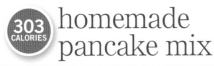

homemade pancake mix

303 CALORIES

PREP/TOTAL TIME: 20 minutes

Wendy Mink | HUNTINGTON, INDIANA

Whole wheat flour easily makes flapjacks more filling. We really like the blueberry-banana variation. It's great to have this mix on hand for busy mornings.

>   4 cups all-purpose flour
>   2 cups whole wheat flour
>   2/3 cup sugar
>   2 tablespoons baking powder
>   1 tablespoon baking soda

ADDITIONAL INGREDIENTS FOR PANCAKES:

>   1 egg
>   3/4 cup whole milk

ADDITIONAL INGREDIENTS FOR BLUEBERRY BANANA PANCAKES:

>   1 egg
>   3/4 cup whole milk
>   1 medium ripe banana, mashed
>   3/4 cup blueberries

- In a large bowl, combine the first five ingredients. Store in an airtight container in a cool dry place for up to 6 months.

YIELD: 6-7 batches of pancakes (about 6-3/4 cups total).

- **To prepare pancakes:** Contents of mix may settle during storage. When preparing recipe, spoon mix into measuring cup. In a small bowl, whisk egg and milk. Whisk in 1 cup pancake mix.

- Pour batter by 1/4 cupfuls onto a lightly greased hot griddle; turn when bubbles form on top of pancakes. Cook until second side is golden brown.

YIELD: about 6 pancakes per batch.

- **To prepare blueberry banana pancakes:** Contents of mix may settle during storage. When preparing recipe, spoon mix into measuring cup. In a large bowl, combine the egg, milk and banana. Whisk in 1 cup pancake mix. Fold in blueberries. Cook as directed above.

YIELD: about 8 pancakes per batch.

NUTRITION FACTS: 3 plain pancakes equals 303 calories, 5 g fat (2 g saturated fat), 98 mg cholesterol, 504 mg sodium, 53 g carbohydrate, 3 g fiber, 11 g protein.

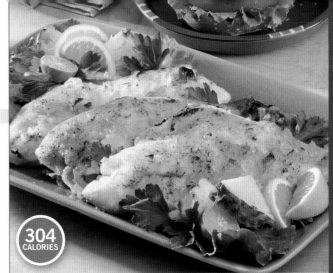

304 CALORIES

SNAPPER WITH SPICY PINEAPPLE GLAZE

snapper with spicy pineapple glaze

PREP: 15 minutes **| COOK:** 15 minutes

Taste of Home Test Kitchen

Ginger and cayenne pepper spice up this tangy treatment for moist red snapper fillets. Sweet pineapple preserves round out the delectable combination of flavors in this unique recipe.

>   1/2 cup pineapple preserves
>   2 tablespoons rice vinegar
>   2 teaspoons minced fresh gingerroot
>   2 garlic cloves, minced
>   3/4 teaspoon salt, *divided*
>   1/4 teaspoon cayenne pepper
>   4 red snapper fillets (6 ounces *each*)
>   3 teaspoons olive oil

- In a small bowl, combine the preserves, vinegar, ginger, garlic, 1/2 teaspoon salt and cayenne; set aside. Place fillets on a broiler pan coated with cooking spray. Spoon oil over both sides of fillets; sprinkle with remaining salt.

- Broil 4-6 in. from the heat for 5 minutes. Baste with half of the glaze. Broil 5-7 minutes longer or until fish flakes easily with a fork. Baste with remaining glaze.

YIELD: 4 servings.

NUTRITION FACTS: 1 fillet equals 304 calories, 6 g fat (1 g saturated fat), 63 mg cholesterol, 552 mg sodium, 27 g carbohydrate, trace fiber, 35 g protein. **DIABETIC EXCHANGES:** 5 lean meat, 2 starch.

20-minute or less prep recipes

312 CALORIES mexican-inspired turkey burgers

PREP: 15 minutes | **COOK:** 10 minutes

Heather Byers | PITTSBURGH, PENNSYLVANIA
We love grilled burgers, but turkey can be bland, and beef can be fatty. These patties balance taco spices and cheese to keep them light and lively.

- 1/2 cup salsa, *divided*
- 1/4 cup shredded reduced-fat cheddar cheese
- 3 teaspoons paprika
- 1 teaspoon dried oregano
- 1 teaspoon ground cumin
- 3/4 teaspoon sugar
- 3/4 teaspoon garlic powder
- 1/2 teaspoon dried thyme
- 1/4 teaspoon *each* salt and cayenne pepper
- 1 pound extra-lean ground turkey
- 1/4 cup reduced-fat sour cream
- 4 hamburger buns, split
- 1/2 cup torn curly endive
- 1 medium tomato, chopped

- In a large bowl, combine 1/4 cup salsa, cheese, paprika, oregano, cumin, sugar, garlic powder, thyme, salt and cayenne. Crumble turkey over mixture and mix well. Shape into four burgers.

- Using long-handled tongs, moisten a paper towel with cooking oil and lightly coat the grill rack. Grill, covered, over medium heat or broil 4 in. from the heat for 5-7 minutes on each side or until a meat thermometer reads 165° and juices run clear.

- In a small bowl, combine sour cream and remaining salsa. Place burgers on buns; top with endive, tomato and sour cream mixture.

YIELD: 4 servings.

NUTRITION FACTS: 1 burger equals 312 calories, 7 g fat (2 g saturated fat), 55 mg cholesterol, 599 mg sodium, 29 g carbohydrate, 3 g fiber, 36 g protein. **DIABETIC EXCHANGES:** 4 lean meat, 2 starch.

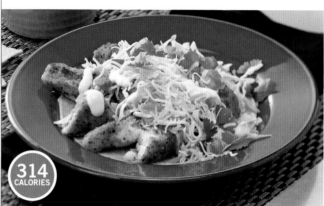

FANTASTIC FISH TACOS

314 CALORIES

fantastic fish tacos

PREP: 15 minutes | **COOK:** 10 minutes

Jennifer Palmer | RANCHO CUCAMONGA, CALIFORNIA
Searching for a lighter substitute to traditional fried fish tacos, I came up with this recipe. It's been a hit with friends and family. The orange roughy fillets are so mild that even non-fish eaters are pleasantly surprised by this tasty entree.

- 1/2 cup fat-free mayonnaise
- 1 tablespoon lime juice
- 2 teaspoons fat-free milk
- 1/3 cup dry bread crumbs
- 2 tablespoons salt-free lemon-pepper seasoning
- 1 egg, lightly beaten
- 1 teaspoon water
- 1 pound orange roughy fillets, cut into 1-inch strips
- 4 corn tortillas (6 inches), warmed
- 1 cup coleslaw mix
- 2 medium tomatoes, diced
- 1 cup (4 ounces) shredded reduced-fat Mexican cheese blend
- 1 tablespoon minced fresh cilantro

- In a small bowl, combine the mayonnaise, lime juice and milk; cover and refrigerate until serving.

- In a shallow bowl, combine bread crumbs and lemon pepper. In another shallow bowl, combine egg and water. Dip fish in egg mixture, then roll in crumbs.

- In a large nonstick skillet coated with cooking spray, cook fish over medium-high heat for 3-4 minutes on each side or until it flakes easily with a fork. Spoon onto tortillas; top with coleslaw mix, tomatoes, cheese and cilantro. Drizzle with mayonnaise mixture.

YIELD: 4 servings.

NUTRITION FACTS: 1 taco equals 314 calories, 10 g fat (4 g saturated fat), 99 mg cholesterol, 659 mg sodium, 32 g carbohydrate, 3 g fiber, 30 g protein. **DIABETIC EXCHANGES:** 4 lean meat, 2 starch.

raspberry chicken salad

PREP: 15 minutes | **COOK:** 15 minutes

Sue Zimonick | GREEN BAY, WISCONSIN

It's so easy to make this pretty summer salad—but it looks as though you toiled much longer. The slightly tart dressing also serves as a basting sauce, giving the thin slices of tender chicken breast a pleasant fruit flavor.

- 1 cup 100% raspberry spreadable fruit
- 1/3 cup raspberry vinegar
- 4 boneless skinless chicken breast halves (4 ounces *each*)
- 8 cups torn mixed salad greens
- 1 small red onion, thinly sliced
- 24 fresh raspberries

RASPBERRY CHICKEN SALAD

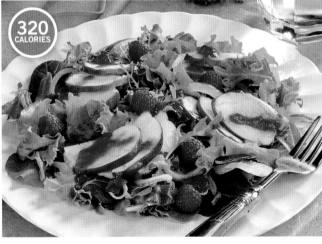

- In a small bowl, combine spreadable fruit and vinegar; set aside 3/4 cup for dressing. Broil chicken 4 in. from the heat for 5-7 minutes on each side or until a meat thermometer reads 170°, basting occasionally with remaining raspberry mixture. Cool for 10 minutes.

- Meanwhile, arrange greens and onion on salad plates. Slice chicken; place over greens. Drizzle with reserved dressing. Garnish with raspberries.

YIELD: 4 servings.

NUTRITION FACTS: 2 cups greens with 1 chicken breast half and 3 tablespoons dressing equals 320 calories, 3 g fat (1 g saturated fat), 63 mg cholesterol, 97 mg sodium, 48 g carbohydrate, 3 g fiber, 25 g protein. **DIABETIC EXCHANGES:** 3 starch, 3 lean meat, 2 vegetable.

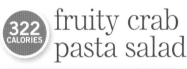

fruity crab pasta salad

PREP: 15 minutes | **COOK:** 15 minutes

Darlene Jurek | FOLEY, MINNESOTA

A sweet ginger dressing spices up this tasty medley of oranges, grapes, crabmeat and pasta. It's an ideal warm-weather entree.

- 3/4 cup uncooked spiral pasta
- 1 package (8 ounces) imitation crabmeat
- 1 snack-size cup (4 ounces) mandarin oranges, drained
- 1/4 cup halved seedless red grapes
- 1/4 cup halved seedless green grapes
- 1/4 cup plain yogurt
- 2 tablespoons mayonnaise
- 1-1/2 teaspoons honey
- 1/4 teaspoon ground ginger

- Cook pasta according to package directions; drain and rinse in cold water. In a small bowl, combine the pasta, crab, oranges and grapes.

- Combine the yogurt, mayonnaise, honey and ginger; pour over salad and toss to coat. Refrigerate until serving.

YIELD: 2 servings.

NUTRITION FACTS: 1-1/2 cups (prepared with reduced-fat yogurt and fat-free mayonnaise) equals 322 calories, 2 g fat (1 g saturated fat), 59 mg cholesterol, 215 mg sodium, 55 g carbohydrate, 2 g fiber, 21 g protein.

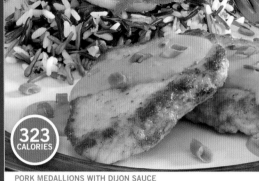

323 CALORIES

PORK MEDALLIONS WITH DIJON SAUCE

pork medallions with dijon sauce

PREP: 15 minutes I **COOK:** 10 minutes

Lois Kinneberg I PHOENIX, ARIZONA
I lightened up this recipe years ago, and I've been using it ever since. I brown pork in a skillet before swiftly stirring up a succulent sauce.

1	pork tenderloin (1 pound)
1/3	cup all-purpose flour
1/4	teaspoon salt
1/4	teaspoon pepper
1	tablespoon butter
3	green onions
1/3	cup white wine *or* chicken broth
1/2	cup fat-free evaporated milk
4	teaspoons Dijon mustard

- Cut pork widthwise into 6 pieces; flatten to 1/4-in. thickness. In a large resealable plastic bag, combine the flour, salt and pepper. Add pork, a few pieces at a time, and shake to coat. In a large nonstick skillet, brown pork in butter over medium-high heat. Remove and keep warm.

- Slice green onions, separating the white and green portions; reserve green portion for garnish. In the same skillet, saute the white portion of green onions for 1 minute. Add wine.

- Bring to a boil; cook until liquid is reduced to about 2 tablespoons. Add milk. Reduce heat; simmer, uncovered, for 1-2 minutes or until slightly thickened. Whisk in mustard. Serve pork with Dijon sauce. Garnish with reserved green onions.

YIELD: 3 servings.

NUTRITION FACTS: 1 serving equals 323 calories, 10 g fat (4 g saturated fat), 96 mg cholesterol, 516 mg sodium, 18 g carbohydrate, 1 g fiber, 35 g protein. **DIABETIC EXCHANGES:** 4 lean meat, 1 starch, 1/2 fat.

325 CALORIES

colorful beef wraps

PREP: 15 minutes I **COOK:** 15 minutes

Robyn Cavallaro I EASTON, PENNSYLVANIA
For an unbeatable sandwich, try the combination of sirloin steak, onions and peppers in these hearty wraps. Spreading a little fat-free ranch salad dressing inside the tortillas really livens up the taste.

1	beef top sirloin steak (1 pound), cut into thin strips
1/4	teaspoon pepper
3	tablespoons reduced-sodium soy sauce, *divided*
3	teaspoons olive oil, *divided*
1	medium red onion, cut into wedges
3	garlic cloves, minced
1	jar (7 ounces) roasted sweet red peppers, drained and cut into strips
1/4	cup dry red wine *or* reduced-sodium beef broth
6	tablespoons fat-free ranch salad dressing
6	flour tortillas (8 inches)
1-1/2	cups torn iceberg lettuce
1	medium tomato, chopped
1/4	cup chopped green onions

- In a large nonstick skillet coated with cooking spray, saute beef, pepper and 2 tablespoons soy sauce in 2 teaspoons oil until meat is no longer pink. Remove and keep warm.

- Saute the onion and garlic in the remaining oil for 1 minute. Stir in the red peppers, wine and remaining soy sauce; bring to a boil. Return beef to the pan; simmer for 5 minutes or until heated through.

- Spread ranch dressing over one side of each tortilla; sprinkle with lettuce, tomato and green onions. Spoon about 3/4 cup beef mixture down the center of each tortilla; roll up.

YIELD: 6 servings.

NUTRITION FACTS: 1 wrap equals 325 calories, 9 g fat (2 g saturated fat), 43 mg cholesterol, 830 mg sodium, 39 g carbohydrate, 1 g fiber, 20 g protein. **DIABETIC EXCHANGES:** 2 starch, 2 lean meat, 1 vegetable, 1 fat.

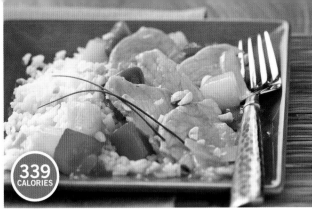

POLYNESIAN STIR-FRY

polynesian stir-fry

PREP: 15 minutes | **COOK:** 15 minutes

Susie Van Etten | CHAPMANSBORO, TENNESSEE
You'll get a restaurant-quality meal when you blend the sweet taste of pineapple and apricot with crunchy veggies and tender pork. I like the peanuts on top.

1 can (8 ounces) unsweetened pineapple chunks
1 tablespoon cornstarch
2 tablespoons cold water
1 tablespoon reduced-sodium soy sauce
2 tablespoons reduced-sugar apricot preserves
1 pork tenderloin (1 pound), thinly sliced
3 teaspoons canola oil, *divided*
1 medium onion, halved and sliced
1 small green pepper, cut into 1-inch pieces
1 small sweet red pepper, cut into 1-inch pieces
2 cups hot cooked rice

Chopped unsalted peanuts, optional

- Drain pineapple, reserving juice; set aside. For sauce, in a small bowl, combine cornstarch and water until smooth. Stir in the soy sauce, preserves and reserved pineapple juice; set aside.

- In a large nonstick skillet or wok, stir-fry the pork in 2 teaspoons oil until no longer pink. Remove; keep warm.

- Stir-fry the onion and peppers in remaining oil for 3 minutes. Add pineapple; stir-fry 2-3 minutes longer or until vegetables are crisp-tender.

- Stir cornstarch mixture and add to the pan. Bring to a boil; cook and stir for 2 minutes or until thickened. Add pork; heat through. Serve with rice. Just before serving, sprinkle each serving with peanuts if desired.

YIELD: 4 servings.

NUTRITION FACTS: 1 cup stir-fry with 1/2 cup rice (calculated without peanuts) equals equals 339 calories, 8 g fat (2 g saturated fat), 63 mg cholesterol, 204 mg sodium, 40 g carbohydrate, 2 g fiber, 26 g protein. **DIABETIC EXCHANGES:** 3 lean meat, 1-1/2 starch, 1 vegetable, 1/2 fruit, 1/2 fat.

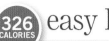 # easy beef stroganoff

PREP: 15 minutes | **COOK:** 15 minutes

Jennifer Riordan | ST. LOUIS, MISSOURI
I lightened my mother-in-law's wonderful stroganoff and came up with this one. My family calls it "special noodles" because this dish is so good.

4-1/2 cups uncooked yolk-free noodles
1 pound lean ground beef (90% lean)
1/2 pound sliced fresh mushrooms
1 large onion, halved and sliced
3 garlic cloves, minced
1 tablespoon reduced-fat butter
2 tablespoons all-purpose flour
1 can (14-1/2 ounces) reduced-sodium beef broth
2 tablespoons tomato paste
1 cup (8 ounces) fat-free sour cream
1/4 teaspoon salt
1/4 teaspoon pepper

- Cook noodles according to package directions. Meanwhile, in a large saucepan, cook the beef, mushrooms and onion over medium heat until meat is no longer pink. Add garlic; cook 1 minute longer. Drain. Remove and keep warm.

- In the same pan, melt butter. Stir in flour until smooth; gradually add broth and tomato paste. Bring to a boil; cook and stir for 2 minutes or until thickened.

- Carefully return beef mixture to the pan. Add the sour cream, salt and pepper; cook and stir until heated through (do not boil). Drain noodles; serve with the beef mixture.

YIELD: 6 servings.

EDITOR'S NOTE: This recipe was tested with Land O'Lakes light stick butter.

NUTRITION FACTS: 2/3 cup beef mixture with 3/4 cup noodles equals 326 calories, 7 g fat (3 g saturated fat), 48 mg cholesterol, 342 mg sodium, 39 g carbohydrate, 3 g fiber, 24 g protein. **DIABETIC EXCHANGES:** 2 starch, 2 lean meat, 1 vegetable.

- Bake, uncovered, at 400° for 20-25 minutes or until chicken is no longer pink and vegetables are tender. Spoon onto tortillas; fold in sides.

YIELD: 6 servings.

NUTRITION FACTS: 2 fajitas equals 340 calories, 8 g fat (1 g saturated fat), 44 mg cholesterol, 330 mg sodium, 41 g carbohydrate, 5 g fiber, 27 g protein. **DIABETIC EXCHANGES:** 2 starch, 2 lean meat, 2 vegetable, 1 fat.

scallops with angel hair

PREP: 15 minutes | **COOK:** 15 minutes

Nancy Mueller | MENOMONEE FALLS, WISCONSIN
Scallops taste extravagant, but they're actually low in fat. This wonderful recipe pairs them with superfine pasta lightly coated with a lively wine, garlic, onion and lemon sauce.

8	ounces uncooked angel hair pasta
3/4	pound bay scallops
2	teaspoons olive oil, *divided*
1	small onion, chopped
2	garlic cloves, minced
1	cup vegetable broth
1/4	cup dry white wine *or* additional vegetable broth
2	tablespoons lemon juice

SCALLOPS WITH ANGEL HAIR

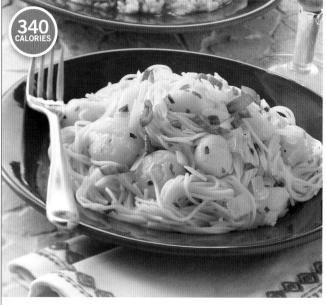

340 CALORIES

BAKED CHICKEN FAJITAS

baked chicken fajitas

PREP: 10 minutes | **COOK:** 20 minutes

Amy Trinkle | MILWAUKEE, WISCONSIN
I can't remember when or where I found this recipe, but I've used it nearly every week since. We like it with hot sauce for added spice.

1	pound boneless skinless chicken breasts, cut into thin strips
1	can (14-1/2 ounces) diced tomatoes and green chilies, drained
1	medium onion, cut into thin strips
1	medium green pepper, cut into thin strips
1	medium sweet red pepper, cut into thin strips
2	tablespoons canola oil
2	teaspoons chili powder
2	teaspoons ground cumin
1/4	teaspoon salt
12	flour tortillas (6 inches), warmed

- In a 13-in. x 9-in. baking dish coated with cooking spray, combine the chicken, tomatoes, onion and peppers. Combine the oil, chili powder, cumin and salt. Drizzle over chicken mixture; toss to coat.

340 CALORIES

> **I work out** on the treadmill in the evenings while watching my favorite TV shows.
> —Mya Hyland

1/4 teaspoon salt

1/8 teaspoon pepper

2 teaspoons cornstarch

2 teaspoons water

1/4 cup minced fresh parsley

Shredded Parmesan cheese and thinly sliced green onions, optional

- Cook pasta according to package directions. Meanwhile, in a large nonstick skillet coated with cooking spray, cook scallops in 1 teaspoon oil over medium heat until firm and opaque; remove and keep warm.

- In the same skillet, saute onion in remaining oil until tender. Add garlic; cook 1 minute longer. Stir in the broth, wine, lemon juice, salt and pepper. Bring to a boil. Combine cornstarch and water until smooth. Gradually stir into the pan. Bring to a boil; cook and stir for 2 minutes or until thickened. Stir in parsley and reserved scallops; heat through.

- Drain pasta; serve with scallops. Sprinkle with cheese and green onions if desired.

YIELD: 4 servings.

NUTRITION FACTS: 1/3 cup scallop mixture with 1 cup pasta (calculated without cheese) equals 340 calories, 4 g fat (1 g saturated fat), 28 mg cholesterol, 527 mg sodium, 50 g carbohydrate, 2 g fiber, 22 g protein.

tortellini primavera

PREP: 15 minutes I **COOK:** 15 minutes

Susie Pietrowski I BELTON, TEXAS

When you make this decadent tortellini with spinach, mushrooms and tomatoes, you're sure to hear compliments on your cooking. Dressed up with fresh Parmesan cheese, no one even notices it's meatless!

1 package (19 ounces) frozen cheese tortellini

1/2 pound sliced fresh mushrooms

1 small onion, chopped

2 teaspoons butter

2 garlic cloves, minced

2/3 cup fat-free milk

1 package (8 ounces) fat-free cream cheese, cubed

1 package (10 ounces) frozen chopped spinach, thawed and squeezed dry

1 teaspoon Italian seasoning

1 large tomato, chopped

1/4 cup shredded Parmesan cheese

- Cook tortellini according to package directions. Meanwhile, in a large nonstick skillet coated with cooking spray, saute mushrooms and onion in butter until tender. Add garlic; cook 1 minute longer. Stir in milk; heat through. Stir in cream cheese until blended. Add spinach and Italian seasoning; heat through.

- Drain tortellini; toss with sauce and tomato. Sprinkle with Parmesan cheese.

YIELD: 5 servings.

NUTRITION FACTS: 1-1/4 cups equals 341 calories, 10 g fat (5 g saturated fat), 28 mg cholesterol, 671 mg sodium, 41 g carbohydrate, 4 g fiber, 23 g protein. **DIABETIC EXCHANGES:** 2-1/2 starch, 2 lean meat, 1 vegetable.

TORTELLINI PRIMAVERA

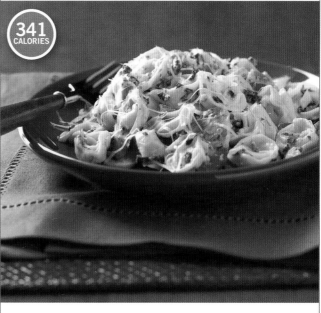

341 CALORIES

349 CALORIES

scallops & shrimp with yellow rice

PREP: 10 minutes | **COOK:** 20 minutes

Lillian Charves | NEW BERN, NORTH CAROLINA
Bright, colorful and weeknight-simple, this seafood entree is special enough to serve company, too.

- 1 large onion, chopped
- 1 tablespoon olive oil
- 1 garlic clove, minced
- 1 cup uncooked long grain rice
- 1/2 teaspoon ground turmeric
- 1 can (14-1/2 ounces) reduced-sodium chicken broth
- 3/4 cup water
- 1/2 pound uncooked medium shrimp, peeled and deveined
- 1/2 pound bay scallops
- 1 cup frozen peas
- 1/4 teaspoon salt
- 1/8 teaspoon pepper

- In a large nonstick skillet, saute onion in oil until tender. Add garlic; cook 1 minute longer. Add rice and turmeric; stir to coat. Stir in broth and water. Bring to a boil. Reduce heat; cover and simmer for 15 minutes or until rice is tender.

- Stir in the remaining ingredients; return to a boil. Reduce heat; cover and simmer for 5 minutes or until shrimp turn pink.

YIELD: 4 servings.

NUTRITION FACTS: 1-1/2 cups equals 349 calories, 5 g fat (1 g saturated fat), 88 mg cholesterol, 646 mg sodium, 48 g carbohydrate, 3 g fiber, 26 g protein. **DIABETIC EXCHANGES:** 3 starch, 3 lean meat, 1/2 fat.

fettuccine with black bean sauce

PREP: 15 minutes | **COOK:** 15 minutes

Marianne Neuman | EAST TROY, WISCONSIN
I had to come up with new ways to get more vegetables into our daily menus. This meatless spaghetti sauce is a winner. It's especially delicious with spinach fettuccine.

- 6 ounces uncooked fettuccine
- 1 small green pepper, chopped
- 1 small onion, chopped
- 1 tablespoon olive oil
- 2 cups garden-style pasta sauce
- 1 can (15 ounces) black beans, rinsed and drained
- 2 tablespoons minced fresh basil *or* 2 teaspoons dried basil
- 1 teaspoon dried oregano
- 1/2 teaspoon fennel seed
- 1/4 teaspoon garlic salt
- 1 cup (4 ounces) shredded part-skim mozzarella cheese

- Cook fettuccine according to package directions. Meanwhile, in a large saucepan, saute green pepper and onion in oil until tender. Stir in the pasta sauce, black beans and seasonings.

- Bring to a boil. Reduce heat; simmer, uncovered, for 5 minutes. Drain fettuccine. Top with sauce and sprinkle with cheese.

YIELD: 5 servings.

NUTRITION FACTS: 3/4 cup pasta with 3/4 cup sauce and 3 tablespoons cheese equals 350 calories, 10 g fat (3 g saturated fat), 17 mg cholesterol, 761 mg sodium, 51 g carbohydrate, 8 g fiber, 16 g protein. **DIABETIC EXCHANGES:** 2-1/2 starch, 2 vegetable, 1 lean meat, 1 fat.

FETTUCCINE WITH BLACK BEAN SAUCE

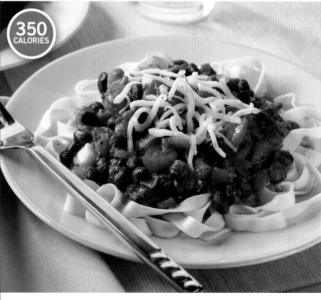

350 CALORIES

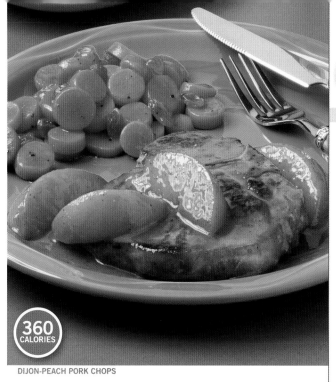

DIJON-PEACH PORK CHOPS

dijon-peach pork chops

PREP: 5 minutes I **COOK:** 20 minutes

Debbie Liberton I BOERNE, TEXAS

I invented this dish one night when I was missing half the ingredients for a pork chop recipe I planned to make. The moist chops in this recipe are swiftly simmered on the stove along with canned peaches, mustard and cloves.

4 bone-in pork loin chops (1/2 inch thick and 7 ounces *each*)
1 can (15-1/4 ounces) sliced peaches, undrained
1/4 cup packed brown sugar
1/4 cup Dijon mustard
1/4 teaspoon ground cloves

- In a large skillet coated with cooking spray, brown pork chops over medium-high heat for 4-5 minutes on each side. Stir in the remaining ingredients. Bring to a boil. Reduce heat; cover and simmer for 10 minutes or until meat is tender.

YIELD: 4 servings.

NUTRITION FACTS: 1 pork chop equals 360 calories, 10 g fat (3 g saturated fat), 86 mg cholesterol, 456 mg sodium, 36 g carbohydrate, 1 g fiber, 31 g protein. **DIABETIC EXCHANGES:** 4 lean meat, 2-1/2 starch.

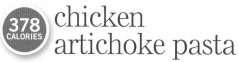

chicken artichoke pasta

PREP: 15 minutes I **COOK:** 15 minutes

Cathy Dick I ROANOKE, VIRGINIA

Here's a colorful, delicious chicken dish that's so easy you'll be making it on busy days and for guests.

2-1/4 cups uncooked ziti *or* 6 ounces uncooked fettuccine
1 pound boneless skinless chicken breasts, cut into thin strips
3 teaspoons olive oil, *divided*
1/2 cup fresh broccoli florets
1/2 cup sliced fresh mushrooms
1/2 cup cherry tomatoes, halved
2 garlic cloves, minced
1 can (14 ounces) water-packed artichoke hearts, rinsed, drained and halved
1/2 teaspoon *each* salt and dried oregano
2 teaspoons all-purpose flour
1/4 cup reduced-sodium chicken broth
1/3 cup white wine *or* additional reduced-sodium chicken broth
1 tablespoon minced fresh parsley
1 tablespoon shredded Parmesan cheese

- Cook ziti according to package directions. Meanwhile, in a large nonstick skillet coated with cooking spray, cook chicken in 2 teaspoons oil over medium heat until no longer pink. Remove and keep warm.

- In the same skillet, cook and stir broccoli in remaining oil for 2 minutes. Stir in the mushrooms, tomatoes and garlic; cook 2 minutes longer. Add the artichokes, salt and oregano; heat through.

- Combine the flour with broth and wine or additional broth until smooth; stir into the pan. Bring to a boil; cook and stir for 1-2 minutes or until thickened. Add parsley and reserved chicken.

- Drain ziti; add to chicken mixture and toss to coat. Sprinkle with cheese.

YIELD: 4 servings.

NUTRITION FACTS: 2 cups equals 378 calories, 8 g fat (2 g saturated fat), 64 mg cholesterol, 668 mg sodium, 41 g carbohydrate, 2 g fiber, 33 g protein. **DIABETIC EXCHANGES:** 3 lean meat, 2 starch, 2 vegetable, 1 fat.

> **I work in our yard** almost every day, raking, trimming, planting flowers and vegetables and transplanting plants. These jobs keep me active.
> —Cynthia Pennington Lowery

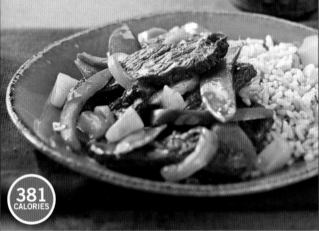

381 CALORIES

PINEAPPLE BEEF STIR-FRY FOR TWO

pineapple beef stir-fry for two

PREP: 20 minutes + marinating | **COOK:** 15 minutes

Jackie Drake | TROUTMAN, NORTH CAROLINA
Packed with veggies, tender beef and pineapple tidbits, this sweet-and-sour stir-fry is ideal for blustery weeknights or activity-packed weekends. I know you'll love the tasty combination of flavors.

for 2

- 1/2 cup unsweetened pineapple juice
- 2 tablespoons white wine *or* reduced-sodium chicken broth
- 1 tablespoon packed brown sugar
- 1 tablespoon reduced-sodium soy sauce
- 1/8 teaspoon cayenne pepper
- 1/2 pound beef top sirloin steak, cut into thin strips
- 1 tablespoon cornstarch
- 3/4 teaspoon olive oil, *divided*
- 1 large carrot, sliced
- 1/2 small onion, halved and sliced
- 1 small green pepper, julienned
- 1/4 cup fresh snow peas
- 1/3 cup unsweetened pineapple tidbits
- 1 cup cooked brown rice

- In a small bowl, combine the first five ingredients. Pour 1/3 cup marinade into a large resealable plastic bag; add the beef. Seal bag and turn to coat; refrigerate for 30 minutes. Cover and refrigerate remaining marinade.

- In a small bowl, combine cornstarch and reserved marinade until smooth; set aside.

- Drain and discard marinade from bag. In a large nonstick skillet or wok, stir-fry beef in 1/2 teaspoon oil for 2-3 minutes or until no longer pink. Remove with a slotted spoon and keep warm.

- Stir-fry carrots and onion in remaining oil for 4 minutes. Add green pepper and snow peas; stir-fry 2-3 minutes longer or until vegetables are crisp-tender.

- Stir cornstarch mixture and add to the pan. Bring to a boil; cook and stir for 2 minutes or until thickened. Add beef and pineapple; heat through. Serve with rice.

YIELD: 2 servings.

NUTRITION FACTS: 1 cup stir-fry with 1/2 cup rice equals 381 calories, 7 g fat (2 g saturated fat), 46 mg cholesterol, 328 mg sodium, 49 g carbohydrate, 4 g fiber, 29 g protein.

portobello burgundy beef

PREP: 20 minutes | **COOK:** 35 minutes

Melanie Coleman | PITTSBURG, CALIFORNIA
Nothing feels light about this rustic dish! Each bite is filled with mushrooms, beef and carrots wrapped in a savory, Burgundy sauce. This dish is real comfort food at its finest!

- 1/4 cup plus 1 tablespoon all-purpose flour, *divided*
- 1 teaspoon dried marjoram, *divided*
- 1/2 teaspoon salt, *divided*
- 1 beef top round steak (1 pound), cut into 1/2-inch cubes
- 1 tablespoon olive oil
- 2 cups sliced baby portobello mushrooms
- 3 garlic cloves, minced

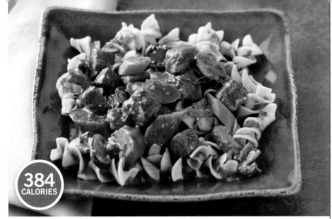

384 CALORIES

PORTOBELLO BURGUNDY BEEF

3 medium carrots, cut into 1/2-inch pieces
1 can (14-1/2 ounces) reduced-sodium beef broth, *divided*
1/2 cup Burgundy wine *or* additional reduced-sodium beef broth
1 bay leaf
4 cups cooked egg noodles

- Place 1/4 cup flour, 1/2 teaspoon marjoram and 1/4 teaspoon salt in a large resealable plastic bag. Add beef, a few pieces at a time, and shake to coat. In a large nonstick skillet coated with cooking spray, brown beef in oil.

- Add mushrooms and garlic; saute until mushrooms are tender. Stir in the carrots, 1-1/2 cups broth, wine, bay leaf, remaining marjoram and salt. Bring to a boil. Reduce heat; cover and simmer for 15-20 minutes or until carrots are tender.

- Combine remaining flour and broth; stir into pan. Bring to a boil; cook and stir for 2 minutes or until thickened. Discard bay leaf. Serve with noodles.

YIELD: 4 servings.

NUTRITION FACTS: 1 cup beef mixture with 1 cup noodles equals 384 calories, 9 g fat (2 g saturated fat), 98 mg cholesterol, 484 mg sodium, 39 g carbohydrate, 3 g fiber, 34 g protein. **DIABETIC EXCHANGES:** 3 lean meat, 2 starch, 1 vegetable, 1/2 fat.

sweet-and-sour beef

PREP: 15 minutes I **COOK:** 15 minutes

Brittany McCloud I KENYON, MINNESOTA
Looking for a new family favorite? Try this healthful stir-fry recipe. I've used a variety of meats and apples and sometimes replace the green onion with yellow onion. It always tastes great—and it always satisfies!

1 pound beef top sirloin steak, cut into 1/2-inch cubes
1 teaspoon salt
1/2 teaspoon pepper
3 teaspoons canola oil, *divided*
1 large green pepper, cut into 1/2-inch pieces
1 large sweet red pepper, cut into 1/2-inch pieces
2 medium tart apples, chopped
1/2 cup plus 2 tablespoons thinly sliced green onions, *divided*
2/3 cup packed brown sugar
1/2 cup cider vinegar
1 tablespoon cornstarch
2 tablespoons cold water
Hot cooked rice, optional

- Sprinkle beef with salt and pepper. In a nonstick skillet or wok coated with cooking spray, stir-fry beef in 2 teaspoons oil until no longer pink. Remove and keep warm.

- In the same pan, stir-fry peppers and apples in remaining oil for 3 minutes. Add 1/2 cup green onions. Stir-fry 2-3 minutes longer or until peppers are crisp-tender. Remove and keep warm.

- Add brown sugar and vinegar to pan; bring to a boil. Combine cornstarch and water until smooth; stir into brown sugar mixture. Return to a boil; cook and stir for 2 minutes or until thickened and bubbly.

- Return beef and vegetable mixture to pan; heat through. Garnish with remaining onions. Serve with rice if desired.

YIELD: 4 servings.

NUTRITION FACTS: 1-1/2 cups (calculated without rice) equals 389 calories, 8 g fat (2 g saturated fat), 46 mg cholesterol, 663 mg sodium, 53 g carbohydrate, 4 g fiber, 25 g protein.

SWEET-AND-SOUR BEEF

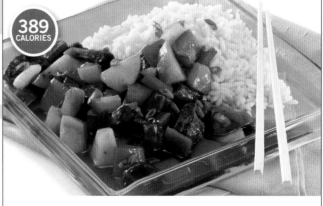

389 CALORIES

389 CALORIES

WEEKNIGHT BEEF SKILLET

weeknight beef skillet

PREP: 20 minutes | **COOK:** 10 minutes

Clara Coulson Minney | WASHINGTON COURT HOUSE, OHIO

Satisfy hearty appetites with this mild but filling dish chock-full of veggies, Italian seasoning and nutrition. It's a quick-and-easy meal that just might become one of your family's new favorites!

- 3 cups uncooked yolk-free whole wheat noodles
- 1 pound lean ground beef (90% lean)
- 1 medium green pepper, finely chopped
- 1 package (16 ounces) frozen mixed vegetables, thawed and drained
- 1 can (15 ounces) tomato sauce
- 1 tablespoon Worcestershire sauce
- 1-1/2 teaspoons Italian seasoning
- 2 teaspoons sugar
- 1/4 teaspoon salt
- 1/4 cup minced fresh parsley

- Cook noodles according to package directions. Meanwhile, in a large nonstick skillet over medium heat, cook beef and pepper until meat is no longer pink; drain.

- Stir in the mixed vegetables, tomato sauce, Worcestershire sauce, Italian seasoning, sugar and salt; heat through. Drain noodles; serve with meat mixture. Sprinkle with parsley.

YIELD: 4 servings.

NUTRITION FACTS: 1-1/4 cups beef mixture with 3/4 cup noodles equals 389 calories, 9 g fat (3 g saturated fat), 56 mg cholesterol, 800 mg sodium, 49 g carbohydrate, 10 g fiber, 31 g protein. **DIABETIC EXCHANGES:** 3 starch, 3 lean meat, 1 vegetable.

---

417 CALORIES

spicy warm chicken salad

PREP: 10 minutes | **COOK:** 20 minutes

Iola Egle | BELLA VISTA, ARKANSAS

This flavorful salad makes a great cool-weather entree. It's tasty, colorful and on the table in half an hour.

- 1 envelope onion soup mix
- 4 boneless skinless chicken breast halves (4 ounces *each*)
- 2 tablespoons olive oil
- 1 can (15 ounces) pinto beans, rinsed and drained
- 1 cup frozen corn
- 1/2 cup picante sauce
- 1 can (4 ounces) chopped green chilies
- 1/4 cup chopped green onions
- 1/2 cup *each* sour cream and jalapeno pepper jelly
- 1 tablespoon lemon juice
- 2 cups chopped iceberg lettuce
- 2 cups torn romaine
- 1 small sweet red pepper, thinly sliced
- 1/4 cup minced fresh cilantro
- 2 jalapeno peppers, seeded and chopped, optional

- Rub soup mix over both sides of chicken. In a large skillet, cook chicken in oil over medium heat for 8-10 minutes on each side or until a meat thermometer reads 170°. Remove and keep warm.

- In the same skillet, combine the beans, corn and picante sauce. Cook and stir over medium heat for 2-3 minutes or until heated through. Stir in chilies and onions; set aside. In a small bowl, combine the sour cream, pepper jelly and lemon juice; set aside.

- Toss lettuce and romaine; divide among four salad plates. Slice chicken; arrange on greens. Place red pepper slices and bean mixture around chicken. Drizzle with sour cream mixture; sprinkle with cilantro. Serve with jalapenos if desired.

YIELD: 4 servings.

EDITOR'S NOTE: We recommend wearing disposable gloves when cutting hot peppers. Avoid touching your face.

NUTRITION FACTS: 1 serving (prepared with reduced-fat sour cream) equals 417 calories, 11 g fat (3 g saturated fat), 26 mg cholesterol, 1,054 mg sodium, 65 g carbohydrate, 8 g fiber, 16 g protein.

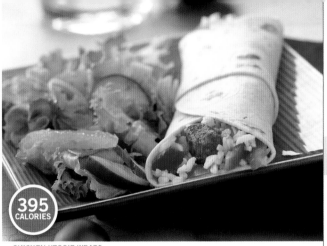

CHICKEN VEGGIE WRAPS

chicken veggie wraps

PREP: 15 minutes | **COOK:** 15 minutes

Kendra Katt | ALBUQUERQUE, NEW MEXICO
I gathered bits and pieces of things I like about Southwest cooking to come up with this economical recipe. Serve with a green salad and vinaigrette dressing for a refreshing meal.

- 1-1/2 cups uncooked instant rice
- 1 medium tomato, chopped
- 2 cans (4 ounces *each*) chopped green chilies
- 7 tablespoons lime juice, *divided*
- 1-1/2 teaspoons chili powder
- 1-1/2 teaspoons ground cumin
- 1/2 teaspoon salt
- 1 pound boneless skinless chicken breasts, cubed
- 3 teaspoons canola oil, *divided*
- 1 large onion, halved and sliced
- 1 large green pepper, julienned
- 1 large sweet red pepper, julienned
- 3 garlic cloves, minced
- 1 tablespoon brown sugar
- 6 flour tortillas (8 inches), warmed

- Cook rice according to package directions. Stir in the tomato, chilies and 3 tablespoons lime juice.

- Meanwhile, combine the chili powder, cumin and salt; sprinkle over chicken. In a large nonstick skillet coated with cooking spray, saute chicken in 2 teaspoons oil until no longer pink. Remove and keep warm.

- In the same skillet, cook onion and peppers in remaining oil until crisp-tender. Add garlic; cook for

1 minute longer. Stir in the brown sugar, chicken and remaining lime juice; heat through.

- Spoon 2/3 cup each of rice mixture and chicken mixture down the center of each tortilla; roll up.

YIELD: 6 servings.

NUTRITION FACTS: 1 wrap equals 395 calories, 8 g fat (1 g saturated fat), 42 mg cholesterol, 646 mg sodium, 59 g carbohydrate, 3 g fiber, 23 g protein.

family-favorite cheeseburger pasta

PREP: 15 minutes | **COOK:** 15 minutes

Raquel Haggard | EDMOND, OKLAHOMA
This recipe was invented to fulfill a cheeseburger craving. What a scrumptious yet healthy classic!

- 1-1/2 cups uncooked whole wheat penne pasta
- 3/4 pound lean ground beef (90% lean)
- 2 tablespoons finely chopped onion
- 1 can (14-1/2 ounces) no-salt-added diced tomatoes
- 2 tablespoons dill pickle relish
- 2 tablespoons *each* prepared mustard and ketchup
- 1 teaspoon steak seasoning
- 1/4 teaspoon seasoned salt
- 3/4 cup shredded reduced-fat cheddar cheese

Chopped green onions, optional

- Cook pasta according to package directions. Meanwhile, in a large skillet, cook beef and onion over medium heat until meat is no longer pink; drain. Drain pasta; add to meat mixture.

- Stir in the tomatoes, relish, mustard, ketchup, steak seasoning and seasoned salt. Bring to a boil. Reduce heat; simmer, uncovered, for 5 minutes.

- Sprinkle with cheese. Remove from the heat; cover and let stand until cheese is melted. Garnish with green onions if desired.

YIELD: 4 servings.

EDITOR'S NOTE: This recipe was tested with McCormick's Montreal Steak Seasoning. Look for it in the spice aisle.

NUTRITION FACTS: 1-1/2 cups equals 391 calories, 12 g fat (6 g saturated fat), 57 mg cholesterol, 759 mg sodium, 43 g carbohydrate, 4 g fiber, 28 g protein. **DIABETIC EXCHANGES:** 3 lean meat, 2 starch, 1 vegetable, 1/2 fat.

do-it-yourself
MEAL PLANNING
worksheet

date: _____

FOOD	CALORIES	FOOD	CALORIES

planned breakfast

_____ _____

_____ _____

_____ _____

_____ _____

PLANNED BREAKFAST TOTAL CALORIES: _____

actual breakfast

_____ _____

_____ _____

_____ _____

_____ _____

ACTUAL BREAKFAST TOTAL CALORIES: _____

planned lunch

_____ _____

_____ _____

_____ _____

_____ _____

PLANNED LUNCH TOTAL CALORIES: _____

actual lunch

_____ _____

_____ _____

_____ _____

_____ _____

ACTUAL LUNCH TOTAL CALORIES: _____

planned dinner

_____ _____

_____ _____

_____ _____

_____ _____

PLANNED DINNER TOTAL CALORIES: _____

actual dinner

_____ _____

_____ _____

_____ _____

_____ _____

ACTUAL DINNER TOTAL CALORIES: _____

planned snacks

_____ _____

_____ _____

PLANNED SNACKS TOTAL CALORIES: _____

actual snacks

_____ _____

_____ _____

ACTUAL SNACKS TOTAL CALORIES: _____

PLANNED TOTAL CALORIES: _____

ACTUAL TOTAL CALORIES: _____

exercise _____

_____

do-it-yourself
MEAL PLANNING
worksheet

date: _____

FOOD	CALORIES	FOOD	CALORIES
planned breakfast		actual breakfast	
_____	_____	_____	_____
_____	_____	_____	_____
_____	_____	_____	_____
_____	_____	_____	_____
PLANNED BREAKFAST TOTAL CALORIES:	_____	**ACTUAL BREAKFAST TOTAL CALORIES:**	_____
planned lunch		actual lunch	
_____	_____	_____	_____
_____	_____	_____	_____
_____	_____	_____	_____
_____	_____	_____	_____
PLANNED LUNCH TOTAL CALORIES:	_____	**ACTUAL LUNCH TOTAL CALORIES:**	_____
planned dinner		actual dinner	
_____	_____	_____	_____
_____	_____	_____	_____
_____	_____	_____	_____
_____	_____	_____	_____
PLANNED DINNER TOTAL CALORIES:	_____	**ACTUAL DINNER TOTAL CALORIES:**	_____
planned snacks		actual snacks	
_____	_____	_____	_____
_____	_____	_____	_____
PLANNED SNACKS TOTAL CALORIES:	_____	**ACTUAL SNACKS TOTAL CALORIES:**	_____
PLANNED TOTAL CALORIES:	_____	**ACTUAL TOTAL CALORIES:**	_____

exercise _____

_____

index by food category

To help you find the perfect dish for your family, we've created four different indexes.

This first one is divided into food and meal categories as well as major ingredients. Use this index when you're looking for recipes that call for a specific item or when you want to find an ideal appetizer, etc.

You'll also notice that major categories are broken down a bit. If you look up "Chicken," for instance, you'll notice that there are sub-categories for lunch dishes and dinner options.

Best of all, every entry in every index offers the calorie count per serving of that item. Planning a healthy meal for your family has never been easier!

APPLES

Apple-Cinnamon Oatmeal Mix
(176 CALORIES), **94**
Apple Cranberry Delight
(70 CALORIES), **238**
Apple Pork Stir-Fry (370 CALORIES), **164**
Apple Skewers (80 CALORIES), **265**
Apple Walnut Pancakes
(208 CALORIES), **95**
Applesauce-Glazed Pork Chops
(291 CALORIES), **259**
Chipotle Sweet Potato and Spiced Apple
Purees (224 CALORIES), **255**

Cranberry Apple Tart
(183 CALORIES), **218**
Cranberry-Stuffed Apples
(136 CALORIES), **227**
Curried Chicken with Apples
(272 CALORIES), **144**
French Toast with Apple Topping
(219 CALORIES), **96**
Puffy Apple Omelet (249 CALORIES), **277**
Turkey with Apple Slices
(263 CALORIES), **138**
Wholesome Apple-Hazelnut Stuffing
(159 CALORIES), **195**

APRICOTS

Apricot-Almond Chicken Breasts
(372 CALORIES), **262**
Apricot Turkey Sandwiches
(338 CALORIES), **116**
Cranberry-Apricot Pork Roast with
Potatoes (433 CALORIES), **235**

ARTICHOKES

Artichoke-Lamb Sandwich Loaves
(239 CALORIES), **105**
Chicken Artichoke Pasta
(378 CALORIES), **289**
Grilled Artichoke-Mushroom Pizza
(283 CALORIES), **146**

ASPARAGUS

Asparagus with Dill Sauce
(76 CALORIES), **179**
Balsamic Asparagus (45 CALORIES), **173**
Ham Asparagus Spirals (49 CALORIES), **80**
Spring Frittata (163 CALORIES), **91**
Springtime Barley (226 CALORIES), **201**

BACON & CANADIAN BACON

Bacon-Broccoli Quiche Cups
(170 CALORIES), **249**
Baked Eggs with Cheddar and Bacon
(107 CALORIES), **267**
Eggs Benedict (216 CALORIES), **96**

BANANAS

Banana Blueberry Smoothies
(99 CALORIES), **88**
Banana Split Cheesecake
(247 CALORIES), **223**

Makeover Frosted Banana Bars
(149 CALORIES), **216**

BARLEY, BULGUR & QUINOA

Barley Beef Skillet (400 CALORIES), **263**
Go for the Grains Casserole
(226 CALORIES), **202**
Great Grain Pilaf (154 CALORIES), **194**
Quinoa Pilaf (198 CALORIES), **272**
Springtime Barley (226 CALORIES), **201**

BEANS (ALSO SEE GREEN BEANS)

Alfresco Bean Salad (146 CALORIES), **192**
Black Bean Chicken Tacos
(267 CALORIES), **141**
Black Bean Chicken with Rice
(400 CALORIES), **263**
Black Bean Taco Pizza
(264 CALORIES), **108**
Corn Bread-Topped Frijoles
(367 CALORIES), **234**
Fettuccine with Black Bean Sauce
(350 CALORIES), **288**
Garbanzo Bean Pitas
(241 CALORIES), **105**
Go for the Grains Casserole
(226 CALORIES), **202**
Heavenly Earth Burgers
(320 CALORIES), **153**
Italian Sausage Bean Soup
(339 CALORIES), **115**
Southwest Black Bean Soup
(273 CALORIES), **109**
White Bean Soup (270 CALORIES), **108**
Zippy Three-Bean Chili
(269 CALORIES), **142**

BEEF (ALSO SEE GROUND BEEF)

LUNCHES
Colorful Beef Wraps (325 CALORIES), **284**
Red, White and Blue Pita Pockets
(351 CALORIES), **116**
Super Flatbread Wraps
(348 CALORIES), **261**

DINNERS
All-American Beef Stew
(324 CALORIES), **155**
Asian Orange Beef (351 CALORIES), **157**
Asian Steak Wraps (402 CALORIES), **169**

Baked Barbecued Brisket
(159 CALORIES), 247
Barley Beef Skillet (400 CALORIES), 263
BBQ Beef Sandwiches
(354 CALORIES), 233
Beef Kabobs with Chutney Sauce
(258 CALORIES), 257
Beef Roast Dinner (245 CALORIES), 230
Beef Tenderloin with Roasted Vegetables
(283 CALORIES), 147
Blue-Cheese Topped Steaks
(228 CALORIES), 132
Braised Southwest Beef Roast
(255 CALORIES), 136
Broiled Sirloin Steaks
(187 CALORIES), 126
Burgundy Beef Stew
(388 CALORIES), 234
Cajun Beef Tenderloin
(172 CALORIES), 124
Colorful Beef Stir-Fry
(318 CALORIES), 152
Flank Steak Pitas (362 CALORIES), 161
Herbed Beef Tenderloin
(198 CALORIES), 253
Home-Style Pot Roast
(341 CALORIES), 260
Hot 'n' Spicy Flank Steak
(201 CALORIES), 128
Hungarian Goulash (310 CALORIES), 151
Moroccan Beef Kabobs
(185 CALORIES), 125
Old-Fashioned Swiss Steak
(359 CALORIES), 160
Pineapple Beef Kabobs
(412 CALORIES), 170
Pineapple Beef Stir-Fry for Two
(381 CALORIES), 290
Portobello Burgundy Beef
(384 CALORIES), 290
Sirloin Roast with Gravy
(185 CALORIES), 227
Sirloin Strips over Rice
(299 CALORIES), 149
Southwestern Beef Stew
(222 CALORIES), 131
Stuffed Steak Spirals
(214 CALORIES), 130
Sweet-and-Sour Beef
(389 CALORIES), 291

Tex-Mex Beef Barbecues
(294 CALORIES), 232
Whiskey Sirloin Steak for Two
(169 CALORIES), 248

BEVERAGES
Banana Blueberry Smoothies
(99 CALORIES), 88
Strawberry Mango Smoothies for 2
(100 CALORIES), 84
Sun-Kissed Smoothies
(100 CALORIES), 85
Three-Fruit Smoothies
(225 CALORIES), 97
Tropical Fruit Smoothies
(97 CALORIES), 87

BLUEBERRIES
Baked Blueberry & Peach Oatmeal
(277 CALORIES), 99
Banana Blueberry Smoothies
(99 CALORIES), 88
Blueberry Oatmeal Pancakes
(171 CALORIES), 270
Blueberry-Stuffed French Toast
(167 CALORIES), 92
Cinnamon Blueberry Sauce
(50 CALORIES), 207

BREAKFASTS (ALSO SEE BEVERAGES; EGGS & EGG SUBSTITUTE)
Apple-Cinnamon Oatmeal Mix
(176 CALORIES), 94
Apple Walnut Pancakes
(208 CALORIES), 95
Baked Blueberry & Peach Oatmeal
(277 CALORIES), 99
Baked Peach Pancake
(157 CALORIES), 246
Blueberry Oatmeal Pancakes
(171 CALORIES), 270
Blueberry-Stuffed French Toast
(167 CALORIES), 92
Brunch Risotto (279 CALORIES), 258
Cafe Mocha Mini Muffins
(81 CALORIES), 266
Caramel Cream Crepes
(206 CALORIES), 95
Chewy Granola Bars (160 CALORIES), 90
Festive French Pancakes (163 CALORIES), 89

French Toast with Apple Topping
(219 CALORIES), 96
Garlic Cheese Grits (186 CALORIES), 94
Granola-to-Go Bars (130 CALORIES), 88
Homemade Pancake Mix
(303 CALORIES), 281
Orange Fruit Cups (80 CALORIES), 87
Turkey Breakfast Sausage
(85 CALORIES), 267
Whole Grain Waffle Mix
(284 CALORIES), 99
Zucchini Pancakes (88 CALORIES), 88

BROCCOLI
Bacon-Broccoli Quiche Cups
(170 CALORIES), 249
Bravo Broccoli (78 CALORIES), 180
Broccoli Brown Rice Pilaf
(202 CALORIES), 198
Broccoli-Cheddar Baked Potatoes
(226 CALORIES), 202
Broccoli-Cheese Stuffed Pizza
(252 CALORIES), 134
Broccoli-Turkey Casserole
(303 CALORIES), 150
Italian Broccoli with Peppers
(55 CALORIES), 174
Italian Vegetable Medley
(79 CALORIES), 180

CARROTS
Glazed Orange Carrots
(132 CALORIES), 191
Herbed Beans and Carrots
(63 CALORIES), 176
Parmesan Roasted Carrots
(82 CALORIES), 181

CHEESE
Baked Eggs with Cheddar and Bacon
(107 CALORIES), 267
Banana Split Cheesecake
(247 CALORIES), 223
Basil-Parmesan Angel Hair
(203 CALORIES), 199
Blue-Cheese Topped Steaks
(228 CALORIES), 132
Broccoli-Cheddar Baked Potatoes
(226 CALORIES), 202

CHEESE *(CONTINUED)*
Broccoli-Cheese Stuffed Pizza
(252 CALORIES), **134**
Cheesecake Phyllo Cups
(46 CALORIES), **80**
Cheesy Pita Crisps (95 CALORIES), **83**
Cheesy Rigatoni Bake
(274 CALORIES), **144**
Colorful Cheese Omelet
(167 CALORIES), **91**
French Cheeseburger Loaf
(277 CALORIES), **145**
Garlic Cheese Grits (186 CALORIES), **94**
Greek Pizzas (320 CALORIES), **155**
Gruyere Mashed Potatoes
(193 CALORIES), **197**
Hawaiian Breakfast Cups
(131 CALORIES), **242**
Hot Swiss Chicken Sandwiches
(218 CALORIES), **104**
Italian Cheese-Stuffed Shells
(351 CALORIES), **158**
Light Chicken Cordon Bleu
(306 CALORIES), **150**
Low-Fat Macaroni and Cheese
(250 CALORIES), **205**
Macaroni 'n' Cheese Italiano
(262 CALORIES), **106**
Monterey Quiche (265 CALORIES), **98**
No-Bake Cheesecake Pie
(141 CALORIES), **214**
Parmesan Cauliflower
(121 CALORIES), **189**
Parmesan Popcorn (49 CALORIES), **81**
Parmesan Pork Medallions
(220 CALORIES), **131**
Parmesan Roasted Carrots
(82 CALORIES), **181**
Southwestern Pasta & Cheese
(240 CALORIES), **204**
Spinach Cheddar Squares
(219 CALORIES), **97**
Spinach-Feta Chicken Rolls
(272 CALORIES), **109**
Veggie Cheese Ravioli (322 CALORIES), **154**
Zucchini Parmesan (81 CALORIES), **266**

CHERRIES
Black Forest Cake (186 CALORIES), **219**

Cherry Chocolate Parfaits
(146 CALORIES), **244**
Coconut-Cherry Cream Squares
(142 CALORIES), **214**
Tart Cherry Pie (174 CALORIES), **251**

CHICKEN
LUNCHES
Chicken Alfredo Veggie Pizza
(317 CALORIES), **113**
Chicken Caesar Pasta Toss
(363 CALORIES), **120**
Chicken Caesar Wraps
(332 CALORIES), **115**
Chicken Fajita Pizza
(382 CALORIES), **120**
Chicken Pesto Pizza (293 CALORIES), **112**
Chicken Veggie Wraps
(395 CALORIES), **293**
Hearty Chipotle Chicken Soup
(287 CALORIES), **111**
Hot Swiss Chicken Sandwiches
(218 CALORIES), **104**
Makeover Curried Chicken Rice Soup
(263 CALORIES), **107**
Raspberry Chicken Salad
(320 CALORIES), **283**
Simple Chicken Soup
(195 CALORIES), **104**
Spicy Warm Chicken Salad
(417 CALORIES), **292**
Spinach-Feta Chicken Rolls
(272 CALORIES), **109**
**Teriyaki Chicken Salad with Poppy Seed
Dressing** (361 CALORIES), **119**
White Bean Soup (270 CALORIES), **108**

DINNERS
Apricot-Almond Chicken Breasts
(372 CALORIES), **262**
Baked Chicken Fajitas
(340 CALORIES), **286**
Black Bean Chicken Tacos
(267 CALORIES), **141**
Black Bean Chicken with Rice
(400 CALORIES), **263**
Bow Ties with Chicken and Shrimp
(399 CALORIES), **168**
Chicken and Shrimp Satay
(190 CALORIES), **128**

Chicken & Vegetable Stir-Fry
(297 CALORIES), **280**
Chicken Artichoke Pasta
(378 CALORIES), **289**
**Chicken Patties with Roasted Tomato
Salsa** (134 CALORIES), **243**
Chicken with Beans and Potatoes
(209 CALORIES), **229**
Country Chicken with Gravy
(274 CALORIES), **278**
Creole Chicken (320 CALORIES), **154**
Crunchy Onion Barbecue Chicken
(286 CALORIES), **258**
Curried Chicken with Apples
(272 CALORIES), **144**
Dijon-Crusted Chicken Breasts
(169 CALORIES), **269**
Grilled Breaded Chicken
(224 CALORIES), **132**
Honey-Lime Roasted Chicken
(197 CALORIES), **252**
Italian Skillet Supper
(248 CALORIES), **277**
Lemon Chicken with Gravy
(195 CALORIES), **228**
Lemon Mushroom Chicken
(213 CALORIES), **273**
Light Chicken Cordon Bleu
(306 CALORIES), **150**
Malibu Chicken Bundles
(400 CALORIES), **167**
Mexican Manicotti
(390 CALORIES), **166**
Mustard-Herb Chicken Breasts
(163 CALORIES), **248**
Presto Chicken Tacos
(215 CALORIES), **273**
Savory Baked Chicken
(210 CALORIES), **272**
Skillet Arroz Con Pollo
(373 CALORIES), **164**
**Spicy Chicken Breasts with Pepper
Peach Relish** (263 CALORIES), **138**
Spicy Chicken Spaghetti
(401 CALORIES), **168**
Thai Restaurant Chicken
(359 CALORIES), **161**
Tuscan Chicken for Two
(217 CALORIES), **274**

CHOCOLATE

Black Forest Cake (186 CALORIES), 219
Blondies with Chips (133 CALORIES), 213
Cafe Mocha Mini Muffins (81 CALORIES), 266
Candy Bar Cupcakes (250 CALORIES), 223
Cappuccino Pudding (105 CALORIES), 210
Cherry Chocolate Parfaits (146 CALORIES), 244
Chocolate Bliss Marble Cake (215 CALORIES), 220
Chocolate Chip Cookies (94 CALORIES), 209
Chocolate Dunk-Shot Biscotti (40 CALORIES), 207
Chocolate Ganache Cake (179 CALORIES), 218
Frozen Yogurt Cookie Dessert (220 CALORIES), 255
Peanut Butter-Chocolate Chip Cookies (75 CALORIES), 208
Peanut Butter S'mores Bars (200 CALORIES), 253
Warm Chocolate Melting Cups (131 CALORIES), 212

CORN & GRITS

Corn Pudding Stuffed Tomatoes (157 CALORIES), 195
Flavorful Corn (116 CALORIES), 188
Garlic Cheese Grits (186 CALORIES), 94
Makeover Corn 'n' Green Bean Bake (241 CALORIES), 204
Mexican Veggies (70 CALORIES), 178
Sauteed Corn with Tomatoes & Basil (85 CALORIES), 182

CORN BREAD & CORNMEAL

Corn Bread-Topped Frijoles (367 CALORIES), 234
Mini Polenta Pizzas (57 CALORIES), 81
Ratatouille with Polenta (195 CALORIES), 271
Sausage Corn Bread Dressing (157 CALORIES), 194

CRANBERRIES

Apple Cranberry Delight (70 CALORIES), 238
Cranberry Apple Tart (183 CALORIES), 218
Cranberry-Apricot Pork Roast with Potatoes (433 CALORIES), 235
Cranberry Couscous (202 CALORIES), 198
Cranberry-Orange Turkey Cutlets (399 CALORIES), 166
Cranberry-Stuffed Apples (136 CALORIES), 227

DESSERTS

Apple Cranberry Delight (70 CALORIES), 238
Banana Split Cheesecake (247 CALORIES), 223
Berries with Sour Cream Sauce (147 CALORIES), 216
Black Forest Cake (186 CALORIES), 219
Blondies with Chips (133 CALORIES), 213
Broiled Fruit Dessert (80 CALORIES), 209
Candy Bar Cupcakes (250 CALORIES), 223
Cappuccino Pudding (105 CALORIES), 210
Cherry Chocolate Parfaits (146 CALORIES), 244
Chocolate Bliss Marble Cake (215 CALORIES), 220
Chocolate Chip Cookies (94 CALORIES), 209
Chocolate Dunk-Shot Biscotti (40 CALORIES), 207
Chocolate Ganache Cake (179 CALORIES), 218
Cinnamon Blueberry Sauce (50 CALORIES), 207
Coconut-Cherry Cream Squares (142 CALORIES), 214
Coconut Custard Pie (214 CALORIES), 254
Colorful Frozen Yogurt (143 CALORIES), 215
Cranberry Apple Tart (183 CALORIES), 218
Cranberry-Stuffed Apples (136 CALORIES), 227
Fresh Fruit Parfaits (149 CALORIES), 216

Frozen Fruit Cups (48 CALORIES), 237
Frozen Pistachio Dessert with Raspberry Sauce (214 CALORIES), 220
Frozen Yogurt Cookie Dessert (220 CALORIES), 255
Fruit Juice Pops (149 CALORIES), 217
Fruit Pizza (216 CALORIES), 221
Ladyfinger Cream Sandwiches (129 CALORIES), 212
Lemon Anise Biscotti (66 CALORIES), 208
Lemon Fluff Dessert (135 CALORIES), 243
Lemon Sorbet (138 CALORIES), 242
Low-Calorie Pumpkin Pie (124 CALORIES), 211
Luscious Lime Angel Squares (139 CALORIES), 244
Makeover Frosted Banana Bars (149 CALORIES), 216
Makeover Oatmeal Bars (127 CALORIES), 211
Mom's Orange-Spice Gelatin (62 CALORIES), 238
No-Bake Cheesecake Pie (141 CALORIES), 214
Peach-Topped Cake (121 CALORIES), 210
Peanut Butter-Chocolate Chip Cookies (75 CALORIES), 208
Peanut Butter S'mores Bars (200 CALORIES), 253
Pecan Kisses (46 CALORIES), 265
Pina Colada Pudding Cups (171 CALORIES), 250
Quick Crisp Snack Bars (144 CALORIES), 268
Raspberry Pie with Oat Crust (167 CALORIES), 249
Rich Peach Ice Cream (140 CALORIES), 213
Strawberry-Raspberry Ice (118 CALORIES), 241
Tart Cherry Pie (174 CALORIES), 251
Tres Leches Cake (233 CALORIES), 224
Triple-Berry Cobbler (235 CALORIES), 222
Tropical Meringue Tarts (145 CALORIES), 215
Vanilla Tapioca Pudding (133 CALORIES), 242
Warm Chocolate Melting Cups (131 CALORIES), 212

DINNERS *(ALSO SEE SANDWICHES; SOUPS & CHILI)*

BEEF AND GROUND BEEF
All-American Beef Stew (324 CALORIES), 155
Asian Orange Beef (351 CALORIES), 157
Baked Barbecued Brisket (159 CALORIES), 247
Barley Beef Skillet (400 CALORIES), 263
Beef Kabobs with Chutney Sauce (258 CALORIES), 257
Beef Roast Dinner (245 CALORIES), 230
Beef Tenderloin with Roasted Vegetables (283 CALORIES), 147
Blue-Cheese Topped Steaks (228 CALORIES), 132
Braised Southwest Beef Roast (255 CALORIES), 136
Broiled Sirloin Steaks (187 CALORIES), 126
Burgundy Beef Stew (388 CALORIES), 234
Cajun Beef Tenderloin (172 CALORIES), 124
Colorful Beef Stir-Fry (318 CALORIES), 152
Easy Beef Stroganoff (326 CALORIES), 285
Enchilada Casser-ole! (357 CALORIES), 159
Family-Favorite Cheeseburger Pasta (391 CALORIES), 293
Hearty Salisbury Steaks (233 CALORIES), 275
Herbed Beef Tenderloin (198 CALORIES), 253
Home-Style Pot Roast (341 CALORIES), 260
Hot 'n' Spicy Flank Steak (201 CALORIES), 128
Hungarian Goulash (310 CALORIES), 151
Italian Beef and Shells (396 CALORIES), 262
Italian Hot Dish (391 CALORIES), 166
Macaroni Scramble (351 CALORIES), 157
Mexican Meat Loaf (266 CALORIES), 140
Moroccan Beef Kabobs (185 CALORIES), 125

Old-Fashioned Swiss Steak (359 CALORIES), 160
Pineapple Beef Kabobs (412 CALORIES), 170
Pineapple Beef Stir-Fry for Two (381 CALORIES), 290
Portobello Burgundy Beef (384 CALORIES), 290
Sirloin Roast with Gravy (185 CALORIES), 227
Sirloin Strips over Rice (299 CALORIES), 149
Southwestern Beef Stew (222 CALORIES), 131
Stuffed Steak Spirals (214 CALORIES), 130
Sweet-and-Sour Beef (389 CALORIES), 291
Weeknight Beef Skillet (389 CALORIES), 292
Whiskey Sirloin Steak for Two (169 CALORIES), 248
Zesty Horseradish Meat Loaf (207 CALORIES), 129
Zippy Spaghetti Sauce (220 CALORIES), 230

CHICKEN
Apricot-Almond Chicken Breasts (372 CALORIES), 262
Baked Chicken Fajitas (340 CALORIES), 286
Black Bean Chicken Tacos (267 CALORIES), 141
Black Bean Chicken with Rice (400 CALORIES), 263
Bow Ties with Chicken and Shrimp (399 CALORIES), 168
Chicken and Shrimp Satay (190 CALORIES), 128
Chicken & Vegetable Stir-Fry (297 CALORIES), 280
Chicken Artichoke Pasta (378 CALORIES), 289
Chicken Patties with Roasted Tomato Salsa (134 CALORIES), 243
Country Chicken with Gravy (274 CALORIES), 278
Creole Chicken (320 CALORIES), 154
Crunchy Onion Barbecue Chicken (286 CALORIES), 258

Curried Chicken with Apples (272 CALORIES), 144
Dijon-Crusted Chicken Breasts (169 CALORIES), 269
Grilled Breaded Chicken (224 CALORIES), 132
Honey-Lime Roasted Chicken (197 CALORIES), 252
Italian Skillet Supper (248 CALORIES), 277
Lemon Chicken with Gravy (195 CALORIES), 228
Lemon Mushroom Chicken (213 CALORIES), 273
Light Chicken Cordon Bleu (306 CALORIES), 150
Malibu Chicken Bundles (400 CALORIES), 167
Mexican Manicotti (390 CALORIES), 166
Mustard-Herb Chicken Breasts (163 CALORIES), 248
Presto Chicken Tacos (215 CALORIES), 273
Savory Baked Chicken (210 CALORIES), 272
Skillet Arroz Con Pollo (373 CALORIES), 164
Spicy Chicken Breasts with Pepper Peach Relish (263 CALORIES), 138
Spicy Chicken Spaghetti (401 CALORIES), 168
Thai Restaurant Chicken (359 CALORIES), 161
Tuscan Chicken for Two (217 CALORIES), 274

FISH AND SEAFOOD
Baked Tilapia (143 CALORIES), 123
Basil Tuna Steaks (214 CALORIES), 130
Bow Ties with Chicken and Shrimp (399 CALORIES), 168
Chicken and Shrimp Satay (190 CALORIES), 128
Chive Crab Cakes (242 CALORIES), 256
Citrus Fish Tacos (411 CALORIES), 169
Fantastic Fish Tacos (314 CALORIES), 282
Fish Tacos (196 CALORIES), 127
Garlic Lemon Shrimp (163 CALORIES), 123

Grilled Tilapia with Lemon Basil Vinaigrette for Two (206 CALORIES), 254
Lemon-Soy Roughy (124 CALORIES), 241
Lime-Marinated Orange Roughy (169 CALORIES), 270
Mediterranean Shrimp 'n' Pasta (368 CALORIES), 163
Red Clam Sauce (305 CALORIES), 232
Scallops & Shrimp with Yellow Rice (349 CALORIES), 288
Scallops with Angel Hair (340 CALORIES), 286
Shrimp & Shiitake Stir-Fry with Crispy Noodles (238 CALORIES), 275
Snapper with Spicy Pineapple Glaze (304 CALORIES), 281
Spanish Fish (251 CALORIES), 135
Tilapia with Grapefruit Salsa (264 CALORIES), 140
Zippy Tomato-Topped Snapper (179 CALORIES), 251

LAMB
Best-Ever Lamb Chops (157 CALORIES), 246
Irish Stew (271 CALORIES), 142

MEATLESS
Asian Vegetable Pasta (358 CALORIES), 159
Broccoli-Cheese Stuffed Pizza (252 CALORIES), 134
Cheesy Rigatoni Bake (274 CALORIES), 144
Corn Bread-Topped Frijoles (367 CALORIES), 234
Fettuccine with Black Bean Sauce (350 CALORIES), 288
Greek Pizzas (320 CALORIES), 155
Grilled Artichoke-Mushroom Pizza (283 CALORIES), 146
Italian Cheese-Stuffed Shells (351 CALORIES), 158
Ratatouille with Polenta (195 CALORIES), 271
Southwest Vegetarian Bake (284 CALORIES), 148

Tortellini Primavera (341 CALORIES), 287
Vegetarian Tex-Mex Peppers (364 CALORIES), 162
Veggie Cheese Ravioli (322 CALORIES), 154
Zucchini Lasagna (272 CALORIES), 143

PORK
Apple Pork Stir-Fry (370 CALORIES), 164
Applesauce-Glazed Pork Chops (291 CALORIES), 259
Cranberry-Apricot Pork Roast with Potatoes (433 CALORIES), 235
Dijon-Peach Pork Chops (360 CALORIES), 289
Glazed Pork Chops (246 CALORIES), 256
Grilled Pork Tenderloin (171 CALORIES), 250
Grilled Spicy Pork Tenderloin (188 CALORIES), 270
Grilled Stuffed Pork Tenderloin (296 CALORIES), 148
Honey-Grilled Pork Tenderloin (298 CALORIES), 260
Onion-Dijon Pork Chops (261 CALORIES), 278
Parmesan Pork Medallions (220 CALORIES), 131
Polynesian Stir-Fry (339 CALORIES), 285
Pork Chop Skillet (360 CALORIES), 162
Pork Medallions with Dijon Sauce (323 CALORIES), 284
Pork Tenderloin with Horseradish Sauce (258 CALORIES), 137

TURKEY AND TURKEY SAUSAGE
Baked Mostaccioli (278 CALORIES), 146
Broccoli-Turkey Casserole (303 CALORIES), 150
Cranberry-Orange Turkey Cutlets (399 CALORIES), 166
Enchilada Lasagna (282 CALORIES), 145
Hearty Pasta Casserole (416 CALORIES), 171
Homemade Spaghetti Sauce (230 CALORIES), 133
Little Kick Jalapeno Burgers (254 CALORIES), 136

Makeover Turkey Biscuit Bake (290 CALORIES), 156
Peppery Grilled Turkey Breast (167 CALORIES), 124
Ragu Bolognese (413 CALORIES), 171
Roast Turkey Breast with Rosemary Gravy (151 CALORIES), 245
Tarragon-Lemon Turkey Breast (162 CALORIES), 247
Turkey Burritos with Fresh Fruit Salsa (371 CALORIES), 165
Turkey Noodle Casserole (357 CALORIES), 158
Turkey Pasta Toss (249 CALORIES), 134
Turkey Pecan Enchiladas (263 CALORIES), 139
Turkey Roulades (184 CALORIES), 126
Turkey with Apple Slices (263 CALORIES), 138
Turkey with Sausage Stuffing (317 CALORIES), 152

EGGS & EGG SUBSTITUTE
Bacon-Broccoli Quiche Cups (170 CALORIES), 249
Baked Eggs with Cheddar and Bacon (107 CALORIES), 267
Colorful Cheese Omelet (167 CALORIES), 91
Crab-Spinach Egg Casserole (163 CALORIES), 90
Eggs Benedict (216 CALORIES), 96
Hard-Cooked Eggs (75 CALORIES), 239
Hawaiian Breakfast Cups (131 CALORIES), 242
Italian Mini Frittatas (172 CALORIES), 93
Monterey Quiche (265 CALORIES), 98
Mushroom Quiche (154 CALORIES), 245
Potato Egg Bake (235 CALORIES), 98
Puffy Apple Omelet (249 CALORIES), 277
Sausage and Egg Pizza (241 CALORIES), 276
Scrambled Egg Muffins (133 CALORIES), 268
Spinach Cheddar Squares (219 CALORIES), 97
Spring Frittata (163 CALORIES), 91

FISH & SEAFOOD

BREAKFAST
Crab-Spinach Egg Casserole
(163 CALORIES), 90

LUNCHES
Floribbean Fish Burgers with Tropical
Sauce (353 CALORIES), 118
Fruity Crab Pasta Salad
(322 CALORIES), 283
Grandma's French Tuna Salad Wraps
(328 CALORIES), 114
Grilled Fish Sandwiches
(241 CALORIES), 276
Makeover Creamy Seafood Soup
(274 CALORIES), 279
Super-Duper Tuna Sandwiches
(291 CALORIES), 112

DINNERS
Baked Tilapia (143 CALORIES), 123
Basil Tuna Steaks (214 CALORIES), 130
Bow Ties with Chicken and Shrimp
(399 CALORIES), 168
Chicken and Shrimp Satay
(190 CALORIES), 128
Chive Crab Cakes (242 CALORIES), 256
Citrus Fish Tacos (411 CALORIES), 169
Fantastic Fish Tacos
(314 CALORIES), 282
Fish Tacos (196 CALORIES), 127
Garlic Lemon Shrimp
(163 CALORIES), 123
Grilled Tilapia with Lemon Basil
Vinaigrette for Two
(206 CALORIES), 254
Lemon-Soy Roughy (124 CALORIES), 241
Lime-Marinated Orange Roughy
(169 CALORIES), 270
Mediterranean Shrimp 'n' Pasta
(368 CALORIES), 163
Red Clam Sauce (305 CALORIES), 232
Scallops & Shrimp with Yellow Rice
(349 CALORIES), 288
Scallops with Angel Hair
(340 CALORIES), 286
Shrimp & Shiitake Stir-Fry with Crispy
Noodles (238 CALORIES), 275
Snapper with Spicy Pineapple Glaze
(304 CALORIES), 281

Spanish Fish (251 CALORIES), 135
Tilapia with Grapefruit Salsa
(264 CALORIES), 140
Veggie Tuna Burgers
(275 CALORIES), 279
Zippy Tomato-Topped Snapper
(179 CALORIES), 251

FRUIT (ALSO SEE SPECIFIC KINDS)
Berries with Sour Cream Sauce
(147 CALORIES), 216
Colorful Frozen Yogurt
(143 CALORIES), 215
Fresh Fruit Parfaits (149 CALORIES), 216
Frozen Fruit Cups (48 CALORIES), 237
Fruit Juice Pops (149 CALORIES), 217
Fruit Pizza (216 CALORIES), 221
Fruity Crab Pasta Salad
(322 CALORIES), 283
Granola-to-Go Bars (130 CALORIES), 88
Holiday Gelatin Mold
(105 CALORIES), 187
Low-Calorie Pumpkin Pie
(124 CALORIES), 211
Melon 'n' Grape Medley
(74 CALORIES), 239
Sangria Gelatin Dessert
(95 CALORIES), 240
Strawberry Mango Smoothies for 2
(100 CALORIES), 84
Strawberry-Raspberry Ice
(118 CALORIES), 241
Sun-Kissed Smoothies
(100 CALORIES), 85
Three-Fruit Smoothies
(225 CALORIES), 97
Triple-Berry Cobbler (235 CALORIES), 222
Tropical Fruit Smoothies
(97 CALORIES), 87
Tropical Meringue Tarts
(145 CALORIES), 215
Turkey Burritos with Fresh Fruit Salsa
(371 CALORIES), 165

GREEN BEANS
Chicken with Beans and Potatoes
(209 CALORIES), 229
Dijon Green Beans (54 CALORIES), 174

Herbed Beans and Carrots
(63 CALORIES), 176
Italian Green Beans (85 CALORIES), 182
Makeover Corn 'n' Green Bean Bake
(241 CALORIES), 204
Makeover Fancy Bean Casserole
(213 CALORIES), 200
Pretty Almond Green Beans
(78 CALORIES), 179

GROUND BEEF

LUNCHES
Chili Beef Quesadillas
(353 CALORIES), 117
Chili Con Carne (299 CALORIES), 113
Lasagna Soup (280 CALORIES), 280

DINNERS
Easy Beef Stroganoff
(326 CALORIES), 285
Enchilada Casser-ole!
(357 CALORIES), 159
Family-Favorite Cheeseburger Pasta
(391 CALORIES), 293
French Cheeseburger Loaf
(277 CALORIES), 145
Hearty Salisbury Steaks
(233 CALORIES), 275
Italian Beef and Shells
(396 CALORIES), 262
Italian Hot Dish (391 CALORIES), 166
Macaroni Scramble (351 CALORIES), 157
Mexican Meat Loaf (266 CALORIES), 140
Weeknight Beef Skillet
(389 CALORIES), 292
Zesty Horseradish Meat Loaf
(207 CALORIES), 129
Zippy Slow-Cooked Chili
(266 CALORIES), 231
Zippy Spaghetti Sauce
(220 CALORIES), 230
Zippy Three-Bean Chili
(269 CALORIES), 142

HAM & PROSCIUTTO
Focaccia Sandwich (113 CALORIES), 101
German Deli Pizza (330 CALORIES), 114
Ham Asparagus Spirals (49 CALORIES), 80

Hawaiian Breakfast Cups
(131 CALORIES), 242
Italian Mini Frittatas (172 CALORIES), 93
Light Chicken Cordon Bleu
(306 CALORIES), 150
Malibu Chicken Bundles
(400 CALORIES), 167

LAMB
Artichoke-Lamb Sandwich Loaves
(239 CALORIES), 105
Best-Ever Lamb Chops
(157 CALORIES), 246
Irish Stew (271 CALORIES), 142

LEMON & LIME
Garlic Lemon Shrimp
(163 CALORIES), 123
Grilled Tilapia with Lemon Basil
Vinaigrette for Two
(206 CALORIES), 254
Honey-Lime Roasted Chicken
(197 CALORIES), 252
Lemon Anise Biscotti
(66 CALORIES), 208
Lemon Fluff Dessert (135 CALORIES), 243
Lemon Garlic Mushrooms
(96 CALORIES), 185
Lemon Mushroom Chicken
(213 CALORIES), 273
Lemon Pepper Pasta (249 CALORIES), 205
Lemon-Pepper Veggies
(75 CALORIES), 178
Lemon Risotto with Peas
(207 CALORIES), 200
Lemon Sorbet (138 CALORIES), 242
Lemon-Soy Roughy (124 CALORIES), 241
Lemony New Potatoes
(118 CALORIES), 189
Lime-Marinated Orange Roughy
(169 CALORIES), 270
Luscious Lime Angel Squares
(139 CALORIES), 244
Tarragon-Lemon Turkey Breast
(162 CALORIES), 247

LUNCHES (ALSO SEE SALADS; SANDWICHES; SOUPS & CHILI)
Black Bean Taco Pizza
(264 CALORIES), 108

Chicken Alfredo Veggie Pizza
(317 CALORIES), 113
Chicken Caesar Pasta Toss
(363 CALORIES), 120
Chicken Fajita Pizza
(382 CALORIES), 120
Chicken Pesto Pizza (293 CALORIES), 112
Chili Beef Quesadillas
(353 CALORIES), 117
German Deli Pizza (330 CALORIES), 114
Macaroni 'n' Cheese Italiano
(262 CALORIES), 106
Turkey Enchiladas (284 CALORIES), 110

MEATLESS ENTREES
Asian Vegetable Pasta
(358 CALORIES), 159
Better Than Egg Salad
(274 CALORIES), 110
Black Bean Taco Pizza
(264 CALORIES), 108
Breaded Eggplant Sandwiches
(288 CALORIES), 111
Broccoli-Cheese Stuffed Pizza
(252 CALORIES), 134
Cheesy Rigatoni Bake
(274 CALORIES), 144
Corn Bread-Topped Frijoles
(367 CALORIES), 234
Fettuccine with Black Bean Sauce
(350 CALORIES), 288
Greek Pizzas (320 CALORIES), 155
Grilled Artichoke-Mushroom Pizza
(283 CALORIES), 146
Grilled Veggie Sandwiches
(231 CALORIES), 274
Heavenly Earth Burgers
(320 CALORIES), 153
Italian Cheese-Stuffed Shells
(351 CALORIES), 158
Macaroni 'n' Cheese Italiano
(262 CALORIES), 106
Monterey Quiche (265 CALORIES), 98
Ratatouille with Polenta
(195 CALORIES), 271
Southwest Vegetarian Bake
(284 CALORIES), 148
Tortellini Primavera
(341 CALORIES), 287

Vegetarian Tex-Mex Peppers
(364 CALORIES), 162
Veggie Cheese Ravioli
(322 CALORIES), 154
Zucchini Lasagna (272 CALORIES), 143

MUSHROOMS
Couscous with Mushrooms
(230 CALORIES), 203
Easy Beef Stroganoff
(326 CALORIES), 285
Grilled Artichoke-Mushroom Pizza
(283 CALORIES), 146
Lemon Garlic Mushrooms (
96 CALORIES), 185
Lemon Mushroom Chicken
(213 CALORIES), 273
Mushroom Quiche (154 CALORIES), 245
Portobello Burgundy Beef
(384 CALORIES), 290
Shrimp & Shiitake Stir-Fry with Crispy
Noodles (238 CALORIES), 275

NUTS & PEANUT BUTTER
Apple Walnut Pancakes
(208 CALORIES), 95
Apricot-Almond Chicken Breasts
(372 CALORIES), 262
Coconut-Pecan Sweet Potatoes
(211 CALORIES), 229
Frozen Pistachio Dessert with Raspberry
Sauce (214 CALORIES), 220
No-Bake Peanut Butter Treats
(70 CALORIES), 82
Nut 'n' Corn Clusters
(43 CALORIES), 79
Peanut Butter-Chocolate Chip Cookies
(75 CALORIES), 208
Peanut Butter S'mores Bars
(200 CALORIES), 253
Pecan Kisses (46 CALORIES), 265
Pretty Almond Green Beans
(78 CALORIES), 179
Quick Crisp Snack Bars
(144 CALORIES), 268
Turkey Pecan Enchiladas
(263 CALORIES), 139
Wholesome Apple-Hazelnut Stuffing
(159 CALORIES), 195

OATS & GRANOLA

Apple-Cinnamon Oatmeal Mix
(176 CALORIES), 94
Baked Blueberry & Peach Oatmeal
(277 CALORIES), 99
Blueberry Oatmeal Pancakes
(171 CALORIES), 270
Chewy Granola Bars (160 CALORIES), 90
Granola-to-Go Bars (130 CALORIES), 88
Makeover Oatmeal Bars
(127 CALORIES), 211
Raspberry Pie with Oat Crust
(167 CALORIES), 249

ONIONS & LEEKS

Baked Onion Rings (98 CALORIES), 186
Crunchy Onion Barbecue Chicken
(286 CALORIES), 258
Onion-Dijon Pork Chops
(261 CALORIES), 278
Spring Frittata (163 CALORIES), 91

ORANGE & GRAPEFRUIT

Asian Orange Beef (351 CALORIES), 157
Citrus Fish Tacos (411 CALORIES), 169
Citrus Spinach Salad
(52 CALORIES), 173
Cranberry-Orange Turkey Cutlets
(399 CALORIES), 166
Glazed Orange Carrots
(132 CALORIES), 191
Mom's Orange-Spice Gelatin
(62 CALORIES), 238
Orange Fruit Cups (80 CALORIES), 87
Tilapia with Grapefruit Salsa
(264 CALORIES), 140

PASTA & NOODLES

Asian Vegetable Pasta
(358 CALORIES), 159
Baked Mostaccioli (278 CALORIES), 146
Basil-Parmesan Angel Hair
(203 CALORIES), 199
Bow Ties with Chicken and Shrimp
(399 CALORIES), 168
Cheesy Rigatoni Bake
(274 CALORIES), 144
Chicken Artichoke Pasta
(378 CALORIES), 289

Chicken Caesar Pasta Toss
(363 CALORIES), 120
Couscous with Mushrooms
(230 CALORIES), 203
Cranberry Couscous (202 CALORIES), 198
Easy Beef Stroganoff
(326 CALORIES), 285
Enchilada Lasagna (282 CALORIES), 145
Family-Favorite Cheeseburger Pasta
(391 CALORIES), 293
Fettuccine with Black Bean Sauce
(350 CALORIES), 288
Garlic-Herb Orzo Pilaf
(227 CALORIES), 203
Hearty Pasta Casserole
(416 CALORIES), 171
Homemade Spaghetti Sauce
(230 CALORIES), 133
Italian Beef and Shells
(396 CALORIES), 262
Italian Cheese-Stuffed Shells
(351 CALORIES), 158
Italian Hot Dish (391 CALORIES), 166
Italian Vegetable Soup
(164 CALORIES), 103
Lasagna Soup (280 CALORIES), 280
Lemon Pepper Pasta
(249 CALORIES), 205
Low-Fat Macaroni and Cheese
(250 CALORIES), 205
Macaroni 'n' Cheese Italiano
(262 CALORIES), 106
Macaroni Scramble (351 CALORIES), 157
Mediterranean Shrimp 'n' Pasta
(368 CALORIES), 163
One-Pot Chili (384 CALORIES), 121
Ragu Bolognese (413 CALORIES), 171
Red Clam Sauce (305 CALORIES), 232
Scallops with Angel Hair
(340 CALORIES), 286
Shrimp & Shiitake Stir-Fry with Crispy
Noodles (238 CALORIES), 275
Southwestern Pasta & Cheese
(240 CALORIES), 204
Spicy Chicken Spaghetti
(401 CALORIES), 168
Tortellini Primavera (341 CALORIES), 287
Turkey Meatball Soup (258 CALORIES), 106

Turkey Noodle Casserole
(357 CALORIES), 158
Turkey Pasta Toss (249 CALORIES), 134
Veggie Cheese Ravioli (322 CALORIES), 154
Weeknight Beef Skillet
(389 CALORIES), 292
Zippy Spaghetti Sauce
(220 CALORIES), 230
Zucchini Lasagna (272 CALORIES), 143

PEACHES

Baked Blueberry & Peach Oatmeal
(277 CALORIES), 99
Baked Peach Pancake
(157 CALORIES), 246
Broiled Fruit Dessert (80 CALORIES), 209
Dijon-Peach Pork Chops
(360 CALORIES), 289
Mom's Orange-Spice Gelatin
(62 CALORIES), 238
Peach-Topped Cake (121 CALORIES), 210
Pineapple Peach Soup
(88 CALORIES), 184
Rich Peach Ice Cream
(140 CALORIES), 213
Roast Pork Sandwiches with Peach
Chutney (357 CALORIES), 118
Spicy Chicken Breasts with Pepper
Peach Relish (263 CALORIES), 138

PEAS

Holiday Peas (87 CALORIES), 183
Lemon Risotto with Peas
(207 CALORIES), 200
Peas a la Francaise (112 CALORIES), 188
Snow Pea Medley (83 CALORIES), 181

PEPPERS

Hearty Chipotle Chicken Soup
(287 CALORIES), 111
Italian Broccoli with Peppers
(55 CALORIES), 174
Lemon Pepper Pasta
(249 CALORIES), 205
Little Kick Jalapeno Burgers
(254 CALORIES), 136
Spicy Chicken Breasts with Pepper
Peach Relish (263 CALORIES), 138
Vegetarian Tex-Mex Peppers
(364 CALORIES), 162

PINEAPPLE

Citrus Fish Tacos (411 CALORIES), 169
Hawaiian Breakfast Cups
(131 CALORIES), 242
Pina Colada Pudding Cups
(171 CALORIES), 250
Pineapple Beef Kabobs
(412 CALORIES), 170
Pineapple Beef Stir-Fry for Two
(381 CALORIES), 290
Pineapple Peach Soup
(88 CALORIES), 184
Polynesian Stir-Fry (339 CALORIES), 285
Snapper with Spicy Pineapple Glaze
(304 CALORIES), 281

PORK (ALSO SEE BACON & CANADIAN BACON; HAM & PROSCIUTTO; SAUSAGE)

Apple Pork Stir-Fry (370 CALORIES), 164
Applesauce-Glazed Pork Chops
(291 CALORIES), 259
Barbecued Pork Sandwiches
(287 CALORIES), 259
Cranberry-Apricot Pork Roast with
Potatoes (433 CALORIES), 235
Dijon-Peach Pork Chops
(360 CALORIES), 289
Glazed Pork Chops (246 CALORIES), 256
Grilled Pork Tenderloin
(171 CALORIES), 250
Grilled Pork Tenderloin Sandwiches
(382 CALORIES), 121
Grilled Spicy Pork Tenderloin
(188 CALORIES), 270
Grilled Stuffed Pork Tenderloin
(296 CALORIES), 148
Honey-Grilled Pork Tenderloin
(298 CALORIES), 260
Onion-Dijon Pork Chops
(261 CALORIES), 278
Parmesan Pork Medallions
(220 CALORIES), 131
Polynesian Stir-Fry (339 CALORIES), 285
Pork Chop Skillet (360 CALORIES), 162
Pork Medallions with Dijon Sauce
(323 CALORIES), 284
Pork Tenderloin with Horseradish Sauce
(258 CALORIES), 137
Roast Pork Sandwiches with Peach
Chutney (357 CALORIES), 118

POTATOES & SWEET POTATOES

Broccoli-Cheddar Baked Potatoes
(226 CALORIES), 202
Chicken with Beans and Potatoes
(209 CALORIES), 229
Chipotle Sweet Potato and Spiced Apple
Purees (224 CALORIES), 255
Coconut-Pecan Sweet Potatoes
(211 CALORIES), 229
Flavorful Mashed Potatoes
(146 CALORIES), 192
Golden au Gratin Potatoes
(167 CALORIES), 196
Gruyere Mashed Potatoes
(193 CALORIES), 197
Herbed Potato Salad
(142 CALORIES), 191
Lemony New Potatoes
(118 CALORIES), 189
Makeover Patrician Potatoes
(207 CALORIES), 199
Mashed Potato Cakes
(147 CALORIES), 193
Potato Egg Bake (235 CALORIES), 98
Potato Smashers (224 CALORIES), 201
Seasoned Yukon Gold Wedges
(121 CALORIES), 190
Sweet Potato Casserole
(186 CALORIES), 197

RASPBERRIES

Caramel Cream Crepes
(206 CALORIES), 95
Chocolate Bliss Marble Cake
(215 CALORIES), 220
Frozen Pistachio Dessert with Raspberry
Sauce (214 CALORIES), 220
Raspberry Chicken Salad
(320 CALORIES), 283
Raspberry Pie with Oat Crust
(167 CALORIES), 249

RICE

Black Bean Chicken with Rice
(400 CALORIES), 263
Broccoli Brown Rice Pilaf
(202 CALORIES), 198
Brunch Risotto (279 CALORIES), 258
Garlic-Herb Orzo Pilaf (227 CALORIES), 203

Great Grain Pilaf (154 CALORIES), 194
Heavenly Earth Burgers
(320 CALORIES), 153
Lemon Risotto with Peas
(207 CALORIES), 200
Makeover Curried Chicken Rice Soup
(263 CALORIES), 107
Rice with Summer Squash
(123 CALORIES), 190
Scallops & Shrimp with Yellow Rice
(349 CALORIES), 288
Sirloin Strips over Rice
(299 CALORIES), 149

SALADS

Alfresco Bean Salad (146 CALORIES), 192
Better Than Egg Salad
(274 CALORIES), 110
Citrus Spinach Salad (52 CALORIES), 173
Fruity Crab Pasta Salad
(322 CALORIES), 283
Herbed Potato Salad
(142 CALORIES), 191
Holiday Gelatin Mold
(105 CALORIES), 187
Home-Style Coleslaw (88 CALORIES), 183
Mediterranean Salad (69 CALORIES), 101
Melon 'n' Grape Medley
(74 CALORIES), 239
Raspberry Chicken Salad
(320 CALORIES), 283
Spicy Warm Chicken Salad
(417 CALORIES), 292
Teriyaki Chicken Salad with Poppy Seed
Dressing (361 CALORIES), 119
Veggie Tossed Salad (62 CALORIES), 176

SANDWICHES

Apricot Turkey Sandwiches
(338 CALORIES), 116
Artichoke-Lamb Sandwich Loaves
(239 CALORIES), 105
Asian Steak Wraps (402 CALORIES), 169
Barbecued Pork Sandwiches
(287 CALORIES), 259
BBQ Beef Sandwiches
(354 CALORIES), 233
Breaded Eggplant Sandwiches
(288 CALORIES), 111
Chicken Caesar Wraps (332 CALORIES), 115

SANDWICHES (CONTINUED)

Chicken Veggie Wraps (395 CALORIES), 293
Chutney Turkey Burgers
(359 CALORIES), 160
Colorful Beef Wraps (325 CALORIES), 284
Flank Steak Pitas (362 CALORIES), 161
Floribbean Fish Burgers with Tropical
Sauce (353 CALORIES), 118
Focaccia Sandwich (113 CALORIES), 101
French Cheeseburger Loaf
(277 CALORIES), 145
Garbanzo Bean Pitas
(241 CALORIES), 105
Garden Turkey Burgers
(156 CALORIES), 269
Grandma's French Tuna Salad Wraps
(328 CALORIES), 114
Grilled Fish Sandwiches
(241 CALORIES), 276
Grilled Pork Tenderloin Sandwiches
(382 CALORIES), 121
Grilled Veggie Sandwiches
(231 CALORIES), 274
Heavenly Earth Burgers
(320 CALORIES), 153
Hot Swiss Chicken Sandwiches
(218 CALORIES), 104
Little Kick Jalapeno Burgers
(254 CALORIES), 136
Mexican-Inspired Turkey Burgers
(312 CALORIES), 282
Red, White and Blue Pita Pockets
(351 CALORIES), 116
Roast Pork Sandwiches with Peach
Chutney (357 CALORIES), 118
Super-Duper Tuna Sandwiches
(291 CALORIES), 112
Super Flatbread Wraps
(348 CALORIES), 261
Tex-Mex Beef Barbecues
(294 CALORIES), 232
Turkey Sloppy Joes
(247 CALORIES), 231
Turkey Tortilla Roll-Ups
(353 CALORIES), 117
Veggie Tuna Burgers
(275 CALORIES), 279

SAUSAGE

Focaccia Sandwich (113 CALORIES), 101
Italian Sausage Bean Soup
(339 CALORIES), 115
Mini Sausage Quiches (66 CALORIES), 82
Sausage Bread Dressing
(166 CALORIES), 196
Sausage Kale Soup (194 CALORIES), 252
Scrambled Egg Muffins
(133 CALORIES), 268
Slow-Cooked Sausage Dressing
(201 CALORIES), 228

SIDE DISHES (ALSO SEE SALADS)

Asparagus with Dill Sauce
(76 CALORIES), 179
Baked Onion Rings (98 CALORIES), 186
Baked Veggie Chips (108 CALORIES), 187
Balsamic Asparagus (45 CALORIES), 173
Basil-Parmesan Angel Hair
(203 CALORIES), 199
Bravo Broccoli (78 CALORIES), 180
Broccoli Brown Rice Pilaf
(202 CALORIES), 198
Broccoli-Cheddar Baked Potatoes
(226 CALORIES), 202
Brunch Risotto (279 CALORIES), 258
Chipotle Sweet Potato and Spiced Apple
Purees (224 CALORIES), 255
Coconut-Pecan Sweet Potatoes
(211 CALORIES), 229
Corn Pudding Stuffed Tomatoes
(157 CALORIES), 195
Couscous with Mushrooms
(230 CALORIES), 203
Cranberry Couscous (202 CALORIES), 198
Dijon Green Beans (54 CALORIES), 174
Dilly Vegetable Medley
(91 CALORIES), 184
Flavorful Corn (116 CALORIES), 188
Flavorful Mashed Potatoes
(146 CALORIES), 192
Garlic-Herb Orzo Pilaf
(227 CALORIES), 203
Glazed Orange Carrots
(132 CALORIES), 191
Go for the Grains Casserole
(226 CALORIES), 202

Golden au Gratin Potatoes
(167 CALORIES), 196
Grandma's Stuffed Yellow Squash
(103 CALORIES), 240
Great Grain Pilaf (154 CALORIES), 194
Gruyere Mashed Potatoes
(193 CALORIES), 197
Herbed Beans and Carrots
(63 CALORIES), 176
Holiday Peas (87 CALORIES), 183
Italian Broccoli with Peppers
(55 CALORIES), 174
Italian Green Beans (85 CALORIES), 182
Italian Squash Casserole
(99 CALORIES), 186
Italian Vegetable Medley
(79 CALORIES), 180
Italian Veggie Skillet (93 CALORIES), 185
Lemon Garlic Mushrooms
(96 CALORIES), 185
Lemon Pepper Pasta
(249 CALORIES), 205
Lemon-Pepper Veggies
(75 CALORIES), 178
Lemon Risotto with Peas
(207 CALORIES), 200
Lemony New Potatoes
(118 CALORIES), 189
Low-Fat Macaroni and Cheese
(250 CALORIES), 205
Makeover Corn 'n' Green Bean Bake
(241 CALORIES), 204
Makeover Fancy Bean Casserole
(213 CALORIES), 200
Makeover Patrician Potatoes
(207 CALORIES), 199
Mashed Potato Cakes
(147 CALORIES), 193
Mediterranean Summer Squash
(69 CALORIES), 177
Mexican Veggies (70 CALORIES), 178
Parmesan Cauliflower
(121 CALORIES), 189
Parmesan Roasted Carrots
(82 CALORIES), 181
Peas a la Francaise (112 CALORIES), 188
Potato Smashers (224 CALORIES), 201
Pretty Almond Green Beans
(78 CALORIES), 179

Quinoa Pilaf (198 CALORIES), 272
Rice with Summer Squash
(123 CALORIES), 190
Roasted Vegetable Medley
(152 CALORIES), 193
Sausage Bread Dressing
(166 CALORIES), 196
Sausage Corn Bread Dressing
(157 CALORIES), 194
Sauteed Corn with Tomatoes & Basil
(85 CALORIES), 182
Seasoned Yukon Gold Wedges
(121 CALORIES), 190
Sesame Vegetable Medley
(60 CALORIES), 175
Slow-Cooked Sausage Dressing
(201 CALORIES), 228
Snow Pea Medley (83 CALORIES), 181
Southwestern Pasta & Cheese
(240 CALORIES), 204
Springtime Barley (226 CALORIES), 201
Sweet Potato Casserole
(186 CALORIES), 197
Wholesome Apple-Hazelnut Stuffing
(159 CALORIES), 195
Wilted Garlic Spinach (66 CALORIES), 177
Winter Vegetables (51 CALORIES), 237
Zucchini Parmesan (81 CALORIES), 266

SLOW COOKER RECIPES

BBQ Beef Sandwiches
(354 CALORIES), 233
Beef Roast Dinner (245 CALORIES), 230
Burgundy Beef Stew
(388 CALORIES), 234
Chicken with Beans and Potatoes
(209 CALORIES), 229
Coconut-Pecan Sweet Potatoes
(211 CALORIES), 229
Corn Bread-Topped Frijoles
(367 CALORIES), 234
Cranberry-Apricot Pork Roast with
Potatoes (433 CALORIES), 235
Cranberry-Stuffed Apples
(136 CALORIES), 227
Family-Pleasing Turkey Chili
(349 CALORIES), 233
Lemon Chicken with Gravy
(195 CALORIES), 228

Red Clam Sauce (305 CALORIES), 232
Sirloin Roast with Gravy
(185 CALORIES), 227
Slow-Cooked Sausage Dressing
(201 CALORIES), 228
Tex-Mex Beef Barbecues
(294 CALORIES), 232
Turkey Sloppy Joes (247 CALORIES), 231
Zippy Slow-Cooked Chili
(266 CALORIES), 231
Zippy Spaghetti Sauce (220 CALORIES), 230

SNACKS

Apple Skewers (80 CALORIES), 265
Cafe Mocha Mini Muffins
(81 CALORIES), 266
Cheesecake Phyllo Cups
(46 CALORIES), 80
Cheesy Pita Crisps (95 CALORIES), 83
Chive Crab Cakes (242 CALORIES), 256
Ham Asparagus Spirals
(49 CALORIES), 80
Mini Polenta Pizzas (57 CALORIES), 81
Mini Sausage Quiches (66 CALORIES), 82
No-Bake Peanut Butter Treats
(70 CALORIES), 82
Nut 'n' Corn Clusters (43 CALORIES), 79
Parmesan Popcorn (49 CALORIES), 81
Party Pretzels (89 CALORIES), 83
Pretzel Bones (98 CALORIES), 84
Quick Crisp Snack Bars
(144 CALORIES), 268
Salt & Garlic Pita Chips
(21 CALORIES), 79
Tex-Mex Popcorn (44 CALORIES), 79

SOUPS & CHILI

Chili Con Carne (299 CALORIES), 113
Family-Pleasing Turkey Chili
(349 CALORIES), 233
Hearty Chipotle Chicken Soup
(287 CALORIES), 111
Italian Sausage Bean Soup
(339 CALORIES), 115
Italian Vegetable Soup
(164 CALORIES), 103
Lasagna Soup (280 CALORIES), 280
Makeover Creamy Seafood Soup
(274 CALORIES), 279

Makeover Curried Chicken Rice Soup
(263 CALORIES), 107
One-Pot Chili (384 CALORIES), 121
Pineapple Peach Soup
(88 CALORIES), 184
Sausage Kale Soup (194 CALORIES), 252
Simple Chicken Soup
(195 CALORIES), 104
Southwest Black Bean Soup
(273 CALORIES), 109
Turkey Meatball Soup
(258 CALORIES), 106
White Bean Soup (270 CALORIES), 108
Winter Harvest Vegetable Soup
(134 CALORIES), 102
Zippy Slow-Cooked Chili
(266 CALORIES), 231
Zippy Three-Bean Chili
(269 CALORIES), 142

SPINACH & KALE

Citrus Spinach Salad (52 CALORIES), 173
Crab-Spinach Egg Casserole
(163 CALORIES), 90
Sausage Kale Soup (194 CALORIES), 252
Spinach Cheddar Squares
(219 CALORIES), 97
Spinach-Feta Chicken Rolls
(272 CALORIES), 109
Wilted Garlic Spinach (66 CALORIES), 177

SQUASH & ZUCCHINI

Grandma's Stuffed Yellow Squash
(103 CALORIES), 240
Italian Squash Casserole (99 CALORIES), 186
Mediterranean Summer Squash
(69 CALORIES), 177
Mexican Veggies (70 CALORIES), 178
Rice with Summer Squash
(123 CALORIES), 190
Zucchini Lasagna
(272 CALORIES), 143
Zucchini Pancakes (88 CALORIES), 88
Zucchini Parmesan
(81 CALORIES), 266

TOFU

Better Than Egg Salad
(274 CALORIES), 110

TOMATOES & SUN-DRIED TOMATOES

Chicken Patties with Roasted Tomato Salsa (134 CALORIES), **243**
Corn Pudding Stuffed Tomatoes (157 CALORIES), **195**
Mini Polenta Pizzas (57 CALORIES), **81**
Sauteed Corn with Tomatoes & Basil (85 CALORIES), **182**
Zippy Tomato-Topped Snapper (179 CALORIES), **251**

TURKEY, TURKEY SAUSAGE & TURKEY BACON

BREAKFASTS
Sausage and Egg Pizza (241 CALORIES), **276**
Turkey Breakfast Sausage (85 CALORIES), **267**

LUNCHES
Apricot Turkey Sandwiches (338 CALORIES), **116**
Focaccia Sandwich (113 CALORIES), **101**
One-Pot Chili (384 CALORIES), **121**
Turkey Enchiladas (284 CALORIES), **110**
Turkey Meatball Soup (258 CALORIES), **106**
Turkey Tortilla Roll-Ups (353 CALORIES), **117**

DINNERS
Baked Mostaccioli (278 CALORIES), **146**
Broccoli-Turkey Casserole (303 CALORIES), **150**
Chutney Turkey Burgers (359 CALORIES), **160**
Cranberry-Orange Turkey Cutlets (399 CALORIES), **166**
Enchilada Lasagna (282 CALORIES), **145**
Family-Pleasing Turkey Chili (349 CALORIES), **233**
Garden Turkey Burgers (156 CALORIES), **269**
Hearty Pasta Casserole (416 CALORIES), **171**

Homemade Spaghetti Sauce (230 CALORIES), **133**
Little Kick Jalapeno Burgers (254 CALORIES), **136**
Makeover Turkey Biscuit Bake (290 CALORIES), **156**
Mexican-Inspired Turkey Burgers (312 CALORIES), **282**
Mexican Meat Loaf (266 CALORIES), **140**
Peppery Grilled Turkey Breast (167 CALORIES), **124**
Ragu Bolognese (413 CALORIES), **171**
Roast Turkey Breast with Rosemary Gravy (151 CALORIES), **245**
Tarragon-Lemon Turkey Breast (162 CALORIES), **247**
Turkey Burritos with Fresh Fruit Salsa (371 CALORIES), **165**
Turkey Noodle Casserole (357 CALORIES), **158**
Turkey Pasta Toss (249 CALORIES), **134**
Turkey Pecan Enchiladas (263 CALORIES), **139**
Turkey Roulades (184 CALORIES), **126**
Turkey Sloppy Joes (247 CALORIES), **231**
Turkey with Apple Slices (263 CALORIES), **138**
Turkey with Sausage Stuffing (317 CALORIES), **152**

SIDE DISH
Sausage Corn Bread Dressing (157 CALORIES), **194**

VEGETABLES *(ALSO SEE SPECIFIC KINDS)*

Asian Vegetable Pasta (358 CALORIES), **159**
Baked Veggie Chips (108 CALORIES), **187**
Beef Tenderloin with Roasted Vegetables (283 CALORIES), **147**
Breaded Eggplant Sandwiches (288 CALORIES), **111**
Chicken & Vegetable Stir-Fry (297 CALORIES), **280**

Chicken Veggie Wraps (395 CALORIES), **293**
Dilly Vegetable Medley (91 CALORIES), **184**
Go for the Grains Casserole (226 CALORIES), **202**
Greek Pizzas (320 CALORIES), **155**
Grilled Veggie Sandwiches (231 CALORIES), **274**
Home-Style Coleslaw (88 CALORIES), **183**
Italian Vegetable Soup (164 CALORIES), **103**
Italian Veggie Skillet (93 CALORIES), **185**
Lemon-Pepper Veggies (75 CALORIES), **178**
Parmesan Cauliflower (121 CALORIES), **189**
Ratatouille with Polenta (195 CALORIES), **271**
Roasted Vegetable Medley (152 CALORIES), **193**
Sesame Vegetable Medley (60 CALORIES), **175**
Tortellini Primavera (341 CALORIES), **287**
Veggie Cheese Ravioli (322 CALORIES), **154**
Veggie Tossed Salad (62 CALORIES), **176**
Veggie Tuna Burgers (275 CALORIES), **279**
Winter Harvest Vegetable Soup (134 CALORIES), **102**
Winter Vegetables (51 CALORIES), **237**

VEGETARIAN MEAT CRUMBLES

Vegetarian Tex-Mex Peppers (364 CALORIES), **162**

alphabetical index

With the *Comfort Food Diet Cookbook*, serving your family healthy and tasty meals is a breeze. This index (organized by recipe title) also offers the per-serving calorie count of every dish.

If you have a hard time remembering the names of all of those family favorites you've prepared from this book, simply begin to highlight those dishes that get thumbs-up approval from your gang. You could also set a blank sticky note on the back of this book and write down the titles of the recipes your family enjoys most.

A

Alfresco Bean Salad
(146 CALORIES), **192**
All-American Beef Stew
(324 CALORIES), **155**
Apple-Cinnamon Oatmeal Mix
(176 CALORIES), **94**
Apple Cranberry Delight
(70 CALORIES), **238**
Apple Pork Stir-Fry (370 CALORIES), **164**
Apple Skewers (80 CALORIES), **265**
Apple Walnut Pancakes
(208 CALORIES), **95**
Applesauce-Glazed Pork Chops
(291 CALORIES), **259**
Apricot-Almond Chicken Breasts
(372 CALORIES), **262**
Apricot Turkey Sandwiches
(338 CALORIES), **116**
Artichoke-Lamb Sandwich Loaves
(239 CALORIES), **105**

Asian Orange Beef
(351 CALORIES), **157**
Asian Steak Wraps (402 CALORIES), **169**
Asian Vegetable Pasta
(358 CALORIES), **159**
Asparagus with Dill Sauce
(76 CALORIES), **179**

B

Bacon-Broccoli Quiche Cups
(170 CALORIES), **249**
Baked Barbecued Brisket
(159 CALORIES), **247**
Baked Blueberry & Peach Oatmeal
(277 CALORIES), **99**
Baked Chicken Fajitas
(340 CALORIES), **286**
Baked Eggs with Cheddar and Bacon
(107 CALORIES), **267**
Baked Mostaccioli (278 CALORIES), **146**
Baked Onion Rings (98 CALORIES), **186**
Baked Peach Pancake
(157 CALORIES), **246**
Baked Tilapia (143 CALORIES), **123**
Baked Veggie Chips
(108 CALORIES), **187**
Balsamic Asparagus (45 CALORIES), **173**
Banana Blueberry Smoothies
(99 CALORIES), **88**
Banana Split Cheesecake
(247 CALORIES), **223**
Barbecued Pork Sandwiches
(287 CALORIES), **259**
Barley Beef Skillet
(400 CALORIES), **263**
Basil-Parmesan Angel Hair
(203 CALORIES), **199**
Basil Tuna Steaks (214 CALORIES), **130**
BBQ Beef Sandwiches
(354 CALORIES), **233**
Beef Kabobs with Chutney Sauce
(258 CALORIES), **257**
Beef Roast Dinner
(245 CALORIES), **230**
Beef Tenderloin with Roasted Vegetables
(283 CALORIES), **147**
Berries with Sour Cream Sauce
(147 CALORIES), **216**
Best-Ever Lamb Chops
(157 CALORIES), **246**

Better Than Egg Salad
(274 CALORIES), **110**
Black Bean Chicken Tacos
(267 CALORIES), **141**
Black Bean Chicken with Rice
(400 CALORIES), **263**
Black Bean Taco Pizza
(264 CALORIES), **108**
Black Forest Cake
(186 CALORIES), **219**
Blondies with Chips
(133 CALORIES), **213**
Blue-Cheese Topped Steaks
(228 CALORIES), **132**
Blueberry Oatmeal Pancakes
(171 CALORIES), **270**
Blueberry-Stuffed French Toast
(167 CALORIES), **92**
Bow Ties with Chicken and Shrimp
(399 CALORIES), **168**
Braised Southwest Beef Roast
(255 CALORIES), **136**
Bravo Broccoli (78 CALORIES), **180**
Breaded Eggplant Sandwiches
(288 CALORIES), **111**
Broccoli Brown Rice Pilaf
(202 CALORIES), **198**
Broccoli-Cheddar Baked Potatoes
(226 CALORIES), **202**
Broccoli-Cheese Stuffed Pizza
(252 CALORIES), **134**
Broccoli-Turkey Casserole
(303 CALORIES), **150**
Broiled Fruit Dessert
(80 CALORIES), **209**
Broiled Sirloin Steaks
(187 CALORIES), **126**
Brunch Risotto (279 CALORIES), **258**
Burgundy Beef Stew
(388 CALORIES), **234**

C

Cafe Mocha Mini Muffins
(81 CALORIES), **266**
Cajun Beef Tenderloin
(172 CALORIES), **124**
Candy Bar Cupcakes
(250 CALORIES), **223**
Cappuccino Pudding
(105 CALORIES), **210**

C (CONTINUED)

Caramel Cream Crepes
(206 CALORIES), 94
Cheesecake Phyllo Cups
(46 CALORIES), 80
Cheesy Pita Crisps (95 CALORIES), 83
Cheesy Rigatoni Bake
(274 CALORIES), 144
Cherry Chocolate Parfaits
(146 CALORIES), 244
Chewy Granola Bars (160 CALORIES), 90
Chicken Alfredo Veggie Pizza
(317 CALORIES), 113
Chicken and Shrimp Satay
(190 CALORIES), 128
Chicken & Vegetable Stir-Fry
(297 CALORIES), 280
Chicken Artichoke Pasta
(378 CALORIES), 289
Chicken Caesar Pasta Toss
(363 CALORIES), 120
Chicken Caesar Wraps
(332 CALORIES), 115
Chicken Fajita Pizza (382 CALORIES), 120
Chicken Patties with Roasted Tomato
Salsa (134 CALORIES), 243
Chicken Pesto Pizza
(293 CALORIES), 112
Chicken Veggie Wraps
(395 CALORIES), 293
Chicken with Beans and Potatoes
(209 CALORIES), 229
Chili Beef Quesadillas
(353 CALORIES), 117
Chili Con Carne (299 CALORIES), 113
Chipotle Sweet Potato and Spiced Apple
Purees (224 CALORIES), 255
Chive Crab Cakes
(242 CALORIES), 256
Chocolate Bliss Marble Cake
(215 CALORIES), 220
Chocolate Chip Cookies
(94 CALORIES), 209
Chocolate Dunk-Shot Biscotti
(40 CALORIES), 207
Chocolate Ganache Cake
(179 CALORIES), 218
Chutney Turkey Burgers
(359 CALORIES), 160

Cinnamon Blueberry Sauce
(50 CALORIES), 207
Citrus Fish Tacos (411 CALORIES), 169
Citrus Spinach Salad (52 CALORIES), 173
Coconut-Cherry Cream Squares
(142 CALORIES), 214
Coconut Custard Pie (214 CALORIES), 254
Coconut-Pecan Sweet Potatoes
(211 CALORIES), 229
Colorful Beef Stir-Fry
(318 CALORIES), 152
Colorful Beef Wraps
(325 CALORIES), 284
Colorful Cheese Omelet
(167 CALORIES), 91
Colorful Frozen Yogurt
(143 CALORIES), 215
Corn Bread-Topped Frijoles
(367 CALORIES), 234
Corn Pudding Stuffed Tomatoes
(157 CALORIES), 195
Country Chicken with Gravy
(274 CALORIES), 278
Couscous with Mushrooms
(230 CALORIES), 203
Crab-Spinach Egg Casserole
(163 CALORIES), 90
Cranberry Apple Tart
(183 CALORIES), 218
Cranberry-Apricot Pork Roast with
Potatoes (433 CALORIES), 235
Cranberry Couscous (202 CALORIES), 198
Cranberry-Orange Turkey Cutlets
(399 CALORIES), 166
Cranberry-Stuffed Apples
(136 CALORIES), 227
Creole Chicken (320 CALORIES), 154
Crunchy Onion Barbecue Chicken
(286 CALORIES), 258
Curried Chicken with Apples
(272 CALORIES), 144

D

Dijon-Crusted Chicken Breasts
(169 CALORIES), 269
Dijon Green Beans (54 CALORIES), 174
Dijon-Peach Pork Chops
(360 CALORIES), 289
Dilly Vegetable Medley
(91 CALORIES), 184

E

Easy Beef Stroganoff
(326 CALORIES), 285
Eggs Benedict (216 CALORIES), 96
Enchilada Casser-ole!
(357 CALORIES), 159
Enchilada Lasagna (282 CALORIES), 145

F

Family-Favorite Cheeseburger Pasta
(391 CALORIES), 293
Family-Pleasing Turkey Chili
(349 CALORIES), 233
Fantastic Fish Tacos
(314 CALORIES), 282
Festive French Pancakes
(163 CALORIES), 89
Fettuccine with Black Bean Sauce
(350 CALORIES), 288
Fish Tacos (196 CALORIES), 127
Flank Steak Pitas (362 CALORIES), 161
Flavorful Corn (116 CALORIES), 188
Flavorful Mashed Potatoes
(146 CALORIES), 192
Floribbean Fish Burgers with Tropical
Sauce (353 CALORIES), 118
Focaccia Sandwich (113 CALORIES), 101
French Cheeseburger Loaf
(277 CALORIES), 145
French Toast with Apple Topping
(219 CALORIES), 96
Fresh Fruit Parfaits
(149 CALORIES), 216
Frozen Fruit Cups (48 CALORIES), 237
Frozen Pistachio Dessert with Raspberry
Sauce (214 CALORIES), 220
Frozen Yogurt Cookie Dessert
(220 CALORIES), 255
Fruit Juice Pops (149 CALORIES), 217
Fruit Pizza (216 CALORIES), 221
Fruity Crab Pasta Salad
(322 CALORIES), 283

G

Garbanzo Bean Pitas
(241 CALORIES), 105
Garden Turkey Burgers
(156 CALORIES), 269
Garlic Cheese Grits (186 CALORIES), 94

Garlic-Herb Orzo Pilaf
(227 CALORIES), 203
Garlic Lemon Shrimp
(163 CALORIES), 123
German Deli Pizza
(330 CALORIES), 114
Glazed Orange Carrots
(132 CALORIES), 191
Glazed Pork Chops
(246 CALORIES), 256
Go for the Grains Casserole
(226 CALORIES), 202
Golden au Gratin Potatoes
(167 CALORIES), 196
Grandma's French Tuna Salad Wraps
(328 CALORIES), 114
Grandma's Stuffed Yellow Squash
(103 CALORIES), 240
Granola-to-Go Bars (130 CALORIES), 88
Great Grain Pilaf (154 CALORIES), 194
Greek Pizzas (320 CALORIES), 155
Grilled Artichoke-Mushroom Pizza
(283 CALORIES), 146
Grilled Breaded Chicken
(224 CALORIES), 132
Grilled Fish Sandwiches
(241 CALORIES), 276
Grilled Pork Tenderloin
(171 CALORIES), 250
Grilled Pork Tenderloin Sandwiches
(382 CALORIES), 121
Grilled Spicy Pork Tenderloin
(188 CALORIES), 270
Grilled Stuffed Pork Tenderloin
(296 CALORIES), 148
Grilled Tilapia with Lemon Basil
Vinaigrette for Two
(206 CALORIES), 254
Grilled Veggie Sandwiches
(231 CALORIES), 274
Gruyere Mashed Potatoes
(193 CALORIES), 197

H

Ham Asparagus Spirals
(49 CALORIES), 80
Hard-Cooked Eggs (75 CALORIES), 239
Hawaiian Breakfast Cups
(131 CALORIES), 242

Hearty Chipotle Chicken Soup
(287 CALORIES), 111
Hearty Pasta Casserole
(416 CALORIES), 171
Hearty Salisbury Steaks
(233 CALORIES), 275
Heavenly Earth Burgers
(320 CALORIES), 153
Herbed Beans and Carrots
(63 CALORIES), 176
Herbed Beef Tenderloin
(198 CALORIES), 253
Herbed Potato Salad
(142 CALORIES), 191
Holiday Gelatin Mold
(105 CALORIES), 187
Holiday Peas (87 CALORIES), 183
Home-Style Coleslaw
(88 CALORIES), 183
Home-Style Pot Roast
(341 CALORIES), 260
Homemade Pancake Mix
(303 CALORIES), 281
Homemade Spaghetti Sauce
(230 CALORIES), 133
Honey-Grilled Pork Tenderloin
(298 CALORIES), 260
Honey-Lime Roasted Chicken
(197 CALORIES), 252
Hot 'n' Spicy Flank Steak
(201 CALORIES), 128
Hot Swiss Chicken Sandwiches
(218 CALORIES), 104
Hungarian Goulash
(310 CALORIES), 151

I

Irish Stew (271 CALORIES), 142
Italian Beef and Shells
(396 CALORIES), 262
Italian Broccoli with Peppers
(55 CALORIES), 174
Italian Cheese-Stuffed Shells
(351 CALORIES), 158
Italian Green Beans
(85 CALORIES), 182
Italian Hot Dish (391 CALORIES), 166
Italian Mini Frittatas
(172 CALORIES), 93

Italian Sausage Bean Soup
(339 CALORIES), 115
Italian Skillet Supper (248 CALORIES), 277
Italian Squash Casserole
(99 CALORIES), 186
Italian Vegetable Medley
(79 CALORIES), 180
Italian Vegetable Soup
(164 CALORIES), 103
Italian Veggie Skillet (93 CALORIES), 185

L

Ladyfinger Cream Sandwiches
(129 CALORIES), 212
Lasagna Soup
(280 CALORIES), 280
Lemon Anise Biscotti
(66 CALORIES), 208
Lemon Chicken with Gravy
(195 CALORIES), 228
Lemon Fluff Dessert
(135 CALORIES), 243
Lemon Garlic Mushrooms
(96 CALORIES), 185
Lemon Mushroom Chicken
(213 CALORIES), 273
Lemon Pepper Pasta
(249 CALORIES), 205
Lemon-Pepper Veggies
(75 CALORIES), 178
Lemon Risotto with Peas
(207 CALORIES), 200
Lemon Sorbet (138 CALORIES), 242
Lemon-Soy Roughy (124 CALORIES), 241
Lemony New Potatoes
(118 CALORIES), 189
Light Chicken Cordon Bleu
(306 CALORIES), 151
Lime-Marinated Orange Roughy
(169 CALORIES), 270
Little Kick Jalapeno Burgers
(254 CALORIES), 136
Low-Calorie Pumpkin Pie
(124 CALORIES), 211
Low-Fat Macaroni and Cheese
(250 CALORIES), 205
Luscious Lime Angel Squares
(139 CALORIES), 244

M

Macaroni 'n' Cheese Italiano
(262 CALORIES), 106

Macaroni Scramble
(351 CALORIES), 157

Makeover Corn 'n' Green Bean Bake
(241 CALORIES), 204

Makeover Creamy Seafood Soup
(274 CALORIES), 279

Makeover Curried Chicken Rice Soup
(263 CALORIES), 107

Makeover Fancy Bean Casserole
(213 CALORIES), 200

Makeover Frosted Banana Bars
(149 CALORIES), 216

Makeover Oatmeal Bars
(127 CALORIES), 211

Makeover Patrician Potatoes
(207 CALORIES), 199

Makeover Turkey Biscuit Bake
(290 CALORIES), 156

Malibu Chicken Bundles
(400 CALORIES), 167

Mashed Potato Cakes
(147 CALORIES), 193

Mediterranean Salad
(69 CALORIES), 101

Mediterranean Shrimp 'n' Pasta
(368 CALORIES), 163

Mediterranean Summer Squash
(69 CALORIES), 177

Melon 'n' Grape Medley
(74 CALORIES), 239

Mexican-Inspired Turkey Burgers
(312 CALORIES), 282

Mexican Manicotti
(390 CALORIES), 166

Mexican Meat Loaf
(266 CALORIES), 140

Mexican Veggies
(70 CALORIES), 178

Mini Polenta Pizzas
(57 CALORIES), 81

Mini Sausage Quiches
(66 CALORIES), 82

Mom's Orange-Spice Gelatin
(62 CALORIES), 238

Monterey Quiche (265 CALORIES), 98

Moroccan Beef Kabobs
(185 CALORIES), 125

Mushroom Quiche
(154 CALORIES), 245

Mustard-Herb Chicken Breasts
(163 CALORIES), 248

N

No-Bake Cheesecake Pie
(141 CALORIES), 214

No-Bake Peanut Butter Treats
(70 CALORIES), 82

Nut 'n' Corn Clusters (43 CALORIES), 79

O

Old-Fashioned Swiss Steak
(359 CALORIES), 160

One-Pot Chili (384 CALORIES), 121

Onion-Dijon Pork Chops
(261 CALORIES), 278

Orange Fruit Cups
(80 CALORIES), 87

P

Parmesan Cauliflower
(121 CALORIES), 189

Parmesan Popcorn
(49 CALORIES), 81

Parmesan Pork Medallions
(220 CALORIES), 131

Parmesan Roasted Carrots
(82 CALORIES), 181

Party Pretzels (89 CALORIES), 83

Peach-Topped Cake
(121 CALORIES), 210

Peanut Butter-Chocolate Chip Cookies
(75 CALORIES), 208

Peanut Butter S'mores Bars
(200 CALORIES), 253

Peas a la Francaise
(112 CALORIES), 188

Pecan Kisses (46 CALORIES), 265

Peppery Grilled Turkey Breast
(167 CALORIES), 124

Pina Colada Pudding Cups
(171 CALORIES), 250

Pineapple Beef Kabobs
(412 CALORIES), 170

Pineapple Beef Stir-Fry for Two
(381 CALORIES), 290

Pineapple Peach Soup
(88 CALORIES), 184

Polynesian Stir-Fry
(339 CALORIES), 285

Pork Chop Skillet
(360 CALORIES), 162

Pork Medallions with Dijon Sauce
(323 CALORIES), 284

Pork Tenderloin with Horseradish Sauce
(258 CALORIES), 137

Portobello Burgundy Beef
(384 CALORIES), 290

Potato Egg Bake
(235 CALORIES), 98

Potato Smashers
(224 CALORIES), 201

Presto Chicken Tacos
(215 CALORIES), 273

Pretty Almond Green Beans
(78 CALORIES), 179

Pretzel Bones (98 CALORIES), 84

Puffy Apple Omelet
(249 CALORIES), 277

Q

Quick Crisp Snack Bars
(144 CALORIES), 268

Quinoa Pilaf (198 CALORIES), 272

R

Ragu Bolognese
(413 CALORIES), 171

Raspberry Chicken Salad
(320 CALORIES), 283

Raspberry Pie with Oat Crust
(167 CALORIES), 249

Ratatouille with Polenta
(195 CALORIES), 271

Red Clam Sauce
(305 CALORIES), 232

Red, White and Blue Pita Pockets
(351 CALORIES), 116

Rice with Summer Squash
(123 CALORIES), 190

Rich Peach Ice Cream
(140 CALORIES), 213

Roast Pork Sandwiches with Peach
Chutney (357 CALORIES), 118

Roast Turkey Breast with Rosemary Gravy (151 CALORIES), 245
Roasted Vegetable Medley (152 CALORIES), 193

S

Salt & Garlic Pita Chips (21 CALORIES), 79
Sangria Gelatin Dessert (95 CALORIES), 240
Sausage and Egg Pizza (241 CALORIES), 276
Sausage Bread Dressing (166 CALORIES), 196
Sausage Corn Bread Dressing (157 CALORIES), 194
Sausage Kale Soup (194 CALORIES), 252
Sauteed Corn with Tomatoes & Basil (85 CALORIES), 182
Savory Baked Chicken (210 CALORIES), 272
Scallops & Shrimp with Yellow Rice (349 CALORIES), 288
Scallops with Angel Hair (340 CALORIES), 286
Scrambled Egg Muffins (133 CALORIES), 268
Seasoned Yukon Gold Wedges (121 CALORIES), 190
Sesame Vegetable Medley (60 CALORIES), 175
Shrimp & Shiitake Stir-Fry with Crispy Noodles (238 CALORIES), 275
Simple Chicken Soup (195 CALORIES), 104
Sirloin Roast with Gravy (185 CALORIES), 227
Sirloin Strips over Rice (299 CALORIES), 149
Skillet Arroz Con Pollo (373 CALORIES), 164
Slow-Cooked Sausage Dressing (201 CALORIES), 228
Snapper with Spicy Pineapple Glaze (304 CALORIES), 281
Snow Pea Medley (83 CALORIES), 181

Southwest Black Bean Soup (273 CALORIES), 109
Southwest Vegetarian Bake (284 CALORIES), 148
Southwestern Beef Stew (222 CALORIES), 131
Southwestern Pasta & Cheese (240 CALORIES), 204
Spanish Fish (251 CALORIES), 135
Spicy Chicken Breasts with Pepper Peach Relish (263 CALORIES), 138
Spicy Chicken Spaghetti (401 CALORIES), 168
Spicy Warm Chicken Salad (417 CALORIES), 292
Spinach Cheddar Squares (219 CALORIES), 97
Spinach-Feta Chicken Rolls (272 CALORIES), 109
Spring Frittata (163 CALORIES), 91
Springtime Barley (226 CALORIES), 201
Strawberry Mango Smoothies for 2 (100 CALORIES), 84
Strawberry-Raspberry Ice (118 CALORIES), 241
Stuffed Steak Spirals (214 CALORIES), 130
Sun-Kissed Smoothies (100 CALORIES), 85
Super-Duper Tuna Sandwiches (291 CALORIES), 112
Super Flatbread Wraps (348 CALORIES), 261
Sweet-and-Sour Beef (389 CALORIES), 291
Sweet Potato Casserole (186 CALORIES), 197

T

Tarragon-Lemon Turkey Breast (162 CALORIES), 247
Tart Cherry Pie (174 CALORIES), 251
Teriyaki Chicken Salad with Poppy Seed Dressing (361 CALORIES), 119
Tex-Mex Beef Barbecues (294 CALORIES), 232
Tex-Mex Popcorn (44 CALORIES), 79

Thai Restaurant Chicken (359 CALORIES), 161
Three-Fruit Smoothies (225 CALORIES), 97
Tilapia with Grapefruit Salsa (264 CALORIES), 140
Tortellini Primavera (341 CALORIES), 287
Tres Leches Cake (233 CALORIES), 224
Triple-Berry Cobbler (235 CALORIES), 222
Tropical Fruit Smoothies (97 CALORIES), 87
Tropical Meringue Tarts (145 CALORIES), 215
Turkey Breakfast Sausage (85 CALORIES), 267
Turkey Burritos with Fresh Fruit Salsa (371 CALORIES), 165
Turkey Enchiladas (284 CALORIES), 110
Turkey Meatball Soup (258 CALORIES), 106
Turkey Noodle Casserole (357 CALORIES), 158
Turkey Pasta Toss (249 CALORIES), 134
Turkey Pecan Enchiladas (263 CALORIES), 139
Turkey Roulades (184 CALORIES), 126
Turkey Sloppy Joes (247 CALORIES), 231
Turkey Tortilla Roll-Ups (353 CALORIES), 117
Turkey with Apple Slices (263 CALORIES), 138
Turkey with Sausage Stuffing (317 CALORIES), 152
Tuscan Chicken for Two (217 CALORIES), 274

V

Vanilla Tapioca Pudding (133 CALORIES), 242
Vegetarian Tex-Mex Peppers (364 CALORIES), 162

V *(CONTINUED)*
Veggie Cheese Ravioli
(322 CALORIES), **154**
Veggie Tossed Salad
(62 CALORIES), **176**
Veggie Tuna Burgers
(275 CALORIES), **279**

W
Warm Chocolate Melting Cups
(131 CALORIES), **212**
Weeknight Beef Skillet
(389 CALORIES), **292**
Whiskey Sirloin Steak for Two
(169 CALORIES), **248**
White Bean Soup (270 CALORIES), **108**
Whole Grain Waffle Mix
(284 CALORIES), **99**
Wholesome Apple-Hazelnut Stuffing
(159 CALORIES), **195**
Wilted Garlic Spinach
(66 CALORIES), **177**
Winter Harvest Vegetable Soup
(134 CALORIES), **102**
Winter Vegetables (51 CALORIES), **237**

Z
Zesty Horseradish Meat Loaf
(207 CALORIES), **129**
Zippy Slow-Cooked Chili
(266 CALORIES), **231**
Zippy Spaghetti Sauce
(220 CALORIES), **230**
Zippy Three-Bean Chili
(269 CALORIES), **142**
Zippy Tomato-Topped Snapper
(179 CALORIES), **251**
Zucchini Lasagna (272 CALORIES), **143**
Zucchini Pancakes (88 CALORIES), **88**
Zucchini Parmesan (81 CALORIES), **266**

index by calories

The Taste of Home Comfort Food Diet success rests on the calories you consume each day. To help you plan your caloric intake and daily menus, this index categorizes recipes by type (snacks, breakfast, dinner, etc.). The items are then broken down into their applicable calorie ranges.

When looking for a dinner that's on the lighter side, see the 53 dishes listed under "Dinners: 250 Calories or Less." If you saved a few more calories for the end of the day, consider the recipes found under "Dinners: 251 to 350 Calories." There you'll find 58 recipes.

With a little help from this index, you'll be amazed at how easy it is to meet your goals and make the Taste of Home Comfort Food Diet a healthy and delicious part of your life.

SNACKS
100 CALORIES OR LESS
Apple Skewers (80 CALORIES), **265**
Cafe Mocha Mini Muffins
(81 CALORIES), **266**
Cheesecake Phyllo Cups
(46 CALORIES), **80**
Cheesy Pita Crisps (95 CALORIES), **83**
Ham Asparagus Spirals
(49 CALORIES), **80**
Mini Polenta Pizzas (57 CALORIES), **81**
Mini Sausage Quiches (66 CALORIES), **82**

No-Bake Peanut Butter Treats
(70 CALORIES), **82**
Nut 'n' Corn Clusters (43 CALORIES), **79**
Parmesan Popcorn (49 CALORIES), **81**
Party Pretzels (89 CALORIES), **83**
Pretzel Bones (98 CALORIES), **84**
Salt & Garlic Pita Chips
(21 CALORIES), **79**
Strawberry Mango Smoothies for 2
(100 CALORIES), **84**
Sun-Kissed Smoothies
(100 CALORIES), **85**
Tex-Mex Popcorn (44 CALORIES), **79**

BREAKFASTS
100 CALORIES OR LESS
Banana Blueberry Smoothies
(99 CALORIES), **88**
Hard-Cooked Eggs (75 CALORIES), **239**
Orange Fruit Cups (80 CALORIES), **87**
Tropical Fruit Smoothies
(97 CALORIES), **87**
Turkey Breakfast Sausage
(85 CALORIES), **267**
Zucchini Pancakes (88 CALORIES), **88**

BREAKFASTS
101 TO 200 CALORIES
Apple-Cinnamon Oatmeal Mix
(176 CALORIES), **94**
Bacon-Broccoli Quiche Cups
(170 CALORIES), **249**
Baked Eggs with Cheddar and Bacon
(107 CALORIES), **267**
Baked Peach Pancake
(157 CALORIES), **246**
Blueberry Oatmeal Pancakes
(171 CALORIES), **270**
Blueberry-Stuffed French Toast
(167 CALORIES), **92**
Chewy Granola Bars (160 CALORIES), **90**
Colorful Cheese Omelet
(167 CALORIES), **91**
Crab-Spinach Egg Casserole
(163 CALORIES), **90**
Festive French Pancakes
(163 CALORIES), **89**
Garlic Cheese Grits (186 CALORIES), **94**
Granola-to-Go Bars (130 CALORIES), **88**

Hawaiian Breakfast Cups
(131 CALORIES), 242
Italian Mini Frittatas (172 CALORIES), 93
Mushroom Quiche (154 CALORIES), 245
Scrambled Egg Muffins
(133 CALORIES), 268
Spring Frittata (163 CALORIES), 91

BREAKFASTS
201 TO 350 CALORIES
Apple Walnut Pancakes
(208 CALORIES), 95
Baked Blueberry & Peach Oatmeal
(277 CALORIES), 99
Brunch Risotto (279 CALORIES), 258
Caramel Cream Crepes
(206 CALORIES), 95
Eggs Benedict (216 CALORIES), 96
French Toast with Apple Topping
(219 CALORIES), 96
Homemade Pancake Mix
(303 CALORIES), 281
Monterey Quiche (265 CALORIES), 98
Potato Egg Bake (235 CALORIES), 98
Puffy Apple Omelet (249 CALORIES), 277
Sausage and Egg Pizza
(241 CALORIES), 276
Spinach Cheddar Squares
(219 CALORIES), 97
Three-Fruit Smoothies
(225 CALORIES), 97
Whole Grain Waffle Mix
(284 CALORIES), 99

LUNCHES
250 CALORIES OR LESS
Artichoke-Lamb Sandwich Loaves
(239 CALORIES), 105
Focaccia Sandwich (113 CALORIES), 101
Garbanzo Bean Pitas
(241 CALORIES), 105
Grilled Fish Sandwiches
(241 CALORIES), 276
Grilled Veggie Sandwiches
(231 CALORIES), 274
Hot Swiss Chicken Sandwiches
(218 CALORIES), 104
Italian Vegetable Soup
(164 CALORIES), 103

Mediterranean Salad (69 CALORIES), 101
Simple Chicken Soup
(195 CALORIES), 104
Winter Harvest Vegetable Soup
(134 CALORIES), 102

LUNCHES
251 TO 350 CALORIES
Apricot Turkey Sandwiches
(338 CALORIES), 116
Better Than Egg Salad
(274 CALORIES), 110
Black Bean Taco Pizza
(264 CALORIES), 108
Breaded Eggplant Sandwiches
(288 CALORIES), 111
Chicken Alfredo Veggie Pizza
(317 CALORIES), 113
Chicken Caesar Wraps
(332 CALORIES), 115
Chicken Pesto Pizza (293 CALORIES), 112
Chili Con Carne (299 CALORIES), 113
Colorful Beef Wraps (325 CALORIES), 284
Fruity Crab Pasta Salad
(322 CALORIES), 283
German Deli Pizza (330 CALORIES), 114
Grandma's French Tuna Salad Wraps
(328 CALORIES), 114
Hearty Chipotle Chicken Soup
(287 CALORIES), 111
Italian Sausage Bean Soup
(339 CALORIES), 115
Lasagna Soup (280 CALORIES), 280
Macaroni 'n' Cheese Italiano
(262 CALORIES), 106
Makeover Creamy Seafood Soup
(274 CALORIES), 279
Makeover Curried Chicken Rice Soup
(263 CALORIES), 107
Mexican-Inspired Turkey Burgers
(312 CALORIES), 282
Raspberry Chicken Salad
(320 CALORIES), 283
Southwest Black Bean Soup
(273 CALORIES), 109
Spinach-Feta Chicken Rolls
(272 CALORIES), 109
Super-Duper Tuna Sandwiches
(291 CALORIES), 112

Super Flatbread Wraps
(348 CALORIES), 261
Turkey Enchiladas (284 CALORIES), 110
Turkey Meatball Soup
(258 CALORIES), 106
Veggie Tuna Burgers
(275 CALORIES), 279
White Bean Soup (270 CALORIES), 108

LUNCHES
351 TO 450 CALORIES
Chicken Caesar Pasta Toss
(363 CALORIES), 120
Chicken Fajita Pizza
(382 CALORIES), 120
Chicken Veggie Wraps
(395 CALORIES), 293
Chili Beef Quesadillas
(353 CALORIES), 117
Floribbean Fish Burgers with Tropical
Sauce (353 CALORIES), 118
Grilled Pork Tenderloin Sandwiches
(382 CALORIES), 121
One-Pot Chili (384 CALORIES), 121
Red, White and Blue Pita Pockets
(351 CALORIES), 116
Roast Pork Sandwiches with Peach
Chutney (357 CALORIES), 118
Spicy Warm Chicken Salad
(417 CALORIES), 292
Teriyaki Chicken Salad with Poppy Seed
Dressing (361 CALORIES), 119
Turkey Tortilla Roll-Ups
(353 CALORIES), 117

DINNERS
250 CALORIES OR LESS
Baked Barbecued Brisket
(159 CALORIES), 247
Baked Tilapia (143 CALORIES), 123
Basil Tuna Steaks (214 CALORIES), 130
Beef Roast Dinner (245 CALORIES), 230
Best-Ever Lamb Chops
(157 CALORIES), 246
Blue-Cheese Topped Steaks
(228 CALORIES), 132
Broiled Sirloin Steaks
(187 CALORIES), 126
Cajun Beef Tenderloin
(172 CALORIES), 124

DINNERS
250 CALORIES OR LESS (CONTINUED)

Chicken and Shrimp Satay
(190 CALORIES), **128**

Chicken Patties with Roasted Tomato
Salsa (134 CALORIES), **243**

Chicken with Beans and Potatoes
(209 CALORIES), **229**

Chive Crab Cakes (242 CALORIES), **256**

Dijon-Crusted Chicken Breasts
(169 CALORIES), **269**

Fish Tacos (196 CALORIES), **127**

Garden Turkey Burgers
(156 CALORIES), **269**

Garlic Lemon Shrimp
(163 CALORIES), **123**

Glazed Pork Chops (246 CALORIES), **256**

Grilled Breaded Chicken
(224 CALORIES), **132**

Grilled Pork Tenderloin
(171 CALORIES), **250**

Grilled Spicy Pork Tenderloin
(188 CALORIES), **270**

Grilled Tilapia with Lemon Basil
Vinaigrette for Two
(206 CALORIES), **254**

Hearty Salisbury Steaks
(233 CALORIES), **275**

Herbed Beef Tenderloin
(198 CALORIES), **253**

Homemade Spaghetti Sauce
(230 CALORIES), **133**

Honey-Lime Roasted Chicken
(197 CALORIES), **252**

Hot 'n' Spicy Flank Steak
(201 CALORIES), **128**

Italian Skillet Supper (248 CALORIES), **277**

Lemon Chicken with Gravy
(195 CALORIES), **228**

Lemon Mushroom Chicken
(213 CALORIES), **273**

Lemon-Soy Roughy
(124 CALORIES), **241**

Lime-Marinated Orange Roughy
(169 CALORIES), **270**

Moroccan Beef Kabobs
(185 CALORIES), **125**

Mustard-Herb Chicken Breasts
(163 CALORIES), **248**

Parmesan Pork Medallions
(220 CALORIES), **131**

Peppery Grilled Turkey Breast
(167 CALORIES), **124**

Presto Chicken Tacos
(215 CALORIES), **273**

Ratatouille with Polenta
(195 CALORIES), **271**

Roast Turkey Breast with Rosemary
Gravy (151 CALORIES), **245**

Sausage Kale Soup (194 CALORIES), **252**

Savory Baked Chicken
(210 CALORIES), **272**

Shrimp & Shiitake Stir-Fry with Crispy
Noodles (238 CALORIES), **275**

Sirloin Roast with Gravy
(185 CALORIES), **227**

Southwestern Beef Stew
(222 CALORIES), **131**

Stuffed Steak Spirals
(214 CALORIES), **130**

Tarragon-Lemon Turkey Breast
(162 CALORIES), **247**

Turkey Pasta Toss (249 CALORIES), **134**

Turkey Roulades (184 CALORIES), **126**

Turkey Sloppy Joes (247 CALORIES), **231**

Tuscan Chicken for Two
(217 CALORIES), **274**

Whiskey Sirloin Steak for Two
(169 CALORIES), **248**

Zesty Horseradish Meat Loaf
(207 CALORIES), **129**

Zippy Spaghetti Sauce
(220 CALORIES), **230**

Zippy Tomato-Topped Snapper
(179 CALORIES), **251**

DINNERS
251 TO 350 CALORIES

All-American Beef Stew
(324 CALORIES), **155**

Applesauce-Glazed Pork Chops
(291 CALORIES), **259**

Baked Chicken Fajitas
(340 CALORIES), **286**

Baked Mostaccioli (278 CALORIES), **146**

Barbecued Pork Sandwiches
(287 CALORIES), **259**

Beef Kabobs with Chutney Sauce
(258 CALORIES), **257**

Beef Tenderloin with Roasted
Vegetables (283 CALORIES), **147**

Black Bean Chicken Tacos
(267 CALORIES), **141**

Braised Southwest Beef Roast
(255 CALORIES), **136**

Broccoli-Cheese Stuffed Pizza
(252 CALORIES), **134**

Broccoli-Turkey Casserole
(303 CALORIES), **150**

Cheesy Rigatoni Bake
(274 CALORIES), **144**

Chicken & Vegetable Stir-Fry
(297 CALORIES), **280**

Colorful Beef Stir-Fry
(318 CALORIES), **152**

Country Chicken with Gravy
(274 CALORIES), **278**

Creole Chicken (320 CALORIES), **154**

Crunchy Onion Barbecue Chicken
(286 CALORIES), **258**

Curried Chicken with Apples
(272 CALORIES), **144**

Easy Beef Stroganoff
(326 CALORIES), **285**

Enchilada Lasagna (282 CALORIES), **145**

Family-Pleasing Turkey Chili
(349 CALORIES), **233**

Fantastic Fish Tacos
(314 CALORIES), **282**

Fettuccine with Black Bean Sauce
(350 CALORIES), **288**

French Cheeseburger Loaf
(277 CALORIES), **145**

Greek Pizzas (320 CALORIES), **155**

Grilled Artichoke-Mushroom Pizza
(283 CALORIES), **146**

Grilled Stuffed Pork Tenderloin
(296 CALORIES), **148**

Heavenly Earth Burgers
(320 CALORIES), **153**

Home-Style Pot Roast
(341 CALORIES), **260**

Honey-Grilled Pork Tenderloin
(298 CALORIES), **260**

Hungarian Goulash (310 CALORIES), **151**

Irish Stew (271 CALORIES), **142**

Light Chicken Cordon Bleu
(306 CALORIES), 151

Little Kick Jalapeno Burgers
(254 CALORIES), 136

Makeover Turkey Biscuit Bake
(290 CALORIES), 156

Mexican Meat Loaf (266 CALORIES), 140

Onion-Dijon Pork Chops
(261 CALORIES), 278

Polynesian Stir-Fry (339 CALORIES), 285

Pork Medallions with Dijon Sauce
(323 CALORIES), 284

Pork Tenderloin with Horseradish Sauce
(258 CALORIES), 137

Red Clam Sauce (305 CALORIES), 232

Scallops & Shrimp with Yellow Rice
(349 CALORIES), 288

Scallops with Angel Hair
(340 CALORIES), 286

Sirloin Strips over Rice (299 CALORIES),
149

Snapper with Spicy Pineapple Glaze
(304 CALORIES), 281

Southwest Vegetarian Bake
(284 CALORIES), 148

Spanish Fish (251 CALORIES), 135

Spicy Chicken Breasts with Pepper
Peach Relish (263 CALORIES), 138

Tex-Mex Beef Barbecues
(294 CALORIES), 232

Tilapia with Grapefruit Salsa
(264 CALORIES), 140

Tortellini Primavera (341 CALORIES), 287

Turkey Pecan Enchiladas
(263 CALORIES), 139

Turkey with Apple Slices
(263 CALORIES), 138

Turkey with Sausage Stuffing
(317 CALORIES), 152

Veggie Cheese Ravioli (322 CALORIES), 154

Zippy Slow-Cooked Chili
(266 CALORIES), 231

Zippy Three-Bean Chili
(269 CALORIES), 142

Zucchini Lasagna (272 CALORIES), 143

DINNERS
351 TO 450 CALORIES

Apple Pork Stir-Fry (370 CALORIES), 164

Apricot-Almond Chicken Breasts
(372 CALORIES), 262

Asian Orange Beef (351 CALORIES), 157

Asian Steak Wraps (402 CALORIES), 169

Asian Vegetable Pasta (358 CALORIES),
159

Barley Beef Skillet (400 CALORIES), 263

BBQ Beef Sandwiches
(354 CALORIES), 233

Black Bean Chicken with Rice
(400 CALORIES), 263

Bow Ties with Chicken and Shrimp
(399 CALORIES), 168

Burgundy Beef Stew
(388 CALORIES), 234

Chicken Artichoke Pasta
(378 CALORIES), 289

Chutney Turkey Burgers
(359 CALORIES), 160

Citrus Fish Tacos (411 CALORIES), 169

Corn Bread-Topped Frijoles
(367 CALORIES), 234

Cranberry-Apricot Pork Roast with
Potatoes (433 CALORIES), 235

Cranberry-Orange Turkey Cutlets
(399 CALORIES), 166

Dijon-Peach Pork Chops
(360 CALORIES), 289

Enchilada Casser-ole!
(357 CALORIES), 159

Family-Favorite Cheeseburger Pasta
(391 CALORIES), 293

Flank Steak Pitas (362 CALORIES), 161

Hearty Pasta Casserole
(416 CALORIES), 171

Italian Beef and Shells
(396 CALORIES), 262

Italian Cheese-Stuffed Shells
(351 CALORIES), 158

Italian Hot Dish (391 CALORIES), 166

Macaroni Scramble (351 CALORIES), 157

Malibu Chicken Bundles
(400 CALORIES), 167

Mediterranean Shrimp 'n' Pasta
(368 CALORIES), 163

Mexican Manicotti (390 CALORIES), 166

Old-Fashioned Swiss Steak
(359 CALORIES), 160

Pineapple Beef Kabobs
(412 CALORIES), 170

Pineapple Beef Stir-Fry for Two
(381 CALORIES), 290

Pork Chop Skillet (360 CALORIES), 162

Portobello Burgundy Beef
(384 CALORIES), 290

Ragu Bolognese (413 CALORIES), 171

Skillet Arroz Con Pollo
(373 CALORIES), 164

Spicy Chicken Spaghetti (
401 CALORIES), 168

Sweet-and-Sour Beef (389 CALORIES), 291

Thai Restaurant Chicken
(359 CALORIES), 161

Turkey Burritos with Fresh Fruit Salsa
(371 CALORIES), 165

Turkey Noodle Casserole
(357 CALORIES), 158

Vegetarian Tex-Mex Peppers
(364 CALORIES), 162

Weeknight Beef Skillet
(389 CALORIES), 292

SIDE DISHES
100 CALORIES OR LESS

Asparagus with Dill Sauce
(76 CALORIES), 179

Baked Onion Rings (98 CALORIES), 186

Balsamic Asparagus (45 CALORIES), 173

Bravo Broccoli (78 CALORIES), 180

Citrus Spinach Salad (52 CALORIES), 173

Dijon Green Beans (54 CALORIES), 174

Dilly Vegetable Medley
(91 CALORIES), 184

Herbed Beans and Carrots
(63 CALORIES), 176

Holiday Peas (87 CALORIES), 183

Home-Style Coleslaw (88 CALORIES), 183

Italian Broccoli with Peppers
(55 CALORIES), 174

Italian Green Beans (85 CALORIES), 182

Italian Squash Casserole
(99 CALORIES), 186

Italian Vegetable Medley
(79 CALORIES), 180

Italian Veggie Skillet (93 CALORIES), 185

Lemon Garlic Mushrooms
(96 CALORIES), 185

SIDE DISHES
100 CALORIES OR LESS (CONTINUED)

Lemon-Pepper Veggies
(75 CALORIES), **178**

Mediterranean Summer Squash
(69 CALORIES), **177**

Melon 'n' Grape Medley
(74 CALORIES), **239**

Mexican Veggies (70 CALORIES), **178**

Parmesan Roasted Carrots
(82 CALORIES), **181**

Pineapple Peach Soup (88 CALORIES), **184**

Pretty Almond Green Beans
(78 CALORIES), **179**

Sauteed Corn with Tomatoes & Basil
(85 CALORIES), **182**

Sesame Vegetable Medley
(60 CALORIES), **175**

Snow Pea Medley (83 CALORIES), **181**

Veggie-Tossed Salad (62 CALORIES), **176**

Wilted Garlic Spinach
(66 CALORIES), **177**

Winter Vegetables (51 CALORIES), **237**

Zucchini Parmesan (81 CALORIES), **266**

SIDE DISHES
101 TO 200 CALORIES

Alfresco Bean Salad (146 CALORIES), **192**

Baked Veggie Chips (108 CALORIES), **187**

Corn Pudding Stuffed Tomatoes
(157 CALORIES), **195**

Flavorful Corn (116 CALORIES), **188**

Flavorful Mashed Potatoes
(146 CALORIES), **192**

Glazed Orange Carrots
(132 CALORIES), **191**

Golden au Gratin Potatoes
(167 CALORIES), **196**

Grandma's Stuffed Yellow Squash
(103 CALORIES), **240**

Great Grain Pilaf (154 CALORIES), **194**

Gruyere Mashed Potatoes
(193 CALORIES), **197**

Herbed Potato Salad (142 CALORIES), **191**

Holiday Gelatin Mold (105 CALORIES), **187**

Lemony New Potatoes
(118 CALORIES), **189**

Mashed Potato Cakes
(147 CALORIES), **193**

Parmesan Cauliflower
(121 CALORIES), **189**

Peas a la Francaise (112 CALORIES), **188**

Quinoa Pilaf (198 CALORIES), **272**

Rice with Summer Squash
(123 CALORIES), **190**

Roasted Vegetable Medley
(152 CALORIES), **193**

Sausage Bread Dressing
(166 CALORIES), **196**

Sausage Corn Bread Dressing
(157 CALORIES), **194**

Seasoned Yukon Gold Wedges
(121 CALORIES), **190**

Sweet Potato Casserole
(186 CALORIES), **197**

Wholesome Apple-Hazelnut Stuffing
(159 CALORIES), **195**

SIDE DISHES
201 TO 250 CALORIES

Basil-Parmesan Angel Hair
(203 CALORIES), **199**

Broccoli Brown Rice Pilaf
(202 CALORIES), **198**

Broccoli-Cheddar Baked Potatoes
(226 CALORIES), **202**

Chipotle Sweet Potato and Spiced Apple
Purees (224 CALORIES), **255**

Coconut-Pecan Sweet Potatoes
(211 CALORIES), **229**

Couscous with Mushrooms
(230 CALORIES), **203**

Cranberry Couscous
(202 CALORIES), **198**

Garlic-Herb Orzo Pilaf
(227 CALORIES), **203**

Go for the Grains Casserole
(226 CALORIES), **202**

Lemon Pepper Pasta (249 CALORIES), **205**

Lemon Risotto with Peas
(207 CALORIES), **200**

Low-Fat Macaroni and Cheese
(250 CALORIES), **205**

Makeover Corn 'n' Green Bean Bake
(241 CALORIES), **204**

Makeover Fancy Bean Casserole
(213 CALORIES), **200**

Makeover Patrician Potatoes
(207 CALORIES), **199**

Potato Smashers (224 CALORIES), **201**

Slow-Cooked Sausage Dressing
(201 CALORIES), **228**

Southwestern Pasta & Cheese
(240 CALORIES), **204**

Springtime Barley (226 CALORIES), **201**

DESSERTS
100 CALORIES OR LESS

Apple Cranberry Delight
(70 CALORIES), **238**

Broiled Fruit Dessert (80 CALORIES), **209**

Chocolate Chip Cookies
(94 CALORIES), **209**

Chocolate Dunk-Shot Biscotti
(40 CALORIES), **207**

Cinnamon Blueberry Sauce
(50 CALORIES), **207**

Frozen Fruit Cups (48 CALORIES), **237**

Lemon Anise Biscotti (66 CALORIES), **208**

Mom's Orange-Spice Gelatin
(62 CALORIES), **238**

Peanut Butter-Chocolate Chip Cookies
(75 CALORIES), **208**

Pecan Kisses (46 CALORIES), **265**

Sangria Gelatin Dessert
(95 CALORIES), **240**

DESSERTS
101 TO 150 CALORIES

Berries with Sour Cream Sauce
(147 CALORIES), **216**

Blondies with Chips (133 CALORIES), **213**

Cappuccino Pudding
(105 CALORIES), **210**

Cherry Chocolate Parfaits
(146 CALORIES), **244**

Coconut-Cherry Cream Squares
(142 CALORIES), **214**

Colorful Frozen Yogurt
(143 CALORIES), **215**

Cranberry-Stuffed Apples
(136 CALORIES), **227**

Fresh Fruit Parfaits (149 CALORIES), **216**

Fruit Juice Pops (149 CALORIES), **217**

Ladyfinger Cream Sandwiches
(129 CALORIES), **212**

Lemon Fluff Dessert (135 CALORIES), **243**

Lemon Sorbet (138 CALORIES), **242**

Low-Calorie Pumpkin Pie
(124 CALORIES), **211**

Luscious Lime Angel Squares
(139 CALORIES), 244
Makeover Frosted Banana Bars
(149 CALORIES), 216
Makeover Oatmeal Bars
(127 CALORIES), 211
No-Bake Cheesecake Pie
(141 CALORIES), 214
Peach-Topped Cake (121 CALORIES), 210
Quick Crisp Snack Bars
(144 CALORIES), 268
Rich Peach Ice Cream
(140 CALORIES), 213
Strawberry-Raspberry Ice
(118 CALORIES), 241
Tropical Meringue Tarts
(145 CALORIES), 215
Vanilla Tapioca Pudding
(133 CALORIES), 242
Warm Chocolate Melting Cups
(131 CALORIES), 212

DESSERTS
151 TO 250 CALORIES
Banana Split Cheesecake
(247 CALORIES), 223
Black Forest Cake (186 CALORIES), 219
Candy Bar Cupcakes
(250 CALORIES), 223
Chocolate Bliss Marble Cake
(215 CALORIES), 220
Chocolate Ganache Cake
(179 CALORIES), 218
Coconut Custard Pie (214 CALORIES), 254
Cranberry Apple Tart
(183 CALORIES), 218
Frozen Pistachio Dessert with Raspberry
Sauce (214 CALORIES), 220
Frozen Yogurt Cookie Dessert
(220 CALORIES), 255
Fruit Pizza (216 CALORIES), 221
Peanut Butter S'mores Bars
(200 CALORIES), 253
Pina Colada Pudding Cups
(171 CALORIES), 250
Raspberry Pie with Oat Crust
(167 CALORIES), 249
Tart Cherry Pie (174 CALORIES), 251
Tres Leches Cake (233 CALORIES), 224
Triple-Berry Cobbler (235 CALORIES), 222

cooking for 2 index

To make it convenient for people who are looking for smaller yield recipes to find them, we've included this Cooking for 2 index. If you regularly cook for just yourself or yourself and one other person, the recipes listed here might be ideal, because you won't have days of leftovers.

If you're a single person living alone, these recipes might also be great because you can enjoy one serving today and save the second serving for another meal tomorrow.

Like these recipes but want to serve four people? Many of them can easily be doubled.

Be sure not to discount other recipes in this book with larger yields if you usually cook for one or two. You could freeze leftovers for handy future meals. See the list of recipes that freeze well on page 41.

BREAKFASTS
Apple-Cinnamon Oatmeal Mix
(176 CALORIES), 94
Bacon-Broccoli Quiche Cups
(170 CALORIES), 249
Baked Eggs with Cheddar and Bacon
(107 CALORIES), 267
Colorful Cheese Omelet
(167 CALORIES), 91
French Toast with Apple Topping
(219 CALORIES), 96
Garlic Cheese Grits
(186 CALORIES), 94
Mushroom Quiche
(154 CALORIES), 245
Puffy Apple Omelet
(249 CALORIES), 277
Strawberry Mango Smoothies for 2
(100 CALORIES), 84

LUNCHES
Apricot Turkey Sandwiches
(338 CALORIES), 116
Chili Con Carne
(299 CALORIES), 113
Fruity Crab Pasta Salad
(322 CALORIES), 283
Grandma's French Tuna Salad Wraps
(328 CALORIES), 114

DINNERS
Creole Chicken
(320 CALORIES), 154
Grilled Tilapia with Lemon Basil
Vinaigrette for Two
(206 CALORIES), 254
Honey-Grilled Pork Tenderloin
(298 CALORIES), 260
Hungarian Goulash
(310 CALORIES), 151
Italian Skillet Supper
(248 CALORIES), 277
Mexican Manicotti
(390 CALORIES), 166
Parmesan Pork Medallions
(220 CALORIES), 131
Pineapple Beef Stir-Fry for Two
(381 CALORIES), 290
Pork Tenderloin with Horseradish Sauce
(258 CALORIES), 137
Savory Baked Chicken
(210 CALORIES), 272
Spicy Chicken Spaghetti
(401 CALORIES), 168
Tilapia with Grapefruit Salsa
(264 CALORIES), 140
Turkey with Apple Slices
(263 CALORIES), 138
Tuscan Chicken for Two
(217 CALORIES), 274

DINNERS
(CONTINUED)

Whiskey Sirloin Steak for Two
(169 CALORIES), **248**

Zippy Tomato-Topped Snapper
(179 CALORIES), **251**

SIDE DISHES

Asparagus with Dill Sauce
(76 CALORIES), **179**

Broccoli-Cheddar Baked Potatoes
(226 CALORIES), **202**

Grandma's Stuffed Yellow Squash
(103 CALORIES), **240**

Italian Green Beans
(85 CALORIES), **182**

Lemon Pepper Pasta
(249 CALORIES), **205**

Lemony New Potatoes
(118 CALORIES), **189**

Mashed Potato Cakes
(147 CALORIES), **193**

Mexican Veggies
(70 CALORIES), **178**

Parmesan Cauliflower
(121 CALORIES), **189**

Parmesan Roasted Carrots
(82 CALORIES), **181**

Potato Smashers
(224 CALORIES), **201**

Snow Pea Medley
(83 CALORIES), **181**

DESSERT

Broiled Fruit Dessert
(80 CALORIES), **209**

PHOTOGRAPHY CREDITS

autumn harvest, page 8
Zvonimir Atletic/Shutterstock.com

lettuce, page 8
David Kay/Shutterstock.com

boxed lunch, page 9
matka_Wariatka/Shutterstock.com

notebook, page 10
Galushko Sergey/Shutterstock.com

yoga posture, page 11
Deklofenak/Shutterstock.com

fresh fruit salad, page 17
Ildi Papp/Shutterstock.com

popcorn, page 17
Jiri Hera/Shutterstock.com

running shoes, page 23
6493866629/Shutterstock.com

stacked apples, page 26
Ultrashock/Shutterstock.com

roasted salmon, page 27
Yuri Arcurs/Shutterstock.com

dairy products, page 27
matka_Wariatka/Shutterstock.com

rice with beans & peppers, page 27
Tobik/Shutterstock.com

myPlate food pyramid, page 28
Basheera Designs/Shutterstock.com

shopping basket, page 32
Yelena Panyukova/Shutterstock.com

cherry tomatoes, page 33
Larina Natalia/Shutterstock.com

fresh blueberries, page 33
Kati Molin/Shutterstock.com

grilled chicken breast, page 33
barbaradudzinska/Shutterstock.com

healthy dip, page 34
Wiktory/Shutterstock.com

shopping list, page 34
Gina Sanders/Shutterstock.com

cupcakes in pan, page 35
Monkey Business Images/Shutterstock.com

salmon with lemon, page 36
DUSAN ZIDAR/Shutterstock.com

peppermint candy, page 36
J. Broadwater/Shutterstock.com

veggies with hummus, page 37
keko64/Shutterstock.com

lunch snack, page 37
Juriah Mosin/Shutterstock.com

frozen berries, page 38
Silvia Bogdanski/Shutterstock.com

plastic containers, page 39
nito/Shutterstock.com

frozen broccoli, page 39
Volosina/Shutterstock.com

frozen peas, page 40
Cogipix/Shutterstock.com

eating on couch, page 42
Luis Camargo/Shutterstock.com

spinach, page 44
Elena Elisseeva/Shutterstock.com

holding blueberries, page 44
Carly Rose Hennigan/Shutterstock.com

oats in bowl, page 44
Olga Miltsova/Shutterstock.com

pistachios, page 45
Volosina/Shutterstock.com

walking on grass, page 46
Rafal Olechowski/Shutterstock.com

walking family, page 47
Dmitriy Shironosov/Shutterstock.com

woman walking, page 47
Christopher Edwin Nuzzaco/Shutterstock.com

woman stretching, page 48
Monalyn Gracia/Corbis

woman hiking, page 49
Jordan Siemens/Getty Images

mixed nuts, page 49
Nadja Antonova/Shutterstock.com

compass, page 49
STILLFX/Shutterstock.com

couple hiking, page 49
Tyler Olson/Shutterstock.com

couple resting by tree, page 49
Tyler Olson/Shutterstock.com

woman cleaning, page 50
Oscar Abrahams/beyond/Corbis

dog art, page 51
sabri deniz kizil/Shutterstock.com

woman walking dog, page 51
Derek E. Rothchild/Getty Images

habanero chili peppers, page 52
Cogipix/Shutterstock.com

cukes, page 52
Teresa Kasprzycka/Shutterstock.com

rucola in bowl, page 52
Cogipix/Shutterstock.com

summer drink, page 53
Tamara Kulikova/Shutterstock.com

PORTRAITS

Pam Holmes image by Daryl & Mitzi Kuszak, page 12

Tami Kuehl's image by Daryl & Mitzi Kuszak, page 14

Richelle Fry's image by Scott Miller, page 16

Kim Bennett's image by Trey Clark, page 18

RDA Milwaukee Group Shot image by Taste of Home Photo Studio, page 20

Jim Palmen's image by Taste of Home Photo Studio, page 22

Marie Parker image by Taste of Home Photo Studio, page 22